T0385355

THE SLEEP ROOM

THE SLEEP ROOM

JON STOCK

The Bridge Street Press

THE BRIDGE STREET PRESS

First published in Great Britain in 2025 by the Bridge Street Press

3 5 7 9 10 8 6 4 2

A CIP catalogue record for this book is available from the British Library.

Hardback ISBN 978-0-349-12889-4
Trade paperback ISBN 978-0-349-12890-0

Typeset in Sabon by M Rules
Printed and bound in Great Britain by
Clays Ltd, Elcograf S.p.A.

Papers used by The Bridge Street Press are from well-managed forests and other responsible sources.

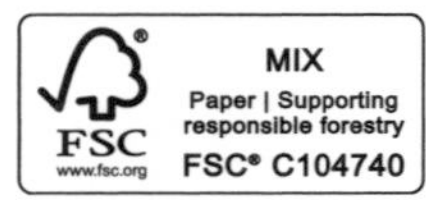

The Bridge Street Press
An imprint of
Little, Brown Book Group
Carmelite House
50 Victoria Embankment
London EC4Y 0DZ

The authorised representative
in the EEA is
Hachette Ireland
8 Castlecourt Centre
Dublin 15, D15 XTP3, Ireland
(email: info@hbgi.ie)

An Hachette UK Company
www.hachette.co.uk

www.littlebrown.co.uk

For all Sargant's patients – those who recovered
and the many who didn't

Contents

Part 2

Part 3

Part 4

Power is in tearing human minds to pieces and putting them together again in new shapes of your own choosing.

GEORGE ORWELL,
Nineteen Eighty-Four

Prologue

The windows were covered with blinds. An Anglepoise in the corner cast an eerie glow across the room. At a desk sat an upright student nurse, trying to ignore the moans and the smell of stale bodies. Occasionally, she glanced at her charges: six young women asleep on low divan beds, wrapped in candlewick covers, small wooden chairs beside them. Were they dreaming? She hoped to God they weren't. Their lives were already a nightmare. Ten minutes earlier, she had checked on each of them in turn, colouring in a sheet of graph paper to record the nature of their sleep: black for deep, grey for shallow, white for awake.

She glanced at her watch. For the six women, day and night no longer held any meaning. Time had long since disappeared into the penumbral half-light, extinguished by a potent cocktail of antipsychotic, sedative and antidepressant drugs. The woman below the window, a young mother of three children, had been admitted with postnatal depression. She had been there for seven weeks now, asleep for at least twenty hours a day. Beside her was a twenty-one-year-old woman, diagnosed with anxiety after a row with her parents over a new boyfriend. When their treatment came to an end these women would barely know who they were. Their memories, the good and the bad, would have been erased for ever. The slate wiped clean.

The nurse checked her watch again, listened to the hum of

London traffic far below on Waterloo Bridge, the sound of the women's slow breathing. Drifting down the corridor, the Beatles' latest hit single, 'Help!'. She looked up at the swing doors. A teenage girl appeared in one of the porthole windows, stared at her and then the women. 'Sleeping beauties' trapped in a twilight world.

In an hour, the nurse would try to wake them, one by one, which was never easy. She had to do it every six hours: wash and feed them, administer enemas, check vital signs. It was even harder to get them to stand without fainting. After recording their blood pressure, which was invariably low, she would help them as they stumbled down the corridor to the bathroom. None could walk unaided. Barely awake, heads lolling, they never recognised her, even though she'd tended to them day and night for weeks. She remained a recurring stranger. And every time she looked into their vacant faces, she wished she were working anywhere but the Sleep Room.

The rattle of a trolley outside; a man's sonorous voice telling patients that they were feeling better. The ward nurses always heard Dr William Sargant long before he arrived. The nurse thought the trolley – a sound she'd come to dread – was due to arrive tomorrow, but she must have lost her own sense of time too. In a moment, it would come rolling through the doors. After the six women had been fed and washed, they would be given electro-convulsive therapy. She could barely watch the procedure, the twisting torsos, haunted by stories of fractured vertebrae and dislocated jaws. Sometimes she was asked to insert a rubber plug into a patient's mouth. It was the protesting that upset her the most, the drug-numbed cries. That and the look of fear in their eyes.

PART 1

1

'Lobotomy would be the next course of treatment for me'

From the reinforced windows of Ward Five, high up in the Edwardian eaves of the Royal Waterloo Hospital for Children and Women, a young Celia Imrie used to stare down on the passing crowds hoping to spot her mother. The 1960s London skyline offered scant comfort for the fourteen-year-old patient: the newly built Shell Centre and the grey maw of Waterloo station, from where she hoped her mother would emerge. 'When I walk past that old, red-brick hospital building today, on my way to the IMAX or the National Theatre,' says Celia, who went on to become a successful actress, 'I can see the window where I would sit waiting for her, and a deep chill passes through me.'

Every day, thousands of commuters and tourists pass beneath the former hospital. Some might look up to admire the terracotta façade, with its ornate colonnades and glazed tile lettering, but few are aware of the medical horrors that took place in one small room on the top floor: the Sleep Room. It was here, on Ward Five, that female patients – they were almost always women – were put to sleep for three to four months (in one case five months), only roused from their beds to be fed, washed and given electro-convulsive therapy (ECT): a shock of up to 110 volts that passed bilaterally through the temporal lobe of the brain, triggering a grand mal seizure.

Fifty years on, Celia and other former patients want to know why they were subjected to such extreme treatments without consent. 'My father was absolutely shattered when he saw me,' remembers Anne White of her time in the Sleep Room. 'He said I just looked like a walking zombie.' 'My memories are like snapshots,' says Mary Thornton. 'One is of the electrodes being attached to the side of my head. I remember the complete, utter terror because I didn't even know who I was.' Staff are reflecting too. Shelley, who worked as a nurse on Ward Five for six months in 1968, recalls the patients' glassy skins. 'They had this dozy, greasy sheen to them. They were like people you just don't see. We knew them all, but not at all really.'

The Royal Waterloo became part of its more famous neighbour, St Thomas' Hospital, in 1948, the year the National Health Service was formed. It was an important year for William Sargant too. An ambitious forty-one-year-old doctor, Sargant was appointed Physician in Charge of the Department of Psychological Medicine at St Thomas', one of the world's most prestigious teaching hospitals. It wasn't long before Ward Five, a psychiatric unit for in-patients, was being referred to as the William Sargant Ward. A brisk ten-minute walk from St Thomas', it was Sargant's personal fiefdom, a place where he could pursue, unchecked, his own mechanistic approach to psychiatry: the brain, like any other organ or limb, was best fixed with physical treatments. If it was damaged, it first needed to be 'splinted'.

Not for him the couch-based therapists who had dominated psychiatry in the early twentieth century – Freudian 'sofa merchants', as he called them. It was, in the words of one of his heroes, Lord Moran, personal doctor to Winston Churchill, time to 'cut the cackle' and allow psychiatry, for so long seen as a Cinderella specialty, to take its rightful place in the medical mainstream. And deep sleep therapy, or continuous narcosis, was his most notorious procedure.

Sleep has long been recognised as a way to calm the distressed – the 'balm of hurt minds', as Shakespeare called it in *Macbeth* – but for Sargant it had another use. The Sleep Room allowed him to administer treatments that his patients might not otherwise agree to, such as intense courses of ECT. Informed consent was implicit rather than sought – the wishes of desperate relatives were often sufficient. 'I am not sure consent forms were in abundant use in the sixties,' remembers one medic who worked on Ward Five in 1968 and wishes to remain anonymous. 'In those days doctors rarely discussed the risks associated with treatments.' It would take the Mental Health Act of 1983 to give patients some legal protection. Narcosis combined with ECT, Sargant believed, broke up set patterns, or circuits, of behaviour and reprogrammed disturbed minds with more positive thoughts. A factory reset. But for many it was a terrifying ordeal that destroyed memories and left them wrestling with existential crises of identity. 'What is also so valuable is that they generally have no memory about the actual length of the treatment or the number of ECT used after the treatment is finished,' Sargant said. 'As a rule the patient does not know how long he has been asleep, or what treatment, even including ECT, he has been given. Under sleep . . . one can now give many kinds of physical treatment, necessary, but often not easily tolerated.'

The ceilings were lower on the top floor of the Royal Waterloo and the windows smaller, giving Ward Five an airless, claustrophobic feel. Access was provided by an old elevator with a sliding grille door big enough for beds to be brought up from the wards below. The sound of babies' cries would often echo up the lift shaft. In 1968, Sargant was filmed for a BBC documentary arriving for his round on the ward. He looks gaunt in a heavy coat, its collar trimmed with black fur. As he emerges from the dark lift, a young nurse takes his coat before he enters the Sleep Room.

'Some people think I'm a marvellous doctor,' he once said. 'Others think I'm the work of the Devil.' It was a rare acknowledgement of what a polarising figure he was in post-war psychiatry. The late Dr Ann Dally, who studied psychiatry under Sargant and had begun to write his biography before she died, observed something similar: 'Of all the twentieth century psychiatrists, he was one of the best loved and most hated.' He was 'Will' to his friends; critics called him 'Bill the Brain Slicer' or 'Sargant the Shock'.

Sargant, who died in 1988, was one of the earliest British psychiatrists to embrace lobotomy (technically referred to as a prefrontal leucotomy in the UK). He also advocated insulin shock therapy, a high-risk treatment that induced near-death hypoglycaemic comas. As for ECT, he claimed to be one of the first to administer it in the UK – he had to buy his own equipment because a disapproving London County Council wouldn't supply him with one. And he administered huge quantities of drugs, including antidepressants and the first generation of antipsychotics, the side effects of which were often worse than the illness.

Few people had the courage to stand up to Sargant. He belonged to an era of unfettered medical authority when doctors, particularly male consultants, exuded a sense of *droit de seigneur*. They were treated like gods, by colleagues as well as by patients, breezing through swing doors, minions trailing behind them. 'He still features in my nightmares,' Celia Imrie says today. 'A proud, incorrigible man with his dark, hard, evil eyes.' A lot of people remember those eyes. Set beneath a prominent, saturnine brow, they were like washed black pebbles. The long sweep of his face, with its firmly sculpted jaw and prominent ears, oozed old school confidence. 'There was a whiff of sulphur about him,' said the late Malcolm Lader, emeritus professor of clinical psychopharmacology at King's College London. He wore immaculate chalk-stripe suits (never a white coat), whether he was presenting TV programmes on the BBC, conducting his rounds or making frequent trips across the Atlantic to lecture. Over six feet tall, he was an imposing physical presence, on the wards as well as the rugby pitch. 'If he'd been a gorilla, he would have been one of those huge male silverbacks,' according to Henry Oakeley, Sargant's registrar in the 1960s.

Almost forgotten today, Sargant was once a household name: the most well-known psychiatrist of his generation and the author of *Battle for the Mind* (1957), a global bestseller about brainwashing. He was the sort of person 'of whom legends are made', according to Lord David Owen, Sargant's registrar in 1965. A man who claimed he could tell if a patient was getting better just by the confidence with which they turned the door handle of his consulting room. When he wasn't appearing on television or hosting cocktail parties at his flat in north London, he was attending to the mental aberrations of the great and the good. Principal dancers from the Royal Ballet as well as politicians,* spies, artists, aristocrats, actors, Middle Eastern royalty – he saw them all, many of them privately. It was nothing short of an honour to be treated by the 'eminent' William Sargant, a step in itself on the road to recovery. At least, that's what GPs up and down the country told their patients when referring them to him.

One of the most disturbing aspects of the Sleep Room was a profound sense of foreboding. Patients were aware that if they didn't

* The controversial Conservative peer Lord Robert Boothby was treated on Ward Five for an apparent drink problem in 1967. Three years earlier, he had been photographed with Ronnie Kray. 'The senior staff were very protective of Boothby,' recalls one nurse. 'He had a raucous laugh and lots of visitors, who used to bring in bottles for him.'

improve an even worse fate awaited them: lobotomy. Sargant had administered narcosis to traumatised soldiers in the Second World War, but admitted it was 'not without its dangers'. He only started to champion the treatment again in the 1960s, when one of his registrars, Chris Walter, noticed that if patients were given ECT, antidepressants *and* narcosis, they did better than those who were just given ECT and antidepressants. As was so often the case in psychiatry, no one was quite sure why. But patients were now sent to the Sleep Room instead of being lobotomised – they would only go under the knife if narcosis failed. The Sleep Room, in other words, had become a last chance saloon.

'Lobotomy was in the air, talked about openly on the ward,' Celia remembers. 'For all I know, that might have been the next treatment for me.' Mary has a similar memory. 'I was absolutely terrified at the prospect of lobotomy,' she says. 'I had it in my head that this was going to happen to me if I didn't pull my socks up.'

Lobotomy might also have been an option for prima ballerina Svetlana Beriosova. During the 1950s and 1960s, she was one of the Royal Ballet's biggest stars. But she began to struggle with alcoholism and failed to respond to psychoanalysis. Her psychiatrist, Donald Winnicott, had been one of Sargant's fiercest critics in the 1950s, accusing him of using lobotomy to treat everything from dermatitis to nervous vomiting, but he still asked Sargant to admit her in the late 1960s. Beriosova, who had once danced *The Sleeping Beauty* for the Sadler's Wells Ballet, was subjected to narcosis and ECT but the treatment failed. She escaped lobotomy – Winnicott would never have allowed it – but her career came to a dramatic end in 1971 during a performance of *Anastasia* at Covent Garden, when she collapsed drunkenly on stage while en pointe.

Sargant encouraged his team to publish papers on Walter's discovery of combined treatments, lending the Sleep Room a veneer of medical respectability. The best results, Sargant claimed, were achieved with patients who were 'severely depressed, anxious and suicidal' and resistant to other treatments. Worthwhile improvements were also achieved in patients with 'obsessional neurosis' (obsessive compulsive disorder) and schizophrenia.

Behind the medical papers, however, the Sleep Room served a more sinister purpose. As the sixties started to swing and Sargant's reputation soared, middle-class parents sent their wayward daughters to the Sleep Room for moral correction. In the mid 1960s, for example, a wealthy businessman contacted Sargant, explaining that his daughter had fallen in love with an 'unsuitable' local man in Europe and wanted to marry him. Could Sargant help? A photo later emerged of Sargant, the father and a heavily sedated daughter standing at the door of the aeroplane that had returned her to the UK. 'Basically, Sargant brought this attractive young woman back at the end of a needle,' recalls a retired professor, who was a student at St Thomas' at the time.

After being admitted to one of the two private rooms on Ward Five, she was given narcosis, together with ECT and a cornucopia of drugs that would have included Largactil, an antipsychotic, and sodium amytal, a sedative, as well as two different types of antidepressant that many colleagues felt shouldn't be combined: Nardil and Tryptizol.

It soon became clear that the main reason for sending the young woman to the Sleep Room was to eradicate all memories of her *folie l'amour* – to wipe her mind clean. A few weeks later, Sargant deemed her sufficiently recovered to be presented at the weekly 'grand teaching round'. He liked to teach by demonstration and his sessions were popular with medical students on their psychiatric 'firm' (a discontinued form of medical apprenticeship). 'It was a bit like the Coliseum,' the retired professor recalls. 'Tiered seating, with the patient and Sargant at the bottom.'

Sargant began by asking the young woman how she was. 'Fine, thank you,' she replied. He then enquired if she still had feelings for her boyfriend. 'Of course,' she said. And what was she going to do about those feelings? 'As soon as I get out of this dump, I'm going to jump on the first plane and marry him,' she replied. Sargant promptly sent her back to the Sleep Room for a further course of narcosis and ECT.

Another St Thomas' medical student, now a retired consultant, vividly remembers the patient locking eyes with him. 'What I think made us uncomfortable was that she was our age and could easily have been in our social circles,' he says. 'One got the impression that Sargant presented her as an illustration of how skilled he was in carrying out her parents' wishes in extracting her from her romance. He was of course certain that he was acting in her best interests, but I will never forget her troubled face.'

There are many disturbing aspects to this story (some details of which have been changed for privacy). One is the use of narcosis and ECT as a form of social correction. Another is the absence of patient consent. The third is that she was, like many of Sargant's patients, an attractive young woman. Other similar cases followed. The BBC radio presenter Alan Keith brought his daughter, Linda, back from America to London, where she was subsequently admitted into the Sleep Room. Linda was a *Vogue* model. After dating the Rolling Stones' Keith Richards for two years, a romance that started when she was seventeen, she left him for Jimi Hendrix and an increasingly destructive life of sex, drugs and rock 'n' roll. By 1969, she was under Sargant's care. 'My father often used to say to me: "You must live within the narrow confines of middle-class society",' Linda remembers today. 'They even drove me past Sargant's house on Hamilton Terrace to persuade me what a great man he was.'

Mary Thornton had a similar experience. Her mother used to turn up at her boyfriend's house to throw milk bottles at him. The stress led to a breakdown and her parents sent Mary to the Sleep Room, aged twenty. 'I was fairly bonny, I suppose,' she says today. 'Years later, I asked my mother why she had signed me up for Sargant. It had been such a vicious, horrible treatment and I wasn't yet twenty-one. She said it was because I was bad. But I was an adult. I wasn't bad! She probably thought Sargant was God.'

In the past fifteen years, websites such as We Were Expendable, The Royal Waterloo Experiment, William Sargant at the Royal Waterloo Hospital and the Ward Five Association have tried to bring survivors together to tell the world what happened to them. It hasn't been easy. Some of the medical records of patients who passed through the Sleep Room, including five who died, have disappeared or been destroyed. And there is still a stigma attached to mental illness. Patients are often reluctant to tell their story, one comparing the shame of her time in the Sleep Room to admitting to a stretch in prison.

Sargant's wasn't the only Sleep Room in the world. There was another based at the Allan Memorial Institute for Psychiatry at McGill University in Montreal in the 1950s and 1960s. In 1979, former State Department analyst John Marks revealed in his book *The Search for the 'Manchurian Candidate'* that it was covertly funded by the CIA as part of the Agency's notorious mind control project, MKULTRA. This Sleep Room was run by Scottish-born psychiatrist Dr Ewen Cameron – a close colleague and personal friend of Sargant's. And then there was Dr Harry Bailey, an Australian disciple of Sargant's who had been inspired by his work with continuous narcosis. In the 1960s and 1970s, twenty-four people died in Bailey's Sleep Room based in a Sydney suburb, a tragedy that was investigated by a royal commission. The US and Australian Sleep Rooms have both been exposed but Sargant's was brushed under the carpet. Perhaps because it took place at the heart of the medical establishment, in the middle of London, and involved a certain class of person with powerful friends – in other words, a very British scandal.

There is still time to establish the true story of the Sleep Room on the top floor of the Royal Waterloo in London. As this book will reveal, the clues are in Sargant's personal papers, left to the Wellcome Collection, and in his own books, including *Battle for the Mind*, and his autobiography, *The Unquiet Mind* (1967), both co-authored by the poet Robert Graves. Through these pages we will explore his failure to become a consultant in general medicine; the unprecedented opportunity to experiment on thousands of traumatised soldiers in the Second World War; his close relationship with Western intelligence services and Big Pharma – and with young female patients, several of whom say they were sexually assaulted by Sargant. Did ambition make him reckless, more concerned with personal reputation than patient welfare? Or did he fit the stereotype of the crazy psychiatrist who was more disturbed that those he sought to cure?

Sargant's surviving patients believe he represented the epitome of patrician arrogance, subjecting them to a pattern of behaviour that echoes how men have, throughout history, exerted control over women's bodies. Suffering from a range of eating disorders, OCD and anxiety, as well as postnatal depression, many were in their teens or early twenties during their treatment, which means that they are now in their seventies. And enough of them are alive and courageous enough to have allowed me to piece together what really happened in Ward Five – and why.

Fifty-year-old recollections can be unreliable, particularly those dimmed by repeated electric shocks and large doses of drugs. And there are those who will argue that memories set down while thoughts are distorted by mental illness are not real and should not be trusted. But the brain is a resilient organ. Sargant underestimated its plasticity, its resistance to being permanently 'repatterned'. For the slate to be wiped clean. And now his patients, for so long neither heard nor believed, are ready to talk, to tell their story in their own words.

2

Celia Imrie

My poor mother used to come and visit me from Guildford every day when I was an anorexia patient on Ward Five at the Royal Waterloo. It was 1966 and I was only fourteen at the time. I used to look out of the fifth-floor window and see her hurrying frantically across the road from the station. There were moments when she sat down beside my bed and I didn't even know who she was. At other times, they wouldn't let me see her, because I was still struggling to eat my midday lunch at 2.30 p.m. It was like being in a prison camp. They are horrible memories, as you can imagine, and sometimes I struggle to recall exactly what happened.

I was brought up in Guildford, the fourth of five siblings. My mother was a true-blue aristocrat; my father was born in a tenement block in Glasgow. He went on to become a successful doctor, dentist and radiologist who worked at the Royal Surrey County Hospital in Guildford. I think it was embarrassing for him to have a daughter who starved herself.

My eating problems started when I applied, aged eleven, to the Royal Ballet School. I was quite stubborn and wilful as a child and had this grand plan to become a ballet dancer. After serving my time in the corps de ballet, I would be discovered and dance in the arms of Rudolf Nureyev, who I worshipped and would hope to marry one day.

I pressed my parents to let me attend ballet classes, and went in for every exam I could, until I was good enough for my teachers to send me to audition for a place at White Lodge, the junior branch of the Royal Ballet School in Richmond. I waited anxiously at home for the results to arrive, yearning for the day when I would be whisked away from our home in Surrey to start my new life as a ballet student. But the letter never came. Sensing that something was wrong, I went searching for it, broke into my mother's bureau, and found it. Hands trembling, I slid the already opened letter from its envelope and read the fatal words: 'Celia is very good and advanced for her age, but sadly she is going to be too big ever to become a dancer.'

Too big? I was shattered, and lost an astonishing amount of weight. I would look at myself in the mirror and, even though I was skeletal, I didn't think I had gone far enough. In fact, I was 5ft 2in and weighed 4 stone. It must have been terribly difficult for my father, but he called in a child psychologist to see me.

I was sent for a brief spell in the local hospital, where staff offered me three meals a day, which I politely refused. After a few weeks, I was released to spend Christmas with my family. I was happy to come home, but I became sly over the following months, knowing that in future I must find ever better ways of avoiding eating. I worked out every means possible to dispose of food, determined to get 'small' enough to be a dancer, and I was soon little more than a carcass with skin.

When I was twelve, I was sent away to Great Ormond Street Hospital for Children. After six weeks or so, two things happened in short succession. First, my dance teacher came to visit me to say goodbye. Miss Hawkesworth had been told that my weight was so low I would not survive the few weeks until Christmas. Apparently, they were thinking of letting me go home because I wouldn't be around for another Christmas. 'I've come to visit you because they told me you would die in two weeks,' she said. For months, people had been telling me to eat: 'If you don't eat, you will fade away. Please eat. Eat. Eat.' And so I hadn't. Now here was someone telling me that I was going to die. Die? How dare anyone tell me what to do. I wasn't going to die just to please them. Whenever I've been issued with an order in life, my instinct has always been the same: do the opposite. Thanks to Miss Hawkesworth, I decided there and then I would not die.

And then, one of the nurses, quite improperly I am sure, said to me one morning, 'You do realise that your selfish act of starving yourself means you are stealing the bed of a truly sick, possibly dying child?' She described other stricken children she had treated at Great Ormond Street – those with polio and cancer. She had no idea, but what she said that day well and truly pricked my conscience and I vowed to get better. I was not going to let anyone think that my selfishness was responsible for depriving a more deserving sick child of treatment.

Back at home, I made a full recovery. But then, a few years later, I began to starve myself again. I really don't know what went wrong or why, but my condition was serious enough for me to be admitted, aged fourteen, to Ward Five at the Royal Waterloo. It was 1966 and I was now at senior school – too old, apparently, for a children's hospital. Once there I was put in the care of a team of doctors, among them Dr John Pollitt and Dr William Sargant, who was then a renowned psychiatrist. My parents must have thought I was being seen by the very best.

The nurses on Ward Five were quite strict with me, even though I was the youngest on the ward. Lunch was always at midday and visitors were allowed from 2.30 p.m., which is why I was sometimes not permitted to see my mother. I had to finish my food if I was to be allowed visitors and there was nowhere to hide it.

I was also put on heavy medication as soon as I arrived. Three doses of liquid Largactil daily. I can remember the tumbler cup quite clearly. The side effects were startling. My hands shook uncontrollably for most of the day, and I'd wake up to find clumps of my hair on the pillow. But the worst consequence was that everything I saw was in double vision. When Sargant came into the room, there were two of him. It was horrific and terrifying. Even simple tasks such as picking up a glass of water became impossible.

I was injected with insulin every day too. Sargant was a big believer in fattening up his patients to get them well and you soon put on weight with insulin. I think I had what was called 'sub-coma shock treatment'– you weren't given enough insulin to induce a hypoglycaemic coma, but it was enough to make you drowsy, weak, sweaty and hungry.

I will never know for sure if I was given electric shocks during my stay. Some years back, I tried to find my hospital records, to see the details of my treatment. Unfortunately, Sargant seems to have taken away a lot of his patients' records, including mine, when he retired from the NHS in 1972. Either that, or they were destroyed. I can't remember ECT happening to me, but I can remember it happening to others.

At one point during my stay, I shared a two-bed room with another woman, and I witnessed her having electric shock treatment right next to me. I vividly recall every sight, sound and smell. The huge rubber plug jammed between her teeth; the strange, almost silent cry, like a sigh of pain, she made as her tormented body shuddered and jerked; the scent of burning hair and flesh. It was a terrible thing for a fourteen-year-old to witness. Afterwards, Sargant came into our room and said in front of the woman, 'Well, if we hadn't caught her, she would have been out of the window.'

The Great Man himself was very grand when he came on his ward rounds, tall with an evil presence. The other doctors and nurses all bowed and scraped – they were in thrall to this self-appointed god of psychiatry. The person who visited me most days was Pollitt, who was actually rather a sweet man – the complete opposite of Sargant.

Sargant still features in my nightmares. He was brusque and cold, and he never talked directly to you. Instead he issued orders over your head, talking about 'this one' and 'that one'. But that was preferable to making eye contact with this proud, incorrigible man with his hard, dark eyes.

When I think of him today, I visualise him like one of the senior doctors in *Dr. Kildare*. He had a face of thunder, like the devil, and had a horrible aura. There was almost something simian about his features, the strong creases and wrinkles, a widow's peak and high forehead. I can see his face now.

After Sargant left the ward, the nurses would start preparing the horrors he'd prescribed for the day, including electro-convulsive therapy. Friends have asked what it was like to have electrodes put either side of your skull before a shock of up to 110 volts was fired through your brain, triggering a grand mal seizure that made you dribble into your pillow and your back arch. But the truth is I don't remember. What I do know is that memory loss is a common side effect of the treatment.

At one point, I do remember having to go over to St Thomas' and be paraded in front of a theatre full of students as part of one of Sargant's 'grand round' presentations. He was there in the middle of everyone, with me, addressing a group of medical students. 'This patient is having blah, blah, blah.' I can't remember exactly what Sargant said, but I suspect he boasted about the insulin I was being given – and possibly the electric shocks. I had to take my clothes off because the students had to see how thin I was, I suppose, but as a child of fourteen, it was a pretty horrific experience.

I also remember going to visit another room on the ward, which had two girls inside. It must have been during the winter months as their room was quite dark. Being taken to the loo is another memory – I clearly wasn't able to walk on my own. And at some point I went down the end of the ward to look at the Sleep Room. I used to peer through the portholes in the swing doors, and gaze at the dead-looking women lying on the floor on grey mattresses, silent in a kind of electrically induced twilight. I can remember the distinctive smell too – the smell of sleep.

People have asked me if I ever spent any time inside that room. I can't be sure, but I can picture it so clearly. And, although I saw many female patients come back to the ward from there, I never saw anyone emerge from the place awake. You went in asleep and you came out asleep, and you were totally unconscious while inside. So you wouldn't necessarily be aware that you'd had the treatment. Who knows? Maybe I was in the Sleep Room. Today, I must accept the very real possibility that I was. Certainly the insulin treatment that I received was often a precursor to narcosis. Like the electric shocks, I have to assume that it might have happened to me, even though I can only recall it happening to others.

I do know that lobotomy – or leucotomy, as the doctors called it – was a very real threat. It was in the air, talked about openly on the ward. People who didn't recover after a course of narcosis in the Sleep Room would go off to be lobotomised. For all I know, that might have been the next treatment for me. I distinctly remember patients on the ward with big bandages on their head, barely able to walk. I'm also sure there were some men on the ward too, which in itself was rather peculiar in those days.

Many years later, I went with friends to see *Coma*. It is a second-rate film starring Michael Douglas and Geneviève Bujold, in which Bujold discovers a ward full of patients suspended in hammocks in drug-induced comas. When we came out into Leicester Square in London, my friends were laughing at the silliness of the plot, but I had the shakes and it took me some days to recover. They probably thought I was coming down with something. In fact, it wasn't until much later that I saw the link and realised why that film had upset me so deeply.

What I find so horrifying is that the doctors increased my

medication so much that I no longer recognised my darling mother. I didn't know who anyone was. In our family, we all had flower names, and our nanny was called Poppy, but my mother said that I kept calling out for 'Bobby'. As a nurse increased the dosage one day, I overheard her saying to the ward sister that I was exhibiting a 'dangerous resistance' to the drugs. Dangerous for whom? The staff or me? Sargant used to say that every dog has his breaking point – the eccentrics just took longer. I suppose my 'dangerous resistance' was what he was talking about. I like to think that I was one of those eccentric dogs he did not manage to break.

Other patients on Ward Five were less fortunate. Most of them were women suffering from depression. From my bed, I watched them howling and moaning, fighting with the nurses. I remember one poor lady who used to run up and down the ward, screaming. I looked at that woman and thought, I don't want to be here any more. It's a madhouse and I don't want to go mad. I came to the conclusion that it was only me who could get myself out of that awful place. I hated every minute of my time there. It must have been later on, when they were taking me down on the Largactil and my mind was starting to clear, but I vowed to get the hell out.

They were only going to discharge me, however, if I ate, so I had to eat. But you have to be so determined. It takes an enormous amount of wilfulness. And whatever Sargant might have thought was going to make me start eating again, the eventual cure from my self-induced anorexia had nothing to do with him or his bizarre techniques. It was my own determination.

I later returned to school, somewhat changed in appearance. During an outpatient consultation with my psychiatrist, I said I would like to have a baby one day, and hoped that would still be possible since my treatment on Ward Five had disrupted the usual order of puberty. Specialists at St Thomas' decided to give me a massive dose of oestrogen to kick-start the process. The trouble was that practically overnight it sent me from being flat chested to a 38-inch double-D cup.

So, resembling a teenage brunette version of Jayne Mansfield in a fright wig, I failed my O levels and left school the day I turned sixteen, the earliest I was legally allowed. Determined to follow a life on stage, preferably one that involved dance, I won a place at the local drama school. I was on my way.

One of the biggest regrets I have today, as I reflect on those years, is what I put my family through: my parents, brother and three sisters. I caused them and my nanny, Poppy, such worry. I do wonder if my mother and father were ever consulted about my treatment on Ward Five. My poor mother was so worried. And she believed in the medical profession – believed in Sargant.

I have gone through my life hoping that I've got over what happened to me all those years ago. It will always be an issue for me, but I love food. I also fear that there is something remaining of Sargant in my psyche. He continues to cast a long shadow over me, sixty years later. I have this thing that I must obey much older men and I sometimes make inexplicable decisions. I was only fourteen and Sargant was fifty-eight when he treated me. It might also be to do with my father being old (he was sixty when he had me, sixty-five when he had my little sister), but I have a feeling that there's an element of Sargant lingering in my brain. The brain is a very fragile thing and I just feel there has to be some legacy that he's left there, like an imprint. Even today, I can still see his face so clearly, his ape-like features. And sometimes I go to the depths of despair for no real reason. Most of the time I manage to pull myself out of it, but there's no question that Sargant damaged me in some way.

Years later, I was talking to a professional dancer, who had appeared with the Royal Ballet. 'A lot of it was hell,' she told me. 'Not at all what I had thought it would be. It often made me very unhappy.' She described the strife and tension, the painful muscles, bleeding toes, rivalry and starvation diets. For the first time in my life, I wondered if I had been fortunate by being forced out of dance and into acting. I felt a tremendous surge of relief and started to wonder what had impelled me to chase a desire that had almost killed me at fourteen. Now, I finally knew that my life had gone the right way. I had taken the best possible path.

As for Sargant, my recovery owed nothing to him or to his barbaric treatments. It was my own sheer determination that got me better, steeled by a desire to escape from a truly horrifying man.*

* This chapter is based on two author interviews with Celia Imrie. It also draws on her account of Sargant in her bestselling memoir, *The Happy Hoofer* (Hodder & Stoughton, 2011).

3

'The full horror of Hanwell was closing in on me'

On a cold December night in 1933, a group of distinguished doctors gathered in a wood-panelled room at the Royal Society of Medicine on Wimpole Street in central London. They were there for an important symposium on neurological complications associated with pernicious anaemia, a condition in which the body doesn't have enough healthy red blood cells. The twenty-six-year-old William Sargant had been invited to speak. It was quite an accolade for such a young doctor, but Sargant had already demonstrated that he was a man in a hurry. The year before, he had been appointed the youngest ever medical superintendent at St Mary's Hospital, Paddington.

One by one, the heavyweights of haematology arrived. But as the symposium got under way, Sargant was noticeable by his absence. It wasn't like him to pass up such an opportunity for self-promotion. At Cambridge, where he'd been president of the university's Medical Society, he'd invited a range of luminaries to address the students, including Sir Humphry Rolleston, physician-in-ordinary to King George V.

Tonight, Sargant was due to speak on what he considered to be a remarkable breakthrough treatment, which he'd first announced in the *Lancet*. (The *Lancet* was edited by his friend Samuel Squire Sprigge, another of the doctors whom he had invited to talk at Cambridge.) Some of the pain, clumsy gait and cognitive impairment that accompanied pernicious anaemia, Sargant argued, could be relieved by a 'massive iron dosage'. Historically, iron had been used in small amounts to treat some forms of anaemia but it was not thought to have had any effect on any related neurological complications.

Sargant's bold hypothesis was part of his goal to become a consultant in general medicine at a leading London teaching hospital. He needed some scientific papers under his belt, but his tentative tone – 'Bearing these considerations in mind, it seemed to me just possible that . . . ' – suggested his findings were based more on a bedside hunch than statistical evidence. He'd followed up with a second article in December 1932 and this time its tone was breathtakingly confident: 'The intention of this paper is to prove that faulty iron metabolism is a cause of the nervous phenomena associated with all forms of anaemia.'

Haematology, the science of blood and its diseases, was an obvious focus for Sargant. In the 1920s and early 1930s, it was one of the most exciting and fashionable branches of medicine. Ingesting large amounts of liver, for example, had only recently been found to control, if not cure, pernicious anaemia. Sargant saw an opportunity to make his mark and duly prescribed vast quantities of iron pills to alleviate the disease's accompanying nervous symptoms. He prescribed as many as forty Blaud's pills a day – more than three times the maximum recommended dose. It was an early glimpse of his prodigious enthusiasm for pill popping. And the first time we see his famous bedside manner in action. Sargant saw himself as something of a holistic healer. He didn't just give patients the iron pills; he told them to get up and walk, persuading them that they *felt* well.

Dr Ann Dally, as his biographer, knew Sargant better than most. She believed that his methods of research into blood disease were remarkably similar to his later work as a psychiatrist. 'He had a powerful personality and a good deal of charisma,' she wrote. '*Everyone* tends to perform better when they have someone urging them on like that. My personal suspicion ... is that – like many bullies and persons of powerful personality – he had an intuitive perception of the patients whom he could dominate and on whom he could impose his ideas and methods – in a way forcing them to improve.'

Back at the Royal Society of Medicine, shortly after 8.30 p.m., Professor Edward Mellanby, secretary of the Medical Research Council, kicked off the symposium. He sat on the fence regarding Sargant's suggested use of Blaud's pills, suggesting instead that nerve degeneration in the spinal cord could be prevented by large amounts of vitamin A.

It was then Sargant's turn to speak but he still hadn't arrived. Dr Edward Carmichael, honorary physician to the National Hospital, Queen's Square, spoke next instead. He also had little time for Sargant's massive iron treatment, stating there 'was no improvement in either the blood picture or nervous symptoms or signs'. Sargant himself was still mysteriously absent and it was left to Frederick Langmead, professor of medicine at St Mary's, to present his findings. Sargant's account was full of the hyperbole and popular flourishes that would later make him such a persuasive communicator with patients and the media. After taking Blaud's pills, his patients made miraculous improvements. 'Reflexes have reappeared ... indecipherable handwriting has again become ordinary.'

Next up was Dr Charles Ungley, from the Royal Victoria Infirmary, Newcastle, who said that Sargant's iron method resulted in 'no significant alteration'. The night was going from bad to worse for Sargant. It was then the turn of Dr Leslie Witts, soon to become professor of haematology at St Bartholomew's.

The two men had history, having recently clashed in the pages of the *British Medical Journal*. Most of the published papers on pernicious anaemia and sub-acute combined degeneration were 'worthless', Witts said. Summing up proceedings, Dr Kinnier Wilson, the chairman, didn't bother to mention Sargant either. His plans to become a consultant in general medicine were in tatters.

'The text from the proceedings of the Royal Society of Medicine is a splendid example of the gentlemanly routines by which the British medical establishment achieves its ends – often without saying what they think at all,' according to Ann Dally. 'But they made it clear that they had no regard for Sargant's work and that he had no future in haematology.'

So where was Sargant that night? Had somebody warned him what sort of reception his iron theory was going to receive? Thanks to Dally's draft chapters of Sargant's early life, which have never been made public before, we now know that Sargant had fallen into a deep depression in December 1933, a condition so severe that he was subsequently admitted as a patient to Hanwell Mental Hospital in Southall, west London. Opened in 1831, Hanwell had been the first purpose-built asylum for 'pauper lunatics' in England, following the Madhouse Act of 1828. By the time Sargant arrived in early 1934, it housed up to three thousand patients, many of whom had languished in their cells for years.

To find out why Sargant had ended up as a patient in a grim asylum, Dally had contacted John Harman, a retired physician and Sargant's oldest friend from Cambridge (also the father of former MP Harriet Harman). This is what John Harman told Dally in a telephone conversation: 'He had his depression and was a patient in Hanwell Mental Asylum. His mother rang me up and told me he had been admitted there. She asked me to visit him as a friend, which I did.'

There is no reason to doubt Dally's or Harman's accounts.

(Dally had alluded to Sargant's depression in her entry on him for the *Dictionary of National Biography*.) We also know, from Sargant's autobiography, that depression played a central role in his life. And significantly, in keeping with his lifelong approach to mental health, he had tried to link it to an underlying physical problem. He begins *The Unquiet Mind* in 1934, when a 'very severe but as yet undiagnosed tuberculosis lung infection' plunged him into such a deep depression that he lost all interest in his medical research at St Mary's Hospital. He had not been on a proper holiday for four years and felt 'tired and ill'.

Sargant hinted further about the nature of what we'd now call a mental breakdown in his last interview, in 1987, the year before he died: 'I was very obsessed with the use of large doses of iron, particularly for sub-acute combined degeneration of the spinal cord, and one was getting quite miraculous results. And then, I suddenly collapsed: I was having this terrific career, and suddenly I couldn't do any more. I remember being nervous even of talking to students of 16, and I just resigned.'

The timeline in both accounts is frustratingly vague, complicated by the fact that Sargant never acknowledged that he was admitted to Hanwell as a patient.* In his autobiography, he wrote about being sent there in 1934 as a locum doctor – which contradicts what Harman, his oldest friend, had told Dally. 'A Hanwell admission in 1934 would have had extreme effects on a proud, ambitious and rather vain man,' according to Ben Spears, who was Sargant's senior registrar (and chief assistant) in psychiatry at St Thomas' from 1969 to 1972. 'It would have afflicted him

* Sargant came close to a public admission that he had been admitted as a patient to Hanwell during a 1968 BBC documentary, *Towards Tomorrow: People Like Us*. In a lively opening discussion with other psychiatrists, he said: 'In 1934, when I went into the old Hanwell, you couldn't get out of Hanwell. You had to have the wisdom of Job to get out.' He then paused, before switching to the third person. 'They stayed there forever.' He could have been referring to his job as a locum, of course, but it was an interesting choice of words.

with the mark of Cain. Words such as "lunacy", "pauper" and "asylum" would have still been in wide usage.'

Both accounts could be right: perhaps Sargant attended Hanwell as a patient *and* as a locum doctor, during two separate three-month stints in 1934. It is more likely, however, that he attended each time as a patient. (It would have been difficult to switch from being a patient to doctor.) There is, however, no clerical evidence of either stay. A thorough search of Hanwell's medical and discharge registers at the London Metropolitan Archives failed to reveal that Sargant had been formally admitted or discharged as a patient on a certified, temporary, permanent or private basis. As a doctor, however, he might have been treated on an informal basis – off the books, as it were. The records also have no trace of Sargant ever having worked at Hanwell as a locum. In 1947, when he was invited to be visiting professor of psychiatry at Duke University in America, his CV included locum work at the Maudsley, but it made no mention of being a locum at Hanwell.

Spears believes Sargant would have been admitted to Hanwell as a 'temporary patient', which would have involved the signature of one or two physicians and a written application from a family member. 'It must have been extreme,' he says. 'Something like a suicide attempt or threat, or a florid psychosis.'

Spears is better placed than most to assess his former boss's state of mind. After three years working with Sargant, he went into private practice in Prince Edward Island, Canada, where he enjoyed a distinguished fifty-year career in psychiatry. During his time at St Thomas', he had got along well with Sargant, admiring his 'clinical courage' and was appreciative of his 'personal kindness'.

Given Sargant's patterns of thought and personal habits, Spears thinks that he had what is known today as attention deficit hyperactivity disorder (ADHD). 'Impulsive, risk-taking behaviour is a frequent concomitant,' he says. One possible sign of Sargant's ADHD was his inability to stop at the correct set of traffic lights in Trafalgar Square. According to Spears, Sargant had so many car accidents that he couldn't get insurance. Eventually, he had to join a trade union in order to qualify under a group insurance policy. 'His issue with traffic lights was pretty typical ADHD behaviour, this impulse to accelerate on a red light.'

In a letter to Robert Graves in 1966, Sargant revealed that he also suffered from another, more unusual, medical condition: porphyria, the hereditary illness that was long thought to be behind George III's insanity. Porphyria affects the liver and nervous system. Symptoms can also be psychiatric, including anxiety, delirium, depression and hallucinations. In rare cases, porphyria can present solely as a psychosis. Spears remembers Sargant referring to a recurrent metabolic disorder. 'He called it "that flu" and talked wistfully about the cocktails he used to have in the past,' Spears says. 'Porphyria was the reason he gave up alcohol.'

Spears also believes that Sargant suffered from bipolar disorder, which often coexists with ADHD. 'If I were asked to tender a diagnosis, we have major depression, type 2 bipolar disorder, ADHD, porphyria and possibly tuberculosis. In fact, none of these are incompatible with the other and they could all be comorbid. Some people might just settle for the proposition that greatness and pathology are often bedmates.'

Depression of one sort or another would haunt Sargant for the rest of his life. Some claim that his condition made him a better psychiatrist. 'He was able to understand that those who were depressed were in many senses far more ill than people with cancer or in severe pain,' according to David Owen. 'His point was that psychiatric illness is very serious and damaging, and that patients can commit suicide from it, therefore you're entitled to take some risks with drug treatment.'

Sargant wouldn't be the first or last psychiatrist to suffer from the same conditions he sought to cure in others. Dr Chloe Beale, consultant liaision psychiatrist at Homerton Hospital, has spoken openly about her own mental illness, five years after becoming a consultant. She doesn't, however, believe that it has given her a greater ability to empathise with all her patients. 'I do not have any first-hand knowledge of many of the social factors that precipitate and perpetuate illness in so many people,' she says. 'I experience illness from a baseline of privilege.'

As a believer in drugs, Sargant was also more than happy to self-medicate, which over time would become a constant prop for him. At one party in the 1960s, the late Dr Eric West, a senior registrar in psychiatry at St Thomas', remembered Sargant refusing cheese and wine because he said he was on Nardil, an antidepressant.

'One of the problems is that Nardil does make patients a bit wild,' according to Peter Tyrer, who was Sargant's house physician at the Royal Waterloo in 1966 and is now emeritus professor of community psychiatry at Imperial College London. 'There's a sort of manic element to these drugs. When they first came out, they used to be called psychic energisers. I felt some of Sargant's behaviour was drug-induced in some ways.'

The Scottish 'anti-psychiatrist' R. D. Laing, one of Sargant's fiercest critics, even suggested that Sargant himself had been treated with ECT. 'There were rumours that he gave himself electric shocks and that he was manic depressive,' Laing said. A former colleague thought that Rudolf Freudenberg, a pioneer of insulin coma therapy, might have given ECT to Sargant at Netherne Hospital in Surrey during the 1950s. (The two men had worked together in the 1930s at Moorcroft House, a private hospital in Middlesex.)

Whatever the cause of Sargant's mental breakdown, Dr G. W. B. James, his boss at St Mary's, was the man responsible for sending him to Hanwell. James was well qualified to diagnose

Sargant's fragile state of mind. Not only was he physician for mental diseases at St Mary's, he also held regular demonstrations for his students at Hanwell. He would have known the staff well enough, perhaps, to ask them to look after one of their own.

Intriguingly, Sargant wrote about his arrival at Hanwell in *The Unquiet Mind*, but the passages resonate with a quite different meaning in the light of Dally's discovery. On his second day, for example, he wrote that he examined a woman who thought she was Queen Mary. To reassure her, he announced himself as the 'Royal Physician come to treat Her Majesty', whereupon she abruptly told him to take his hands out of his pockets. Was this an example of Sargant's empathetic bedside manner as a doctor? Or a description of his own psychosis, sharing delusions of grandeur with a fellow patient? A textbook *folie à deux*?

After his second stint at Hanwell in the summer of 1934, Sargant could bear the place no longer. 'The full horror of Hanwell was closing in on me.' He left to assist his brother-in-law at his general practice in Nottingham. But Hanwell had left an indelible mark, inspiring him to become a psychiatrist. In particular, he became increasingly convinced that 'insanity' would one day be perceived as a series of 'physically treatable disorders'.

More than thirty years later, Sargant's publisher would describe his autobiography as 'frank and forthright reminiscences', and praise its 'startling candour', but we now know its narrator was unreliable. Despite a lifetime claiming to reduce the stigma of mental health, Sargant had felt unable to admit to the real nature of his own illness.

4

'Thrashed time after time'

Sargant made only one direct reference to his mother in *The Unquiet Mind*. Colleagues rarely heard him mention her either. Nor did she feature much in his journalism, except in one article on pornography, written for *The Times* in 1976. 'My mother, who had eight children, always felt that intercourse was something a woman had to undergo to prevent her husband from going to women waiting round the corner to oblige.'

It's as if Sargant was wary of putting himself on the couch. He was almost apologetic for including a chapter on his early years in his autobiography. If it had been up to him (and not Robert Graves, who edited and substantially re-wrote the book), he might have focused more on his self-styled quest to relieve mental suffering. Either that or rugby, about which he wrote at length.

Sargant's father, Norman, was the dominant force in his upbringing, a serious and intense Methodist. He had been obliged to take on the family's merchant business after his own father had been killed in a carriage accident. The large family home was on Hornsey Lane in Highgate, where Norman liked to entertain members of the Church. John James Sainsbury, founder of the supermarket chain, was their neighbour.

His grandfather and father swung between considerable fortune and near bankruptcy. Norman made a lot of money in Indian rubber but would go on to lose it all in the Great Depression. Before his fall from grace, he had met and married the daughter of a Welsh Methodist preacher. Alice was one of fifteen children and she in turn bore eight (four girls, three boys – one child died young). Money was not a problem in Sargant's childhood, but he felt bad being driven around London in a large Wolseley car amid poverty and unemployment during the First World War.

Sargant's older brother, Tom, would become the founding secretary of Justice, the law reform and human rights charity. The two brothers nearly fell out when Tom wrote an article about the hydrogen bomb and communism in the 1950s, arguing that both were the products of the divorce of religion from science and politics respectively. (William thought it would damage his own reputation, calling his brother 'delusional'; Tom accused William of 'unpardonable pride'.) Their younger brother, Norman, continued the family tradition and entered the Church. He was consecrated as the second bishop in the Church of South India's Diocese of Mysore, where he was known for his zeal and evangelism.

A month after the outbreak of war in 1914, Sargant was dispatched to board at St Wilfrid's, in Seaford, Sussex. This stretch of southern England was once full of boys' prep schools, many of which have since closed, including St Wilfrid's, amid allegations of sexual abuse. Sargant revealed little about his own time there except that he was 'thrashed time after time' for his rebelliousness. His behaviour only improved when his younger brother Norman arrived. He went on to be become head of school and captain of football.

Ann Dally had an interesting professional take on the constant beatings. 'For so young a boy to be sent away from home and "thrashed time after time" and then to describe it in so casual a way suggests that he experienced considerable unhappiness and denial of feeling.' According to Dally, there is psychiatric and anecdotal evidence that this kind of trauma can lead to sado-masochistic fantasies and practices. 'Was he already experiencing masochistic satisfaction from being hurt and humiliated, then emerging unbowed?'

Most of Sargant's friends went on from St Wilfrid's to Eton or Harrow. Sargant's father, however, insisted that he attended the Leys School in Cambridge. If he was bitter, he didn't show it. At the Leys, Sargant was poor at Greek and gave up classics. He didn't fancy being a teacher and felt 'unworthy' to become a parson. Although he had attended Archway Methodist Church up to three times every Sunday as a child, Sargant lost what faith he had as he grew older. But his father and his Methodist upbringing made an undeniable impression on him and his brothers. They should dedicate their lives to helping others.

Medicine called, but so too did sport. Sargant captained the school's football, hockey and cricket teams, and played for the rugby XV. He did just enough work to pass exams and spent his spare time reading history. During his first year at St John's College, Cambridge, he did even less work, preferring instead to join numerous societies and play sport every day. Anatomy exams proved a struggle. He had bursts of what he called 'almost hypomanic activity', aware that the joys of university life could not last for ever, and seemed most concerned with getting the rugby blue that always eluded him. (He was on the bench for the Varsity Match.) He would continue to play rugby at St Mary's, where he starred in the hospital team. He also played for Middlesex and turned out three times for the Barbarians, the elite invitation touring team.

In his last year at Cambridge, he was elected to the committee of the Union Society, where he began to show a skill for networking. Perhaps his most significant contact was Selwyn Lloyd, who would go on to become Foreign Secretary and Chancellor of the Exchequer.

The Great Depression was already looming in 1928, and by the time Sargant came down from Cambridge in 1929, his father was close to bankruptcy. Sargant found himself £150 in the red. Just as he considered giving up medicine altogether, the dean of St Mary's Hospital, Dr Charles Wilson, later Lord Moran, offered him a £200 scholarship, a reward more for Sargant's rugby prowess than his academic acumen.

In his autobiography, Sargant justified '"games" scholarships' by citing Wilson's belief that success in medicine required more than intelligence. 'A bright academic boy might end up in a mental hospital suffering from schizophrenia, whereas the rugger man, unless a plain fool, would somehow fight his way over the medical touchline.' It's an interesting justification, given Sargant's own admission to Hanwell. By portraying himself as a rugby-playing student, it's as if he was consciously distancing himself from the academic high achiever, a personality type that was allegedly more prone to breakdown.

Sargant's early years at St Mary's were unhappy. He was broke and could no longer turn to his parents for money. They were soon forced to leave their home on Hornsey Lane and let it out as a hostel, moving back into the small house in Highgate where Sargant had been born on 24 April 1907, and where he now returned to live. The threat of bankruptcy hung heavy and his parents still had three children to educate.

His first job at St Mary's was as an unpaid house surgeon. He had to earn his money from coroners' inquests, begging ambulance drivers to bring dead bodies to St Mary's rather than to St George's in south London. He was also starting to drink and smoke heavily. His father had promised him a sum of money if he didn't smoke before going to university. Sargant had cashed the cheque on his first day at Cambridge and within a fortnight had become hooked, going on to become a forty-a-day man. 'Wine, women and song' characterised his time at St Mary's, which included stitching up a patient's bleeding gum while drunk on champagne and gin.

At the remarkably young age of twenty-five, he became medical superintendent at St Mary's, a role that gave him complete control over in-patient admission, as well oversight of house physicians, house surgeons and nursing staff. He had also published his ill-fated paper in the *Lancet* about the benefits of iron for anaemic patients with neurological symptoms. He was living near Baker Street, away from his family, and had passed his Royal College of Physicians membership exam at the first attempt. But all was not well. He was stressed from his job and word must have reached him in advance that his paper on anaemia was about to go down badly with the people who mattered. As the pressure mounted and his appearance at Wimpole Street in December 1933 drew near, he collapsed.

5

'Took first dose, wrote this story'

History does not record what the animals at London's famous Zoological Gardens made of the man in a smart suit strolling energetically around Regent's Park one Saturday afternoon in 1936. Sargant had taken a break from the Maudsley psychiatric hospital in south London where he was now working to head up to the zoo. Giraffes had arrived that year – the first time they had been seen in England – and had caused a public sensation. Sargant was on a special visit to see them. He was also on another kind of trip. Before setting out, he had taken a Benzedrine sulphate tablet, an amphetamine more commonly known today as speed. Much like the giraffes, he was feeling sixteen feet tall.

He returned to the hospital and worked hard all evening, still full of confidence and vigour. It was possible his 'top-of-the-world' feeling was down to something else, but he began to wonder if Benzedrine might help him pass his examinations.

Sargant had joined the Maudsley the previous year, after working with his brother-in-law in Nottingham. It was his old friend at St Mary's, Dr James, who had fixed him up with a job back in London, still convinced that Sargant's future lay in psychiatry, despite (or because of) his experience at Hanwell. Benzedrine, the first amphetamine to be commercially branded, had been patented a couple of years earlier by Smith, Kline & French (SKF), who had initially sold it as a decongestant spray. SKF was interested in other uses and offered to send Benzedrine sulphate tablets to doctors to trial. The company targeted psychiatrists in particular, believing that the drug was a mood improver. Soon it was being recommended to treat mild depression and narcolepsy, as well as chronic fatigue, hyperactivity, loss of libido and obesity. For now, though, Sargant was more concerned about his own medical exams and thought that he'd stumbled on a potent performance enhancer.

He popped another pill before sitting his Diploma of Psychological Medicine exam and did surprisingly well. Fearing, however, that the Benzedrine might have given him a false sense of confidence, he double-checked with the examiner afterwards on his marks. They were very good. Encouraged by the results, Sargant set up an intelligence test for patients at the Maudsley and found that the drug boosted the confidence of those suffering from mild depression. It hadn't necessarily increased their intelligence, but they scored higher marks. In a sign of things to come, Sargant hastily wrote up his testing methodology and results in the *Lancet*. He concluded that Benzedrine improved intelligence test scores by 'approximately 8 per cent'.

Sargant's test group had not been drawn from ordinary members of the public. It had comprised sick patients at a psychiatric hospital. One patient suffering from 'a depressive state with anxiety features' thought he'd done badly in the tests, but his results improved by fourteen points after he'd taken a 30mg tablet. 'Only one schizophrenic' – how many were there? – showed a large improvement after taking Benzedrine.

The consequences of the *Lancet* article were dire and immediate. By now, the tablets were available at chemists without prescription and word soon spread that they supposedly improved intelligence. No side effects had been considered, let alone the drug's addictive qualities. 'Imprudent people began using Benzedrine at random, often with disastrous results,' Sargant wrote later. One woman, for example, leapt from the window of a London hotel after consuming a large amount of Benzedrine with alcohol.

Benzedrine cocktails became fashionable, and students began taking the drug before exams. For some it worked. Others failed exams that they might otherwise have passed. As Sargant himself explained, Benzedrine generally inspired confidence and lessened fatigue and minor worries, but if an examinee panicked during an exam, the drug would exacerbate his anxiety.*

Sargant conveniently overlooked his own role in the subsequent surge in amphetamine use in 1930s Britain. He claimed that he had 'begged' SKF, which marketed the pills, to stop selling them until further trials had been carried out, but his protests ring hollow. In 1937, he published a second article about Benzedrine, this time in the *British Medical Journal*. Writing with Erich Guttmann, also from the Maudsley, he said that given the drug's properties had yet to be fully investigated, it was inadvisable that the drug be sold without a prescription. But Sargant still went on to extol its many apparent qualities, including its ability to 'remove mental fatigue brought on by excessive work or worry'. Medical colleagues, he added, said that it helped in lectures and interviews, giving them confidence and the ability to think quickly and talk convincingly.

Once again, the press had a field day. An unnamed staff reporter on the *Daily Express* wrote a tongue-in-cheek article with the headline 'New Superiority Drug Is Tried Out – Took First Dose, Wrote This Story'. Filing his copy two hours after taking 15mg of Benzedrine, the reporter began: 'By now I should have

---

* Benzedrine has since been shown to induce amphetamine psychosis in some vulnerable people, increasing underlying anxieties.

extra confidence and initiative. I should be able to make quick decisions and feel at least like a magnate.' The reporter went on to say that his local chemist, who supplied him with his 'superiority complex' pill, didn't know what the drug was for, but thought that it should be taken by prescription. To which the reporter replied: 'I took it by the prescription of Doctors Guttmann and Sargent [sic].'

Sargant's enthusiasm for amphetamines was typical of his time at the Maudsley and of a broader pharmacological optimism that was sweeping through medicine. (It was only eight years earlier that Alexander Fleming had discovered penicillin at St Mary's.) He had found the work in Nottingham claustrophobic, but it had opened his eyes to the benefits of tranquilisers. An 'ounce of phenobarbitone' was usually more effective than 'a hundred-weight of persuasive talk'. Edward Mapother, medical superintendent of the Maudsley, would go on to become Sargant's lifelong ideological hero ('the greatest psychiatrist I have ever met'), not least because of his disdain for the psychotherapeutic claims of the Tavistock Institute. More pragmatist than visionary, Mapother was keen to address psychiatry's low standing in general medicine, insisting that permanent staff were members of the Royal College of Physicians. At the time, he was assembling a team of psychiatrists who had experience in general medicine. He also refused to employ any doctor who had spent more than two years working at a psychiatric hospital, believing them to have become immune to patients' suffering.

Tipped off by Dr James, Mapother duly offered Sargant a locum job as a junior assistant medical officer. On his first day at the Maudsley, a patient took one look at Sargant, walked out of the hospital and killed himself. 'It was not a good start,' Sargant conceded. But he was delighted to be working for Mapother, someone who believed that the torpor of therapeutic nihilism needed to be replaced by therapeutic enthusiasm. And no one would prove more enthusiastic than Sargant when it came to celebrating the smorgasbord of 'shock' treatments that were being developed in Europe in the 1920s and 1930s: insulin coma therapy, convulsive therapy, narcosis and, later, lobotomy, all of which would later lead to the creation of the Sleep Room. As Dr Jonathan Miller, satirist, stage director and physician, observed: 'Shamed by the advances in every other field of medicine, the psychiatric profession was eager to appropriate anything that gave the impression of decisive scientific action.'

Sargant would embrace them all with a decisiveness that he believed was heroic and others felt was cavalier. He would also continue to champion them throughout his career, long after they had been widely condemned and superseded by safer treatments. It's easy for his modern critics to dismiss what were once seen as pioneering treatments in an era of experimentation in psychiatry. Much harder to explain is Sargant's persistence with extreme physical therapies in the face of mounting evidence *at the time* of their dangers. Was it dogmatic stubbornness or something else in his character, a sadomasochistic recklessness forged at his prep school and in the back wards of Hanwell mental asylum?

6

'With skilful handling death should be avoided'

Sargant was never too concerned about why something might improve a patient's mental wellbeing. All that interested him was results. For him, appalling side effects – including the risk of death – were an acceptable trade-off. Few things were riskier for a patient than to be given so much insulin that the body shut down for want of sugar and went into a hypoglycaemic coma. But that's exactly what Manfred Sakel, a doctor in Vienna, was doing to schizophrenic patients in 1935. It was one of the earliest of psychiatry's shock therapies – also known as 'heroic' therapies, because they were high-risk, extreme treatments, comparable historically to bloodletting. (Doctors might have considered their own interventions heroic, but the real heroes were often the patients who survived them.)

Sakel had discovered the treatment in the 1920s, while working as an intern at a Berlin sanatorium. He had given an accidental overdose of insulin to a detoxing morphine addict, who fell into a coma and convulsed violently. When the patient awoke, however, his morphine withdrawal symptoms had diminished and he experienced a period of unprecedented mental clarity. Sakel experimented further with insulin on animals at his kitchen table, and eventually persuaded colleagues at Vienna University's neuropsychiatric clinic to give insulin to schizophrenic patients. The results were dramatic. By 1935, he claimed an 88 per cent improvement rate and word soon reached the Maudsley. Sargant, however, initially baulked at the idea, which struck him as too simple and dangerous. The empirical treatment was also at odds with everything that was known about schizophrenia, and he was 'tempted to greet it with derision'.

It was only when Professor Pötzl, the distinguished head of Vienna University Psychiatric Unit, endorsed Sakel's treatment that Sargant was keen to try it. Mapother, however, was unwilling to risk killing patients or attract the attention of the local coroner, and forbade Sargant from administering the treatment at the Maudsley. It took a further two years and official approval from Dr Isobel Wilson, a commissioner on the English Board of Control for Lunacy and Mental Deficiency, before Sargant was finally given the go-ahead in 1930. This was despite the acknowledged risks of irreversible coma, brain damage, amnesia and hypoglycaemic aftershocks. (Contemporary reports of mortality rates were as high as 4.5 per cent.)

In practice, the treatment was acutely distressing for the patient. According to an article in the *BMJ* in April 1937, 'within about half an hour he becomes restless, tossing from side to side ... He leaps up in bed, staring and crying out aloud ... He may beat his head and hands and feet frantically ... Coma follows and the patient lies shrunken into his bed, profoundly collapsed ... and must be laid on his side to allow the saliva to run out.'

What appealed most to Sakel – and to Sargant – was the fleeting period of lucidity that followed even in highly disturbed patients. It was as if the storm clouds of their psychosis had momentarily cleared. Sakel believed that these brief delusion-free interludes would become longer and longer until the patient had fully recovered. In reality, such moments of clarity were all too short, but the prospect of a cure for schizophrenia – the holy grail of psychiatry – was irresistible for someone with Sargant's ambition.

As with other 'miraculous' cures for mental illness, no one was able to shed much light on why it might work. A few years earlier, another equally bizarre physical treatment had been hailed as a cure for general paralysis of the insane (GPI), a severe mental disorder caused by late-stage syphilis. In 1917, Julius Wagner-Jauregg, an Austrian doctor, had injected blood taken from a malarial patient into two people suffering from GPI. He'd had a hunch that a spiking fever might be therapeutic in some cases of psychosis – the original shock treatment. Some signs of improvement were noted, and it wasn't long before Horton Asylum in Epsom had become a national centre for breeding malarial mosquitoes, which were duly dispatched to hospitals around the UK.

The theory behind Sakel's treatment was that an insulin-induced coma, caused by temporary loss of sugar in the bloodstream, had some sort of beneficial effect on the brain. Acting like a firebreak, it gave the patient a time-out from the inferno of their troubled thoughts. Nobody really knew why. Perhaps it was a subconscious death wish? A 'physiological lobotomy'? Or a sense of being mothered during and after the coma? According to Sargant, 'One unit went so far as to recommend nurses with big breasts so that when the patient came out of his death-like coma, he or she was greeted on rebirth with this invitingly maternal sight.'

Sakel himself admitted that he didn't know how or why his cure worked. Clinical accomplishments were, at this stage, more important than theoretical foundations. In truth, patients probably just felt better, at least in the short term, because they were the focus of a lot of suggestive attention from a large and dedicated team of doctors and nurses. One conservative estimate at the time suggested that patients were given fifty to a hundred times as much medical care and nursing care, measured by the clock, as non-insulin patients.

Insulin coma (or shock) therapy would soon become a staple of Sargant's therapeutic armamentarium, often administered prior to narcosis. Sargant was one of its most vocal champions but other psychiatrists in Britain were also quick to embrace the technique. By 1938, it was being used in thirty-one hospitals in England and Wales to treat schizophrenia. It was equally well received in America, where Sakel had emigrated in 1936.

Sargant maintained that to administer insulin coma therapy required a skill that only a few doctors possessed. He, of course, had exactly what it took. 'It is clear that there is an art of treatment, in which some will be more adept than others', adding, with a touch of bravura, that 'with skilful handling death should be avoided'. Sargant dedicated the entire opening chapter of the first edition of *An Introduction to Physical Methods of Treatment in Psychiatry* (1944) to insulin coma therapy and it continued to feature in all four subsequent editions, including the last, which came out in 1972.

As early as the mid 1950s, however, the treatment was being widely discredited, and was soon replaced by ECT and Largactil, the first antipsychotic drug. 'The Insulin Myth', a coruscating article in the *Lancet* in 1953, had concluded that 'insulin offers the schizophrenic no long-term benefits'. The author was Harold Bourne, a courageous thirty-year-old junior doctor who was subjected to the equivalent of a social media pile-on in the letters page of the *Lancet* for taking on the insulin coma therapy old guard. Four years later, however, another critical article in the *Lancet* was (for most people) the final nail in the coffin.

Sargant, however, continued to give insulin coma therapy to his patients throughout his career. Ultimately, it was the treatment's hands-on physicality that most appealed. It allowed Sargant to address a mental health issue while appearing to perform like a brain surgeon in a bustling operating theatre, supported by a large team of nurses. A far cry from a Freudian chat with a patient about their mother.

Charles Burlingame, an American psychiatrist, described the treatment as a 'skilful sparring with death'. Harold Bourne took a less complimentary view: 'It meant that psychiatrists had something to do. It made them feel like real doctors instead of just institutional attendants.' Peter Tyrer remembers the treatment all too well. His very first job as Sargant's house physician had been to administer insulin coma therapy to a patient. When Tyrer raised the issue of consent, Sargant reassured him that he would take all responsibility, dismissing the 'pen pushers' at the Department of Health. 'No one said anything about ethics,' Tyrer recalls.

'I went on to have the most strange, out-of-world experience giving this man insulin. The interesting thing is, if you give a small amount of insulin to most people, they go unconscious. People with schizophrenia, because they're so highly aroused, you have to give them absolutely piles of insulin before they go unconscious. We did that and then he wouldn't come round. And I thought, Goodness gracious me, my first job, I'm going to be in court for murder!'

The patient didn't die. His condition improved – initially, at least – and his delighted parents gave Sargant a cheque, which he handed on to Tyrer, urging him to buy some books. 'In the short term, Sargant's patients did come out remarkably positively,' says Tyrer, 'but what happens immediately is absolutely useless in predicting the long term.'

As so often with Sargant's treatments, a quick, miracle recovery often disguised a subsequent relapse. And yet, despite so much evidence of its ineffectiveness, let alone its dangers, Sargant persisted with the treatment. In 1972, he wrote, almost nostalgically, that insulin coma was no longer what it once was, the treatment *par excellence* of schizophrenia, but rightly used with other measures 'it can still save years of suffering in otherwise resistant patients'. It was only a year before he died that he finally admitted the limitations of what he had once called a wonder drug. 'One saw people getting better very quickly, but you couldn't keep them better.'

7

'Roasted alive in a white-hot furnace'

While Sargant had been waiting to get permission to administer insulin coma therapy at the Maudsley, word had reached him and his colleagues of another shock treatment making waves in Europe. Ladislas Meduna, a Hungarian neuropsychiatrist, observed that if schizophrenics suffered seizures, they were relieved of their psychosis. Similarly, if an epileptic developed schizophrenia, they had fewer seizures. (Today, epileptics are thought to be more, rather than less, prone to psychosis.) Meduna duly decided to induce an epileptic fit in a schizophrenic – 'as if it were casting out one devil by the aid of another,' Sargant noted.

Meduna initially used camphor to induce seizures but then turned to Cardiazol, a respiratory stimulant. By all accounts, it caused deeply unpleasant symptoms in the fifteen minutes it took from injection to convulsion. The main problem was an overwhelming fear of imminent death, even as the Cardiazol was being injected, combined with a curious aura that often occurs before a seizure. Feelings of strangeness soon gave way to perplexity and dread, a choking sensation, the taste of burnt matches and eventually to an intense existential terror that was only relieved by unconsciousness when the convulsion started.

Understandably, patients did all they could to avoid the treatment. One plunged headlong out of a window to escape what he described as being 'roasted alive in a white-hot furnace'. Worse still, patients could recall the intense fear that had immediately followed the injection (but not the convulsive fit itself). It was no surprise that the Soviets were quick to see its potential in interrogations: the mere threat of Cardiazol was enough to persuade prisoners to talk. There was a gruesome physical legacy to the seizures too. Hairline fractures of the spinal vertebrae, dislocated jaws, shoulders and hips, as well as fractured femurs were not uncommon.

Sargant was unconcerned about physical damage to patients, believing that the treatment was less dangerous, if more unpleasant, than insulin coma therapy. He also felt it would benefit depressives better than schizophrenics, on one occasion lying to a colleague in order to get a depressed patient treated with Cardiazol – effectively an off-label prescription. 'I have always unblushingly resorted to every device or trick that would help by-pass heartless medical authoritarianism,' he admitted.

Meanwhile, over in Italy, Ugo Cerletti, professor of psychiatry at the University of Rome, was more concerned than Sargant by the profound sense of dread that Cardiazol induced in patients. As part of his ongoing research into epilepsy and schizophrenia, he was keen to find a way to induce a seizure quickly, without any prolonged period of fear. To that end, he had started to experiment with electricity and dogs. Most of the time, the animals died.

What happened next was a landmark moment in twentieth-century psychiatry, leading to tens of thousands of patients around the world being treated with an electric shock to the brain – a controversial treatment that is still given today in a considerably modified form.

Not surprisingly, the exact circumstances of the experiments in Rome have become the subject of much debate. Cerletti's account differs in some detail to what his assistant professor at the clinic, Lucio Bini, recorded in his own notebooks. On the advice of a colleague, Cerletti (or perhaps Bini, who was an expert at making electrical devices) visited an abattoir in Rome, as he had heard that 'electric slaughtering' was being used to kill pigs. When he arrived, however, he observed that the shock-induced convulsions stunned the animals into unconsciousness before the butcher's knife went to work. This realisation encouraged Cerletti (or Bini) to investigate electricity further. He duly got permission from the abattoir director to test various methods of electrocution on pigs and concluded that while a current passing across the chest was liable to kill the animal, 'a passage of the current across the head, even for long durations, did not have serious consequences'. The margin of safety was also quite high: 120 volts was sufficient to induce convulsions, but it took 400 volts to kill the animal. Similarly, it would take between 60 and 150 seconds for a dose to be fatal. Could a short-lasting, relatively low voltage be given safely to humans?

Cerletti still had misgivings – 'In everyone's minds was the spectre of "the electric chair".' *Frankenstein* was probably in everyone's minds too. Seven years earlier, the most famous film adaptation of Mary Shelley's story had featured Boris Karloff as a creature brought to life by an electrical device. Cerletti's experiments on pigs, however, had left him satisfied that he wasn't going to kill anyone, let alone create a monster. Where, though, would he find his first patient?

Serendipitously, the local police had just picked up Enrico, a thirty-nine-year-old engineer from Milan, at Rome railway station. He was in an agitated and confused state and was delivered to Cerletti's clinic to be kept under observation. Speaking gibberish, he didn't know who he was and believed he was telepathic. An ideal candidate, in other words, to be the world's first ECT patient.

At 11.15 a.m. on 11 April 1938, Cerletti and Bini, 'as was our custom with dogs', used an elastic band to apply two electrodes, wet with salt solution, to Enrico's temples. An electric shock of 80 volts was administered for a quarter of a second. Enrico, who was lying supine on a bed with his arms tied, tensed his muscles, collapsed and started to sing at the top of his voice. He did not, however, convulse. Ten minutes later, the procedure was repeated, this time for half a second. More singing, still no convulsions.

After much discussion, it was decided to let Enrico rest for a few days before Cerletti tried again. Tensions were running high. It was one thing to electrocute a pig, but it took a considerable leap of faith to pass an electric current through a human brain. As preparations were made for a second attempt, Enrico, hitherto incomprehensible, suddenly sat up on his bed and expressed, clearly and solemnly, what he thought about the prospect of more electric shocks: 'Not another one! It's deadly!' ('*Non una seconda. Mortifera!*') Cerletti was spooked by the patient's clarity of expression but decided to press on and administer another 80-volt shock. Again, no convulsions or loss of consciousness. The world's first attempt at electro-convulsive therapy had failed.

A week later, on 20 April, Cerletti tried again. Turning up the dial to 92 volts, he applied the shock for half a second. This time, it was enough to induce a grand mal seizure. Contraction of the limbs lasted for eighty seconds. Enrico ejaculated, and stopped breathing for 105 seconds – each second counted out aloud by Bini. The atmosphere in the room must have been unbearable. 'The apnea of the spontaneous epileptic convulsion is always impressive, but at that moment it seemed to all of us painfully endless,' Cerletti wrote. After five minutes, Enrico finally opened his eyes. A further five minutes later, the convulsions ceased and he regained consciousness. When Cerletti asked what had happened to him, Enrico replied: 'I don't know; perhaps I've been to sleep . . . ' Cerletti said later, with one eye firmly on professional immortality: 'Thus occurred the first electrically produced convulsion in man, which I at once named "electroshock"'.

Cerletti proceeded to give Enrico another eleven treatments, each one announced in the clinic with two blasts on a trumpet. Rows of spectators were three deep. As for Enrico, he was allowed to return to his family in Milan three weeks later, in 'good condition and well orientated; ideation and memory perfect'. In what would become an all too familiar pattern, however, Enrico relapsed two years later, and was readmitted to the Mombello psychiatric hospital in Milan.

Cerletti administered shocks to a further twenty patients between May and September 1938. The media reception was ecstatic. 'Madness Cured with Electricity' said one national newspaper. Cerletti also coined the term '*zapare*' for the actual process. His findings were published in a book, which became the bible for anyone who wished to know how to give the treatment – until Sargant's own manual was published in 1944.

Sargant, of course, had been desperate to get his hands on a 'shock box', as they were soon known, but he was on a one-year Rockefeller travelling fellowship in psychiatry at Massachusetts General Hospital, affiliated to Harvard Medical School. On his return in October 1939, he did all he could to promote ECT. 'I think I was the second or third person in Britain to use it,' he said. 'I well remember the first time I pressed the button.' Initially, the authorities were reluctant to permit its use. Sargant was not to be deterred. As he crowed later, 'We generally got our own way in the end.' His name would soon become synonymous with ECT – hence his moniker, 'Sargant the Shock' – and by the early 1960s, the psychiatric outpatients department at St Thomas' was administering ECT to hundreds of NHS patients a week. 'There was just too much of it,' remembers Pippa Ecclestone, who worked as a student nurse on psychiatry in 1967 during her fourth year of training. 'Appalling whole days of ECT. They can't have all been the right thing to be done. It was horrifying.'

Catherine Mountain was a second-year student nurse in 1965. She remembers the rows of 'scared patients' waiting to undergo ECT, the 'jerking and convulsing of their anaesthetised bodies', and the routine of prepping the outpatient department for the sessions. 'It was like a conveyor belt. We'd prepare all the syringes – twenty or thirty – drawing them up, just getting it all ready. It was obviously greatly reduced from a full grand mal fit, but the body still arched and shook.'

'Ruth Chadwick' (not her real name) was treated as an outpatient at St Thomas' when she was twenty-one. The ECT destroyed much of her memory, which had once been 'practically photographic', and friends said she underwent a personality change. 'The effects on me were appalling and permanent,' she says. 'For a while I couldn't even remember my own name. The worst thing was how it affected my memory of myself.' It was as if her childhood had happened to someone else. Eventually, she became a teacher, working with children with learning difficulties. She also married and has two children and a grandchild. When she later told her GP what had happened, the doctor said, 'I'd like to offer an apology on behalf of the medical profession.'

Sargant, however, remained fiercely unrepentant, keeping an old shock box in the corner of his Harley Street room until the day he retired.

8

Mary Thornton

My memories of Ward Five are a series of detached snapshots. Electrodes attached to the side of my head; being given a general anaesthetic; seeing an image of myself in the mirror one day, a strange face staring back at me. It was early 1971 and I was barely twenty. I understood that I was being treated for an acute anxiety state on the top floor of the Royal Waterloo. And, as part of that treatment, Dr Sargant would give me continuous narcosis to help my head have a nice long rest.

Initially I stayed in a single room along a narrow corridor. Ward Five was mostly for female psychiatric patients, but I can distinctly recall a tall, thin man wandering up and down, singing 'Hello, Dolly!' endlessly. I was given ECT soon after my arrival. I was also given Largactil – we used to call it the liquid cosh – and Haldol, another antipsychotic.

My parents used to bring me cigarettes – extra-long Dunhills – and I was allowed two during meals. There was never enough time to smoke those damn things. I remember the baths too, because the doors had a horrible peepy hole in them so that the nurse could take a look at you while you were having a bath. I also remember being given sodium pentothal, or maybe sodium amytal. I had recently trained as a nurse and was familiar with the names. Why were they using a truth drug on me? I had nothing to tell.

In the early days, my boyfriend John would come and take me out for a walk on the Embankment. We'd even go for a coffee in the Royal Festival Hall. But that was before things escalated. One day John came in and I didn't recognise him. I had no idea who he was. The ECT and drugs had destroyed my memories of him. He was so upset that he stormed into the great man's office to confront him. Reaching across Sargant's desk, he tried to strangle him, shouting, 'What the fuck have you done to my girlfriend?' Sargant must have pressed a panic button, because John was grabbed by two beefy orderlies, who threw him out onto the embankment and told him never to return. After that, I forgot all about John. And he tried to forget all about me, as he thought he'd never see me again.

It was then, I think, that Sargant decided it was time to move me into the Sleep Room. During narcosis, we slept continuously, only woken every six hours for meals, washing and toileting. We were also given an anaesthetic followed by ECT, but I have no memory of this – it's what I've since read and been told. As for the Sleep Room itself, I can clearly recall the darkened ward. It was dimly lit and there were bodies in the beds that were asleep all the time and I was one of them. I can actually remember lying in the dark in that horrible room. I can remember the smell. The stink. I think the nurses must have been quite kind and sympathetic. There were six divan beds, low on the ground. I was in the one on the left-hand side. I just remember, I don't know how or why.

I was on Ward Five for twelve weeks in all, and received ECT throughout my stay. Waking up after a dose of ECT was absolutely terrifying. I felt complete and utter terror because I didn't even know who I was, or what my name was . . . I remember rubbing my temples and feeling these sort of dry salt patches where they put the electrodes on either side of my head. Apparently, Sargant used to give it to people in my state at least twice a week, so I could have had as many as twenty-four shocks. I can't be certain, though, as my memory was obliterated by the treatment. I have tried in vain to track down my records. For six to eight of those twelve weeks, I was in the Sleep Room. I remember the end of my bed being up on bricks, and some kind of enema being dripped in, very, very slowly. What was that all about?

I didn't like Sargant in person at all. He was a big man, sitting behind his big desk. His office was near the stairs. Power just seemed to emanate from his pores. I got the impression that he was powerful, rather than he had a million brain cells. His face is etched in my memory. I could never forget it. He was a handsome man. Leonine. And he had a very, very arrogant manner. He didn't discuss things with you. He told you. He talked at you, but he didn't really listen to what you might have to say. In fact, I can't ever remember saying anything much to him.

Incredibly, he only lost five of his patients through his inhumane narcosis treatment. But there must have been patients with other complications, intestinal ones, for example, if they were kept asleep, without exercise, for months on end. In later life I certainly had horrible problems with my gut, and with various obstructions, which led to me losing half my bowel and ending up with an ileostomy.

Was Sargant responsible for my subsequent medical problems? I can't go on retrospectively blaming what happened on Ward Five, where I had so much ECT, but I can't help feeling that my time in the Sleep Room is at least partly responsible. They're a legacy of that treatment. I've had three mended cracks in three vertebrae, and I've had surgery on my back five times now, including a botched operation. My gut stopped working because we lay in bed for so long. I also have osteoporosis, but I might have had it anyway.

So yes, I've had terrible medical problems, but I don't like this blame culture. That's why I feel so guilty telling tales about my mother. I'm sure she didn't mean to be so awful, but she was. As a child, I'd had a very poor relationship with her, as did most of my four brothers. We were quite a sad family. Dad was gentle and ineffectual. My mother was violent and aggressive. With hindsight, I believe she had a poorly treated thyroid complaint. She was the youngest of ten children and had come over to Britain from a smallholding in Kerry, in the south-west of Ireland, to study nursing and escape looking after her ageing parents.

It was around this time, just as the Second World War started, that my mother met my father. They had to conduct their courting around London during the Blitz. Eventually they married, and my eldest brother was born in 1941. Dad went abroad with the Royal Engineers for four years, and my mother returned to Ireland to be in a safer place. After the war, they set up home together in Hertfordshire, and brothers numbers two and three were born, and then myself in 1950, followed by my younger brother in 1955. (My adopted sister joined us much later.)

In those days life was quite hard. Although Dad had a good job as a bank manager, my mother always seemed to worry what the neighbours would think, whether we were good enough. She was ashamed of my dad because he was stooped, which made him look old, and he had a Yorkshire accent. She'd lost her own Irish accent on the boat over. I used to dread weekends because they would invariably end up with my mother yelling and shouting at my father, or worse. Her temper was uncontrollable, foul.

When she had no money, my father would say, in his mild way, 'God will provide', and that would send her right over the edge. One time she threw some bank notes into the fire. We were especially hard up that month. Another time she became so frustrated with Dad that she hurled eggs at him. I can remember the egg yolk sliding slowly down the wall. The worst episode for me was when she attacked Dad with a large kitchen knife, which he managed to deflect.

I used to lie in my bed upstairs listening to her voice, wishing that she were out of my life for ever. Periodically she left home and would disappear for days on end. Then my father would receive a telephone call from her. She had run out of money and was stranded with no way of getting home. In all honesty my childhood has more dark than light memories, and to this day it makes me very sad.

When I was eleven, I went away to Farnborough Hill, a posh all-girls Catholic boarding school in Hampshire. It was my mother's decision to send me – I think she preferred having young children to teenagers. Home life was difficult so I went gladly, but I was always worried because I knew that they could not afford the fees. The school, set in a hundred acres of countryside, was a rather grand country house, with many beautiful paintings.

I relished the whole experience until one day, when I was fifteen, Dad said to me, 'Look, I'm sorry, your brother needs to go prep school in Windsor. Do you mind leaving your school?' And I said, 'No, of course I don't mind.' But I minded hugely. I wasn't that happy at home and I was very happy at boarding school. My father didn't have the funds to afford two sets of school fees, and in those days boys were more important than girls. My younger brother's turn had come, and he was very clever. So I was pulled out of Farnborough and sent to a horrible red-brick school in Reading. No grass, all concrete, and I hated the place. To this day, I've resented what my parents did – I've always treated my kids equally.

So I found myself living at home once more, and had to travel on the bus, on the top deck, where I learned how to smoke Number 6 cigarettes – a habit I was unable to kick for the next thirty years. I then had to walk about a mile from the bus stop, putting up with jibes from the local boys, who called us 'shit and custard', as my new uniform was brown and yellow.

After I'd been away to stay with relatives, my mother said, 'My God, they fed you well in Ireland.' A delightful boy had just asked me out and I realised I was overweight. From that day, I went on to have problems with my food for the rest of my life. I stopped eating when my mother said those words, because I was so unhappy. I wasn't even sixteen.

I knew no one at my new school and although I begged my parents to let me study art, I was pointed in the direction of the sciences. I needed to go to medical school and become a doctor or a dentist – my older brother was already studying dentistry at Guy's. I did really badly in my O levels, but I also applied to Guy's for a place to study dentistry. Amazingly, I was accepted. I just needed to get three Ds in my A levels . . .

Results day was dreadful. The only alternative was to go into nursing. Aged nineteen, I was accepted onto a fast-track course for bright students at the Westminster Hospital, beginning in January 1970, and skipped all the way down the road with my little suitcase. I was leaving home and delighted.

And then, just before I started at the Westminster, I met John. He was over from Dublin, and I fancied him the minute I set eyes on him. Shortly afterwards, I brought him home to introduce him to my parents. Unfortunately, it was hate at first sight – my mother in particular disliked John intensely. She never gave him a chance. He had a good job in computers, but his hair was a bit long and he had a beard – she thought he was a pot-smoking hippy.

John moved to Reading for work as our relationship became stronger. I used to come down from London on the train, but my mother would always find out from someone and there would be hell to pay. It was awful. My relationship with her rapidly deteriorated. And then one day it all came to a head. I was spending a sneaky weekend with John at his flat and my parents came round. My mother picked up the milk bottles that were outside his front door and threw them at John. She was absolutely awful! His family, on the other hand, were lovely. (They still are.)

My parents, who liked to be seen as churchgoing, quiet and seemly people, eventually had enough and forbade me to see John. We were Catholics. They even contacted John's mother in

Dublin, and his parish priest, to tell him of the sinful goings on between a son of the parish and a convent girl from the Home Counties.

Meanwhile, back at the Westminster Hospital, I wasn't coping well with all this stress in my life. My mother had been going on at me so much that in the end I had a wobbly. I stopped eating as well. I was living in nursing accommodation at 88 Vauxhall Bridge Road when it happened. I had four fantastic friends – they remain my best friends to this day – and I was around at their flat in Pimlico one night, fagging it – we all smoked in those days – and I just cracked up. It was almost like I wasn't in this world any more. It was as if I had been smoking pot, but I hadn't been. After that I don't remember anything. I ended up in the nurses' sickbay under the care of Dr Peter Dally,* consultant psychiatrist at the Westminster, which was significant, as he specialised in anorexia.

I was under his care for a few weeks and set fire to my bed a couple of times. You were allowed to smoke in hospital – one of my jobs as a nurse was going around emptying all the bedside ashtrays – but I must have fallen asleep with a fag in my hand. I guess they were getting sick of me: what are we going to do with her next? I remember a young girl in the bed next to me, fagging it, with an oxygen mask in her other hand. And I thought, My God, she's going to kill us all.

I can remember Dally very clearly. He was very sweet and gentle, kind and quietly spoken, and had a limp. In my mind, he was a pleasant fellow, with a great intellect and empathy. He had a fascination with Virginia Woolf. I still can't understand to this day why he sold me down the river to a monster like Sargant. He was so opposed to Sargant's way of treating people. And then I discovered that he'd once studied with him at St Thomas'. Was that why I found myself on a trolley, cold raindrops on my face, waiting

* Peter Dally had been married to Ann Dally, Sargant's biographer, but they divorced in 1969. They continued to work in private practice together until 1994.

for an ambulance to take me across the Thames to Sargant's Sleep Room? I will never know.

One memory of the Sleep Room that I used to think was false and imagined, but I now know to be true, was that if the ECT and narcosis were to fail, I would be given a lobotomy. That would be the next course of treatment for me. I was absolutely terrified at the prospect. I had it in my head that this was going to happen if I didn't pull my socks up, and fast. I also took a look at myself in the mirror one day. I had quite nice, long dark hair in those days. I was fairly bonny, I suppose. But on that day I looked awful. My hair was in rats' tails. And I thought, I'm never going to get out of here. This is dreadful. I'd better pull myself together.

They had tried to persuade me to visit occupational therapy, which was in a very attractive semicircular room below the Sleep Room, but I had never wanted to go. I hated stuff like making baskets and fiddling around with bits and pieces. But then I thought, If I don't play ball, I'll never get out of this place; they'll just hang on to me. So I made a very conscious decision to go along with what I thought were horrible therapy sessions. (I only remember one: learning how to put on make-up. I looked like a freak when I saw myself in the mirror.) Otherwise, I might never have escaped. I have no recollection of leaving there after three months, or who came to get me, or anything. It must have been my parents. My memory was in pieces completely. I had even forgotten I had a boyfriend, which was very convenient, as they had told him he was never to attempt to see me again. But it wasn't the end of my story.

After I was finally released, I was sent to my eldest brother in Yorkshire. He was a dentist and had five children at the time. I certainly wouldn't have wanted to go and stay with my parents, and they wouldn't have had me. I would have embarrassed and shamed them. One day, at my brother's house, I suddenly remembered there was someone in my life called John. I must have found his phone number in my luggage or something. I rang him and said, 'Can you meet me at King's Cross station?' It must have been a big shock for him because he'd been told I'd never come out of hospital. He never thought he'd see me again. John just said he'd meet me at King's Cross. And he did! And, thankfully, I recognised him. He picked up my luggage and we went to look for accommodation, ending up in Holland Park.

John said later that I had been like a zombie in Ward Five. He'd visited me four times in hospital before he was thrown out by Sargant's security staff. My brother said I was like a zombie in there too. What I didn't know was that John had got another girlfriend and was going to work on a kibbutz with her, but he never told me any of that. Later, she turned up on our doorstep. 'You must be Mary,' she said. 'You must be Wendy!' I replied. She was all right about everything; there was never any unpleasantness.

After that, things are a little hazy. I kept in touch with my father off and on, but I didn't speak to my mother again for seven or eight years. I think I went briefly back into nursing, night duty, but I soon turned my back on the profession. After a happy six months together, John and I decided to get married and put my whole Sleep Room experience behind us. We got married in Kensington Church Street, but not before the old priest had done his research. 'I was a bit concerned about what I had heard from your parents,' he said. 'They'd told me that you weren't fit to get married – that you were mentally ill. So we sent a delegation down to your home in Wokingham before I agreed to marry you. Two nuns and a priest, to find out what exactly what was going on. And we decided that your mother was the mad one.'

Years later, when I was talking to my mother and I had my own children, I asked her why she had signed me over to Sargant's care. It had been such a vicious, horrible treatment and I wasn't yet twenty-one. She said it was because I was bad. But I was an adult. I wasn't bad! She probably thought Sargant was God. I never really connected with my mother. Until the day she died, she continued to give me grief.

After we were married, John carried on working with computers, but we decided that we didn't want to have a family in London. So we threw all our stuff in a van, including a piano, and went to Kendal and applied to train as teachers in Newcastle. Teaching jobs were very hard to find back in the seventies, and not well paid, so John ended up working offshore, painting rust spots on oil rigs and earning considerably more than he could as a teacher.

We brought up four children in Brampton, Cumbria. John earned good money, but his job was very hard on all of us. He worked away from home for over thirty years, all over the world, sometimes in very dangerous situations. I couldn't work when John was away as I needed to be at home for the children, so for a few years I ran an antique shop from my house before going into teaching. For fifteen years, I also taught children with special educational needs and was head of my own department.

Anxieties have haunted me for most of my life, but I don't get depressed. And I've always had an interesting relationship with food – it's a lot better now than it used to be. But I can't deny that I have had a life of pain since I left the Sleep Room. For over fifteen years, I was addicted to fentanyl. That's another story, and one that's made me angry for a long time. Withdrawal was horrible.

These days, I take nothing. I have stopped all opioids, and pain-killers, without help, and without difficulty. I have quit smoking (a long time ago) and alcohol. I don't miss any of it at all. I could do with being better organised, though. The only thing I occasionally have at night is a tiny bit of cannabis oil (on prescription).

Sadly, John died in June 2021 after many years of fighting cancer heroically, and I miss him dreadfully. My house feels so big and empty, but I don't want to leave as I've been here for forty-four years and I like it here. I spend my time now visiting my children down south, going to the theatre and galleries in London. I went to a play at the National Theatre recently and walked past the old Royal Waterloo Hospital. I always get an odd feeling when I go near that place, even now.

For many years, I carried the nightmare of the Sleep Room around with me, mostly under wraps. Only my close friends, including my late husband, who supported me throughout, knew that I'd had a breakdown of sorts in the early seventies. And then I saw Sargant on television, just before he died, and I became very upset. My (then) teenage daughter had no idea why, and I told myself I had to stop allowing this man to have such a hold over my emotions. So I did, but it took a while.

Now I can honestly say that I have had a wonderful life. I could not wish for a better family – and that includes my Irish relatives. If I were to meet William Sargant today, would I say anything to him? No. Nothing at all. I was unbelievably bitter for a very long time, but it's all gone, thank goodness. As Jung once said, 'We cannot change anything until we accept it.'

9

'Wizardry of Surgery Restores Sanity to Fifty Raving Maniacs'

When Sargant had first heard about Manfred Sakel and his insulin coma therapy, he'd been tempted to treat the idea with derision, before embracing it wholeheartedly. His response was similar when word reached him about a new surgical operation on the brain. Egas Moniz, a Portuguese neurologist and former foreign minister, claimed to have cured mental disorders by drilling two holes into the skull and severing the frontal lobes, thought by some to be the seat of the human psyche. Sargant had roared with laughter. Again, it seemed too simple a treatment for such a complex illness as schizophrenia and struck him as 'utterly ridiculous'.

Much can be learned from Sargant's response to each emerging shock treatment. Initially he reacted with horror, but then something else kicked in. A glint in those pebble-dark eyes, perhaps. Sensing an opportunity to become the consultant physician in general medicine that he'd always wanted to be, he was soon defying medical authority to administer lobotomies.

Sargant would go on to champion the operation with as much

enthusiasm as he showed for ECT and insulin coma therapy, still referring people for the operation as late as 1977. At the fifth Congrès International de Neurologie, held in Lisbon in September 1953, Sargant would ask Moniz, the host, to sign his dinner card. He would even boast that his car was washed by one of his lobotomised patients every Thursday. Thanks largely to Sargant, Britain carried out more lobotomies per capita than any other country in the world. 'I don't think he should escape hellfire for all the damage he did,' according to the late forensic psychiatrist Dr Henry Rollin.

This primitive psychosurgical intervention continues to haunt medicine and popular culture even today. As Dr Jonathan Miller once said, it was akin to a 'Passchendaele of the mind'. The word 'lobotomised' has become shorthand for someone deprived of their mental faculties, their individualism removed. Tens of thousands of people were lobotomised in the UK and America in the 1940s and 1950s. Later Sargant would use the Sleep Room as an alternative to surgery, although months of narcosis, ECT and drugs often left patients feeling as if they had had part of their brains removed anyway.

Moniz believed that psychiatric problems were caused by 'fixed' or repetitive thoughts that had become locked into abnormally stabilised neural pathways in the prefrontal cortex (often described today as the personality centre of the brain). And it was only by cutting these pathways, which connected the frontal lobes with a deeper part of the brain, the thalamus, that those fixed patterns of thought could be disrupted. Thanks to a neurologist called Walter Freeman, who soon adapted and cleverly marketed Moniz's technique in America ('lobotomy gets them home'), it quickly became one of the most popular neurosurgical treatments for mental disorders in the Western world. Freeman and Sargant became firm friends too. In their bid to empty overcrowded asylums, agitated patients weren't so much cured as curtailed, their personalities flattened, in some cases extinguished.

Remarkably, Sargant claimed in 1964 that lobotomy not only relieved anxiety and 'tortured self-concern', but caused 'no observable undesirable change in the general personality of correctly chosen patients. And certainly no change, except for the better, is seen in the patient's intelligence.' He continued to advocate lobotomy in the fifth and final edition of *An Introduction to Physical Methods of Treatment in Psychiatry* (1972) – the book he had first written in 1944. In one now notorious paragraph, he recommended a lobotomy, instead of divorce or separation, for unhappy wives: 'A depressed woman, for instance, may owe her illness to a psychopathic husband who cannot change and will not accept treatment. Separation might be the answer, but ... we have seen patients enabled by a leucotomy to return to the difficult environment and cope with it in a way which had hitherto been impossible.'

Moniz would win a Nobel Prize in 1949 for inventing the procedure, arguably its most controversial winner ever. (There was an unsuccessful campaign twenty years ago to strip him of the award, launched by lobotomy victims and doctors.) But he was by no means the first person to realise that humans could continue to function after the removal of considerable chunks of their brain. On 13 September 1848, Phineas Gage, a foreman working on the Rutland & Burlington Railroad in Vermont, was setting explosive charges in rock. Distracted by his gang of co-workers, the strapping twenty-five-year-old accidentally triggered an explosion that propelled his tamping rod through his head, leaving a large hole. Remarkably, he was conscious and talking within minutes, despite missing part of his brain. He survived for another thirteen years but his personality had changed dramatically. He was 'no longer Gage' and was 'a child in his intellectual capacity'.

Gage's incredible tale lived on long after he did, making him a macabre poster boy for later devotees of lobotomy such as Sargant. More importantly, it suggested that the brain could take a huge hit and still operate on some level.

*

It wasn't until 12 November 1935, at the Santa Marta Hospital in Lisbon, that the world's first lobotomy was performed. Moniz instructed Almeida Lima, an Oxford-educated neurosurgeon, to drill two holes into the skull of a sixty-three-year-old woman who was suffering from anxiety, paranoia and hallucinations. Holes had been drilled into human heads before to relieve mental suffering – there is archaeological evidence of trepanation dating back ten thousand years – but this was another momentous landmark in twentieth-century psychiatry. As we now know, it was also tragically misguided. Lima duly injected absolute alcohol (ethanol) into the woman's brain to destroy the frontal lobes. The doctors had practised the procedure beforehand, using a brain brought up from the morgue and a fountain pen, which Moniz inserted into the cortex several times to confirm the precise positioning of the hypodermic needle.

Within days, Moniz declared his first lobotomy to be a 'clinical cure'. The woman still cried, but with less intensity. Barely two months later, she was deemed calm, if 'slightly sad', well orientated and her 'conscience, intelligence and behaviour intact'. Not intact enough, it seems, for her ever to leave the asylum.

Seven further patients had their frontal lobes destroyed with alcohol before Moniz abandoned the technique in favour of an instrument that he had developed called a 'leucotome' (from *leuko* and *tome*, the Greek for white and a cut or slice). It was sharp and narrow, with an extendable wire loop at one end, operated by a plunger. Once the leucotome had been inserted into the skull, Lima pressed the plunger to extend the wire and twisted the instrument, cutting complete spheres (measuring 1 centimetre in diameter) out of the fibrous brain matter in a procedure Moniz described as 'simple and safe', and not unlike coring an apple.

Moniz and Lima initially operated on twenty patients from local asylums, including one agitated woman who pulled out the needle that was meant to anaesthetise her, groaned when the leucotome was turned in her head (a piece had broken off inside) and ripped off her bandages afterwards. In March 1936, Moniz announced in Paris that seven patients in total had been cured, seven had improved significantly and six were unchanged. He also coined the word 'psychosurgery', a term that would later become synonymous with Sargant.

The findings caused a stir globally and were widely praised, not least by Walter Freeman, who published a fawning review. The operation's importance could 'scarcely be overestimated', even though the patients' long-term fate was unknown. The results were not picked up by anyone in Britain and it would be another two years before Sargant heard about them – and duly roared with laughter.

Freeman, meanwhile, ordered two leucotomes from Moniz's manufacturer in Paris and enlisted the help of a young neurosurgeon called James Watts, who had recently joined the staff of the George Washington Hospital, where Freeman was professor of neurology. Freeman wasn't a surgeon and, like Moniz, needed someone to wield the knife for him. (Moniz's own hands had been deformed by gout.)

His first patient was a sixty-three-year-old woman from Texas. Agitated and depressed, Alice Hammatt nearly pulled out of the treatment when she heard that her hair would need to be shaved off. Freeman reassured her that her curls would be safe and duly went ahead on 14 September 1936, instructing Watts to cut six cores on either side of her head. Immediately afterwards, Hammatt was less agitated and calmer. She was also no longer concerned about her hair. Freeman hailed the result as spectacular. Hammatt died five years later of pneumonia, having suffered from epileptic seizures.

Freeman and Watts initially operated on twenty patients. The results were disastrous. One patient committed suicide, another attempted to do the same, and two died within three months. Other patients were left with 'extreme flattening of emotional life', 'a sterile intellectual life' and 'frequent convulsions and incontinence'. One woman became 'fat, jolly and unspoken'. Seventeen out of the twenty patients were female, and eleven of them were housewives, a gender imbalance that was to persist in both the US and the UK.

Freeman and Watts soon adjusted their technique, believing that they needed to remove more rather than less brain tissue. ('Double the dose!' as Sargant liked to say.) Moniz's leucotome was swapped for a blade that was used like a butter knife to make sweeping cuts across the frontal lobes. Ironically, they called their new approach a 'precision' lobotomy. Sargant would go on to adopt their technique in the UK, where it was known as the 'Freeman-Watts' cut.

The close alliance that was subsequently forged between Sargant and Freeman would prove central to the popularity of the operation in the UK. Later, in a macabre demonstration of friendship, Freeman sent Sargant a pair of sharp lobotomy instruments, now housed in the Wellcome Collection. But it wasn't just Freeman's passion for psychosurgery that attracted Sargant. He was a performer. The American was an eccentric showman, sporting a cane, Texas sombrero and goatee beard. During his neurology lectures and brain dissections – so popular that students brought along their girlfriends – he often drew on the blackboard with both hands. On Saturday mornings, he would wheel out troubled patients and discuss their neurological diseases in front of them, sometimes even imitating their gait. A few years earlier, in 1933, Freeman had had a nervous breakdown while writing a book on neuropathology. Waking at 4.30 a.m. every day to write, he'd complained his brain was on fire. For the rest of his life, he was on Nembutal, a barbiturate.

Freeman, like Sargant, was a savvy media operator. As early as June 1937, the *New York Times* referred to the operation as the new 'surgery of the soul'. A local newspaper headline proclaimed

'Wizardry of Surgery Restores Sanity to Fifty Raving Maniacs'. Freeman told one journalist in 1941, 'We want a little indifference, a little laziness, a little joy of living that patients have sought in vain for so long.'

His story bears uncanny similarities to Sargant's: the nervous breakdown, the dependency on drugs, a coldness beneath the charm, and the heartless public demonstrations of patients. And, like Sargant, Freeman was also a zealous advocate of organic treatments for psychiatric illness, quick to embrace shock therapies. It was against this backdrop that Sargant first encountered him in 1938, when on his Rockefeller travelling fellowship and keen to make connections. In fact, he had begun to network long before his ship had even docked, introducing himself to a young American passenger called Eleanor Roosevelt II. Her aunt, also called Eleanor, just happened to be married to Franklin D. Roosevelt, the President of the United States.

Eleanor was returning to America for the season of debutante balls in Boston and hoped that Sargant would attend some of them. He demurred, feeling too old. She was only eighteen, almost half his age. He soon changed his mind, however, when he discovered that Eleanor's coming-out ball would be held at the White House, preceded by a private dinner with the President. On 27 December 1938, Sargant found himself being frisked at the entrance to the White House. At dinner, he was seated one place away from President Roosevelt, who later asked Sargant all about British medicine and 'seemed greatly interested'.

The one catch for Sargant, who liked a drink, was that there was no alcohol served at the dinner. (The President's brother-in-law, Hall Roosevelt, later gave him a stiff whisky.) For the next two days, Sargant was driven around Washington on a sightseeing tour in White House cars and his name appeared in the newspapers. Not a bad start for an ambitious British psychiatrist. But was his encounter with Roosevelt as fortuitous as he claimed? Or had he travelled across the Atlantic with an introduction already in his pocket? Either way, it would prove to be the beginning of a long association between Sargant and some of the most powerful people in America.

Sargant had clearly been much taken with young Eleanor – she was 'as intelligent as she was kind-hearted' – but he felt less enamoured with the psychiatry department at Massachusetts General Hospital, where he was based for his fellowship. The department leaned firmly towards Freudian psychoanalysis: the use of Cardiazol and insulin coma therapy was frowned upon. So Sargant's joy must have been unbridled when he heard that Walter Freeman and James Watts had managed to successfully replicate Moniz's lobotomy.

He promptly rang Freeman, who was in Washington, keen to examine three of his patients. Sargant 'came away in a state of great excitement', echoing Freeman's original enthusiastic response to Moniz's lobotomies, even if the first patient, an alcoholic, had failed to impress Sargant with his boast that he could now get twice as drunk on half the amount of whisky.

The second patient, a schizophrenic, continued to hear voices but she was no longer troubled by them and was 'reasonably happy'. And the third patient, a chronic melancholic, said she felt 'remarkably better'. Sargant was convinced that Freeman had found a way to cure chronic anxiety and obsessive tension rather than schizophrenia. 'We had, in fact, witnessed a preliminary skirmish in a surgical attack on the supposed "soul" of man.'

Two years later, in November 1941, Freeman was contacted by Joseph P. Kennedy, Sr, father of John, Robert, Ted – and Rosemary. His eldest daughter was twenty-three and prone to mood swings, violent rages and seizures. She'd also been a slow learner at school. Without consulting his wife, Kennedy arranged for Freeman and Watts to give her a lobotomy.

The operation was a disaster. Asking Rosemary to count backwards and sing 'God Bless America', they severed her frontal lobes under local anaesthetic until she became incoherent. At that point they stopped, but it was too late. Rosemary, who was already considered an embarrassment to the Kennedy family by her father, now had the mental capacity of a two-year-old and would be institutionalised until she died, aged eighty-six.

10

'The Versailles of the New York rich'

Sargant was itching to develop and prescribe his own lobotomies in Britain – but he would have to wait until 1941. Back in Boston, he made one other very important connection before returning to Britain. In many respects, Alfred Lee Loomis would have made a perfect Bond villain. A Yale-educated mathematician, amateur physicist and successful Wall Street investment banker, he had presciently converted all his investments into gold in 1928, just before the Wall Street Crash. Subsequently, he used some of his considerable fortune to build a private laboratory in a crumbling mock Tudor mansion called the Tower House, on the edge of Tuxedo Park, a gilded and gated enclave outside New York City where he lived (and which gave its name to the Tuxedo jacket, first worn at the Tuxedo Club).

It was here, in the late 1930s, that Loomis gathered together some of the world's most talented scientists: Albert Einstein, quantum physicists Werner Heisenberg and Niels Bohr, and Enrico Fermi, who created the first nuclear reactor. They worked on a range of projects, including electromagnetic radiation, electrical activity in the brain, the precise measurement of time, spectroscopy (the study of light), powerful radar systems and nuclear fission. It was also where Loomis had his own Sleep Room.

Sargant had first met Loomis in 1939, when the American dropped into the laboratory at Massachusetts General Hospital. The two got talking about research that Sargant was conducting on overbreathing. He had already published two papers on hyperventilation, including one in which he had put a hysterical patient into a trance state with subsequent amnesia, 'without telling the patient he is to be hypnotised'. After two to four minutes of overbreathing, the patient began to feel 'dizzy and confused', with increased suggestibility. Sargant found the treatment particularly useful when treating outpatients with hysterical amnesia who turned up with no knowledge of their own name or address. Once hypnotised, they began to reveal personal details. The military potential was obvious. More than thirty years later, Sargant's work on non-consensual hypnosis would be cited in another paper, 'The Potential Uses of Hypnosis in Interrogation', which was partly funded by the CIA.

Loomis was intrigued and invited Sargant up to Tuxedo Park, apparently to develop a better machine to measure carbon monoxide. They clearly hit it off – 'I made a most valuable and charming permanent friend,' Sargant wrote – and for three weeks he lived a life of luxury, working in the lab in the morning, playing tennis and fishing on the lake in the afternoon, and dining with Loomis in his modern summerhouse in the evening. Not for nothing was Tuxedo Park considered by its residents to be 'the Versailles of the New York rich'.

During his luxurious stay, Sargant often found himself in the presence of eminent scientists and was once privy to 'a secret discussion' on using radar to locate aeroplanes. What he doesn't dwell on in his autobiography is the recent work that Loomis had been carrying out on brain waves during sleep, after reading the work of Hans Berger, a German psychiatrist who had invented electroencephalography (EEG) to record the electrical activity of the brain.

Loomis was obsessed with brain waves and published various papers of his own between 1935 and 1939. In one corner of the basement of the Tower House, he had built a soundproofed 'sleeping room', in which friends, family and guests were regularly encouraged to put on electrodes and take an afternoon nap. Later, he would measure people's brain waves while they slept for the whole night, identifying five distinct types, and established that someone under hypnosis was not actually asleep. Using his sixteen-year-old son, Henry, as a guinea pig, he also tested for the effects of emotional trauma on sleep. While Henry dozed one afternoon, his father whispered into his ear that his brother's sailing boat was on fire. Henry's normal brain wave pattern was interrupted, a finding that Loomis excitedly wrote up. It's hard to imagine that Sargant wasn't deeply interested in these experiments, but he only mentions them in passing in *The Unquiet Mind*.

Loomis' array of distinguished guests was also recruited as volunteers for his experiments, along with their wives and any visiting houseguests. Not surprisingly, he was the focus of a lot of 'mad scientist' stories in the popular press about his exploits at the Tower House – a place that Einstein once called 'the Palace of Science'. His experiments on brain waves in the late 1930s were attracting particular interest from psychiatrists and neurologists interested in electroencephalography.

At the end of Sargant's time at Tuxedo Park, Loomis offered to finance him to work at any American university of his choice for two years. But war loomed and Sargant returned to Britain, staying for one last night of luxury before taking the passenger ship back to Southampton.

He would remain lifelong friends with Loomis and it would prove to be a significant connection. In the summer of 1940, the

FBI and the Naval Intelligence Unit asked Loomis how to 'mark certain confidential documents for the purposes of catching a person they suspected of being a spy'. Loomis, liaising with the nuclear physicist Ernest Lawrence, suggested that a few drops of a radioactive substance (radio-yttrium) could be placed on the documents and detected with a portable Geiger counter at the exit if someone tried to steal them. A cloak and dagger trap worthy of a le Carré novel.

In September 1940, during the Battle of Britain, Loomis played a more pivotal role. He was asked to meet a secret delegation of scientists from Britain, led by Sir Henry Tizard, a mercurial government scientist dubbed 'Tizard the Wizard'. The British had come to share various technological advances in return for America's help in the war. The jewel in Tizard's crown was the airborne cavity magnetron, a recent breakthrough in radar technology later described by an American historian as 'the most valuable cargo ever brought to our shores'. It could generate very short wavelength (10 cm) radio waves and was a potential game changer against the Nazis. Unfortunately, Britain didn't have the ability to produce it at scale.

Loomis moved his laboratory from Tuxedo Park to a site on the Massachusetts Institute of Technology (MIT) campus in Cambridge, where he set up the Radiation Laboratory, better known as the 'Rad Lab'. In a race against time – Britain was taking a beating in the Blitz – Loomis developed an airborne interception radar that could be used by fighter planes to combat German bombers at night. The results were spectacular. As Lee DuBridge, director of the Rad Lab, later said: 'Radar won the war, the atom bomb ended it.' Robert Oppenheimer would turn to the same Rad Lab scientists when he was assembling his team for the Manhattan Project to develop the nuclear bomb.

Although Loomis became a recluse in later life, leaders in government continued to seek his advice. In May 1951, according to an internal CIA memo, he was considered for chairman or director of the Psychological Strategy Board (PSB), a new organisation set up to coordinate America's approach to psychological warfare in the Cold War. Loomis had a 'thorough knowledge of the Soviet Union' and 'few people could surpass him in originality and productivity of thought'. The memo was copied to Allen Dulles, the CIA's Deputy Director for Plans (overseeing covert operations) and a future Director of the Agency. Loomis turned down the job, but his son Henry did choose to join the PSB as a consultant in 1951, while working for the CIA and the Pentagon.

Sargant had found an ally at the heart of America's deep state. 'Loomis moved in intelligence circles,' says his biographer, Jennet Conant. 'He had the Yale and Stimson connections, was a blue blood, and was well connected socially, which was how it all worked back then.' Loomis had also spent time and money researching sleep, including the effects of trauma. Twenty years later, Sargant would have his own Sleep Room which, as we shall see, was possibly funded by the intelligence services. And so would Ewen Cameron, whose Sleep Room in Montreal was definitely financed by the CIA. Sargant's Sleep Room wouldn't be in the basement of a mansion outside New York, or in a psychiatric hospital in Montreal, but on the top floor of an NHS hospital in the heart of central London.

11

'A fifth nurse would hold the head'

By the time Sargant arrived in Southampton on 29 September 1939, Hitler had invaded Poland and Britain was at war. At the Maudsley, the staff had been split in two. Half had been dispatched to Mill Hill School in north London. The other half, including Sargant, had been allocated to Sutton Emergency Hospital, a converted former workhouse in Belmont, Surrey.* His first night at Belmont, a blackout, must have been quite a comedown from the gilded world of Alfred Loomis.

To Sargant, the split in the Maudsley reflected a major ideological schism in British psychiatry: the 'talkers' had gone to Mill Hill, the 'doers' to Belmont. And he saw the rivalry that existed between them as an opportunity to prove the benefits of his own physical approach to mental health.

The chief competition was between Sargant and Aubrey

* In 1946, Sutton Emergency Hospital became Belmont Hospital, the name used throughout this book.

Lewis, clinical director of Mill Hill, who much to Sargant's dismay would later succeed Edward Mapother as head of the Maudsley. Lewis was a stickler for statistics and follow-up studies, neither of which were priorities for Sargant, but their differences weren't just professional. After he had retired, Sargant would confide in a letter to a former colleague: 'I remain remarkably free from hatreds in this world (except Aubrey, who I thought was a wicked man).' Lewis banned insulin coma therapy and leucotomies at Mill Hill – two of Sargant's go-to treatments.

The first person to be given ECT in Britain, in December 1939, was a patient at the Burden Neurological Institute in Bristol. The procedure took place under the guidance of its director, Frederick Golla, and W. Grey Walter, who had assembled a basic electrical device to administer the shocks. A more practical machine was soon developed by Angus MacPhail and Dr Eric Strauss, who treated day patients with ECT at St Bartholomew's Hospital in London.

Sargant was itching to get his hands on a MacPhail-Strauss device, but the London County Council refused to provide him with one. Sargant was incensed by what he saw as 'medical bureaucratic obstructionism' and lobbied the administrator of a private charity in the City of London for the necessary £40 (c. £2,750 today) to purchase a MacPhail-Strauss machine.

The Ministry of Health and the LCC's medical advisers, who had joint oversight of Belmont, were concerned by reports of ECT causing bone fractures and other injuries as patients were restrained: dislocated jaws, shattered teeth, lacerated tongues and broken long bones (arms and legs), as well as fractured vertebrae, were not uncommon. It would be a few years before patients were given muscle relaxants to mitigate the violent spasms.

Similar concerns had, of course, been raised over Cardiazol-induced seizures. It was hoped, however, that electrically induced fits might cause less pain and damage. Those hopes proved unfounded. Sargant admitted that ECT caused just as many hairline fractures in the vertebrae as chemically induced fits, but he once again maintained there was no cause for alarm: the fractures seldom gave the patient any great discomfort and proved to be 'of relative unimportance'.

Years later, in May 1963, an old colleague from Duke Medical School in America wrote to Sargant. She was concerned about a family member's ongoing ECT treatment, after he'd suffered some sort of bone fracture. Understandably, she was anxious about him continuing the treatment, but Sargant seemed remarkably ambivalent about the need for a muscle relaxant. In England, he replied, muscle relaxants were now used 'almost routinely'. And even if a patient got a crush fracture in hospitals where they weren't used, treatment could still be continued and the condition rarely worsened. 'Therefore, if —— needs further shock treatment, he should certainly have it, if possible with muscle relaxants.'

Back in 1941, the LCC had also refused to allow St Ebba's Mental Hospital in Epsom to use a shock box. The medical superintendent duly contacted Sargant, who now had his own private MacPhail-Strauss equipment, asking him to come over to treat a schizophrenic boy. Sargant didn't need to be asked twice, but even he decided that the young patient was too emaciated and that ECT could cause 'multiple bone fractures'.

One can almost picture Sargant, shock box in hand, as disappointed as a child who's been told he can't play with a new toy. Were there, perhaps, any other depressed patients in better physical condition? The superintendent led Sargant through to a ward of forty patients with severe depression. Sargant quickly set to work, giving the treatment to almost everyone on the ward. Bodies would have contorted violently, backs arcing, and even Sargant admitted that 'our sending of an electric current through the patient's head was always an anxious event for us'.

He claimed that more than thirty of the patients made a quick recovery and were able to leave St Ebba's (he doesn't say if they were later readmitted), but very few of them were checked for fractures. Unless patients complained persistently, he refrained from X-raying their spines. He knew that if they revealed any fractures, 'the orthopaedic surgeons would make a fuss and put everyone into plaster jackets'.

Sargant could barely conceal his contempt for his colleagues in orthopaedics, but they had good grounds for concern, as Sargant's instructions in 1944 for inducing a fit make clear. The patient had to remove his false teeth before entering the treatment room. He then lay on a hard but padded couch, ready to receive 70 volts for 0.35 seconds from a MacPhail-Strauss machine, going up gradually to a maximum of 110 volts if a fit was not initially induced.

The patient would be 'put into a specially constructed jacket restraining his movements during the fit,' he explained, having forgotten that the use of a straitjacket to restrain patients was exactly the sort of treatment that he had professed to abhor in asylums. It was copied and modified from an ordinary straitjacket but was not always enough to contain a patient. Sometimes a team of five nurses would be deployed instead: 'One holds the feet in close adduction. One applies the whole of her weight to the pelvis, pressing it firmly to the couch. Two more stand on each side of the shoulders, and with their weight transmitted through their forearms keep the shoulders pressed to the couch ... A fifth nurse will control the head.'

A nurse was also tasked with washing the patient's forehead with soap and saline, before a rubber band was used to keep the electrodes in place at the temples. A dog's rubber bone was recommended as a mouth gag, the chin held firmly in place to avoid dislocation of the jaw. It was only then that the doctor, having checked all his nurses were in position, would give a final word of warning – and flick the switch.

12

'Sara'*

Twenty years ago, I couldn't have talked about what happened to me on the top floor of the Royal Waterloo, but I can now, anonymously. I have accepted that it's a chapter of my life, that I was part of a medical experiment. My second husband, Mark, has no idea what I went through, or that I once couldn't cope, and we've been very happily together since 2006. I prefer it that way. No disrespect to him, it just proves that I'm OK now.

My son Paul, from my first marriage, doesn't know either. He's now in his late forties – I fear he might think I'm a weaker person if I told him. It's awful that one should feel ashamed about being admitted to a psychiatric hospital, but, psychologically, it does almost feel like a prison sentence. Thankfully, I've got through to the other side. And, although I would never wish suffering on anyone, it somehow makes it better knowing that other people were treated in a similar way. It wasn't just me.

I grew up very happily in the southern Home Counties. My father was a stockbroker in London and my mother did volunteer

* Some names have been changed, including Sara's, for privacy.

work for the RNLI. I had a sister, Jen, who was ten years older than me, and we lived in a lovely house. Life was pretty good. And then, when I was thirteen, my school closed down overnight. I was devastated – I was a boarder there and so happy, with lots of friends. My parents obviously had to find me another school and they finally settled on a very grand place about forty miles from our home.

To be honest, I felt out of my depth from the day I arrived. Most of the girls in my year were daughters of earls, top actors, maharajas and diplomats, and their families were all exceptionally rich. At the beginning of term, they would be dropped off in Rolls-Royces. My family had an old Morris Traveller. I made some friends and managed to do quite well academically, despite a challenging change in curriculum, and I finally achieved seven O levels.

It was just after I'd completed the French O level oral exam, which I'd taken early, when I was called to the office of the headmistress – always a nervous moment. The school doctor was also present, which I thought was a bit odd. The doctor told me that, following his recent medical examination of me, I had to go into hospital for a sinus operation and I would be leaving school the next day. I was not happy, to put it mildly. The end of term was in a few days, and I would miss the leaving party with all my friends.

The next morning a taxi arrived, and the school nurse accompanied me to the hospital. I can still picture my friends all lined up on the school drive, waving as the car drove away through the gates. And then I can remember the taxi going down this very long drive and approaching the front door of a huge Victorian mansion. I asked the nurse where we were, and she said it was the hospital. I learned later that it was in fact Holloway Sanatorium – for the mentally insane. As far as I was concerned, I was going for an operation on my sinuses. I wasn't mentally ill. I was also only fifteen.

No other patients were around as I was shown down a long corridor. I was taken to a single room on the ground floor and told to unpack. There was a small glass observation panel in the top of the door – just like they have in prison cells. A stable-type door led outside to a small garden patio.

A doctor soon came in to see me, took my temperature and blood pressure. He returned after I'd eaten a meal, and said he was going to give me an injection, which would make me sleepy. When I came round in my room, which seemed like ages later, I was told to get dressed. I felt dizzy and confused, with a severe headache and a feeling of not knowing where I was. I just presumed that I had been given a general anaesthetic. Not for one moment did I think that I'd had electro-convulsive therapy – I was too young and had never even heard of it. Years later, I discovered that ECT was exactly what I had received.

I was given some reading material, drawing paper and pencils and, as it was summer, I was told I could sit in the small garden outside my room and draw, but it was very difficult to concentrate and focus on anything. I felt very lonely and missed my family and school friends. After about two days – again it seemed so much longer – my family came to see me. My mother and sister were in floods of tears, and I had no idea why. I just assumed I'd had a sinus operation. My father was beside himself with anger and they took me away immediately. I still thought it was a normal hospital. It was only later that I was told I had been taken there without my parents' permission.

I was honestly not aware that I had even been diagnosed with depression. Looking back, I may have been overworking and stressed at the time of taking my O levels, like a lot of my friends. We'd all worked hard for our exams. I had also been very worried about my father, who was in and out of hospital for major operations on his legs.

I went home with my family but the strong sedatives and ECT that I had received left me feeling very withdrawn. I just remember lying in my bedroom, feeling that I was in a bubble and isolated. My self-confidence was zero and I felt a burden and worry to my family, that they would be better off without me. Everyone else was 'normal' and I wasn't. One day, I swallowed lots of pills and tried to commit suicide. Thankfully, I survived, but I must have caused a lot of anguish to my parents. Our family GP referred me to a consultant psychiatrist, Dr Pollitt, who worked closely with Dr Sargant at St Thomas'. He saw me as an outpatient and put me on Largactil, an antipsychotic, and Tryptizol, an antidepressant.

Pollitt then arranged for me to be admitted to Ward Five at the Royal Waterloo Hospital. He told my parents that this was the best place to 'get her right' and back to how I was before I left school. It was early October 1964 and I was still only fifteen. There were patients of all ages and sexes on Ward Five, but they were mostly women. Some walked up and down the long corridor in their dressing gowns and slippers, others were dressed. There was little expression in their faces and they looked sad and serious. I remember the Sleep Room on the left of the ward entrance: it was very dark in there, with what I can only describe as a strange, musty, oppressive smell emanating from it. The room had large swing doors with porthole windows.

I certainly seemed to be the youngest on the ward. To begin with, I was allowed to remain dressed, but I felt incredibly sleepy all the time. Like most of the other patients under the care of Sargant and Pollitt, I was given injections of insulin followed by ECT shock treatment, combined with strong sedatives, including lithium carbonate. A hideous cocktail of drugs that kept us all in a zombie state as we waited to be given narcosis. Because the ECT affected my memory and I was so drugged up, I cannot be 100 per cent certain that I was eventually admitted into the Sleep Room itself. Ironically, I'm not sure I would actually remember if I had been.

My parents and sister visited me when they could. I later discovered that I was an inpatient on Ward Five for about three months and was 'released' to go home in time for Christmas in December 1964. I was still on Largactil and heavily sedated. Despite all the drugs, I was absolutely determined to get better. I was well enough to go to a boarding college near Windsor for a year in 1965 to learn cooking, flower arranging, dressmaking and typing.

I was happy and stable during this time and had a steady boyfriend, whom I had known since I was fourteen. In January 1966, I went up to London and shared a flat with three other girls my age. I was then a debutante and attended lots of cocktail parties, dinners and dances. Later that year, I got a job with a porcelain and glass company and ended up working there for three years. My father wanted me to work for Christie's but my self-confidence was low and I felt secure where I was.

My happiness was shattered on 1 July 1968, when my father had a severe heart attack. As a child, he'd contracted rheumatic fever, which had weakened his heart. He'd also had two major operations at St Thomas' to replace the arteries in both legs and had been resting and convalescing at home. I remember it was a very hot summer that year, but he loved his job and was determined to get back to the office. He hired a taxi to take him to his London flat in Little St James's Street and suffered a massive heart attack on the way. The taxi driver rushed him to St George's Hospital, where he was pronounced dead on arrival.

We were all in total shock. Although my father had been ill for many years, his death was sudden, and we just felt completely numb and empty. It was an awful time. My sister Jen and I eventually went back to our jobs in London and, with the support of family and friends, our mother coped well at home.

In 1969, I met a boyfriend through one of my flatmates. Jon was a surgeon at St Bart's and was kind, loving and caring. He had a grey convertible MG sports car, and most weekends I stayed with his parents or my mother. We had lovely holidays together and were very much in love. And then, on the last day of a holiday, Jon told me that he felt we had no future together. He needed to focus on his career as a doctor and surgeon. I was stunned. I had no idea there was anything wrong with our relationship.

I really struggled in the following year to cope without Jon in my life and became very depressed while on a holiday with my mother in South Africa. I flew back to London with her in early December and was immediately re-admitted to Ward Five. I was twenty-two. Once again, I can't be certain if I was treated with narcosis in the Sleep Room, or 'just' with ECT, lithium therapy, Largactil and Tryptizol. That's the problem with these treatments – they destroy your memory. I certainly recall having a tongue suppressant inserted into my mouth as the anaesthetist nurse put an intravenous drip into the back of my hand, just before I was given ECT.

When I woke up, I did not know where I was or what had happened. I recall a horrible metallic taste in my mouth, a sore throat and tongue. The nurse gave me water because I was so thirsty too. The ECT has definitely affected my early memories, especially my school years and a lot of my young childhood. Seeing old photos helps to remind me. Perhaps my biggest regret, though, has been the loss of my artistic ability. Ever since I was young, I was good at drawing and painting in watercolours, but after my trip to Holloway Sanatorium, my artistic talent weakened considerably. A natural talent that I've never got back.

I also remember spending a lot of time on Ward Five in bed in my room, which I shared with another woman. The window looked out towards the old Shell Centre. When I was really bored, I used to count the number of windows on the building. And I remember the consultation meetings with Sargant. Pollitt and a staff nurse would be present to report on my condition, whether there had been any progress with treating my depression.

Sargant was a large, serious man in a broad-striped suit and smart tie, with brown eyes and dark eyebrows. He had a presence – you just knew he was an important person, like a 1960s bank manager or lawyer. He was the type of man who I trusted to give me the best treatment to help my anxiety and depression, and I didn't feel I could query his prescribed treatment plan for me.

Sargant and Pollitt worked very closely together as a team,

but Sargant was clearly the boss. He was quite abrupt and didn't appear to spend any length of time with a patient. Pollitt seemed kinder and made me feel that the treatment they were giving me was really going to help me get better. During my progress meetings, the two of them always explained that they would not let me leave Ward Five until my monthly period had arrived – if a woman was in the pre-menstruation cycle, they were more prone to depression and less likely to cope with life at home or in the outside world. Pollitt also said that winter was the worst time of the year for my particular type of depression. In retrospect, I believe that this was just an excuse to keep women in Ward Five longer, for their ongoing medical experiments.

My mother came to visit me when she could. Friends visited too sometimes. One day, Pollitt finally discharged me, but I went on seeing him as an outpatient until the end of 1976. He was, however, handing me over for my day-to-day care to our family GP, who would continue to administer the same medicines I had on Ward Five.

I went home to live with my mother in early 1971 and worked locally as a receptionist. And then, in May 1972, I met Bill at a local Conservative Club disco. Bill was a biochemist, divorced, and had two lovely young children. We married in May 1973. I told Bill about Ward Five and he was generally supportive and helpful, accompanying me to my outpatient appointments in London. But he was an export manager and travelled all over the world, leaving me home alone a lot of the time.

I desperately wanted a family of our own and was determined to stop taking the lithium carbonate that Sargant and Pollitt had given me. With the support of our family GP, I gradually ceased taking it and, in February 1976, our son, Paul, was born. Pollitt got involved and arranged for the hospital to give me progesterone injections for seven days to prevent me suffering from postnatal depression, but I really didn't manage very well during this time. My depression and feelings of isolation returned with a vengeance.

Our GP advised that I should be sterilised and have my fallopian tubes tied because my postnatal depression was so severe. I was devastated. Bill and I were hoping to have two children, but I went ahead. At the time, I was still not really in the right frame of mind to make a decision, and I was told the operation was reversible.

I was determined to get better, but then, in early 1981, Bill was made redundant and my world and self-confidence once more came crashing down. He ended up taking a biochemist job in war-torn Iraq. We rented out our cottage and all our belongings were in storage crates. It was a particularly unsettling time for me as I shuttled between my mother's house and my in-laws', waiting to join him in Iraq.

One very icy evening in December 1981, when I was driving to my mother's, the car was slipping and sliding all over the place. There were snowdrifts piling up at the side of the road – nightmare driving conditions. Finally, we reached my mother's and I gave my son his supper, read books to him and put him to bed. I then had supper with my mother and went to bed too. I was shattered – the drive over had been so stressful. For reasons that I still find hard to explain – a mix of extreme confusion, tiredness, stress, lack of confidence – I swallowed all the pills I had with me that night. Before I became sleepy, I managed to ring Bill, who was at his parents', to tell him what I had done. I was panicking, still lucid and needed his help, but I was not expecting him to come over. While my mother and son were asleep, I went out to the log shed in the garden, where it was freezing cold and snowy, and attempted to set fire to my long winter nightdress, given to me by my mother-in-law. It was made from very old-fashioned winceyette-type material, floral with long sleeves, and by some miracle it was flameproof. Someone was looking after me that night.

Within thirty minutes, two policemen with a sniffer spaniel had arrived, thanks to Bill, who had called them. Mercifully, our son slept through everything. My mother had woken up and was obviously concerned. She was also very understanding and could see that I needed to get to the local hospital. The policemen offered to take me there straight away. Like two saints, they drove me with a flashing light, chatting in the car about their children as I told them about Paul.

I fell unconscious in A&E and had to have an emergency stomach pump. The next day I woke up in a single room, with the reassuring sight of my sister and brother-in-law at my bedside. I was well enough to go home that afternoon. My family GP duly increased my lithium dose – and I was at my mother's in time for a family Christmas with Bill and our son.

I will always feel awful about my suicide attempt. If those two police officers had not turned up, I wouldn't be here today. It was a huge shock to me that my young son could have been orphaned and I know that the cocktail of pills prescribed by Pollitt was the main cause of my confusion and depression. I often wonder how many former patients of Ward Five committed suicide as a result of their treatment and experience in that dreadful place. Maybe we will never know.

In 1997, Bill and I decided to move to Devon with our two dogs, having lost my sister to cancer, aged just fifty, and my mother. We bought a lovely house in a village with a large garden near the sea. I was very homesick, however, and recall sitting on the stairs hugging my Border collie and crying into the dog's furry neck. I found a job quite quickly as a legal secretary in the local town, but Bill struggled to find work because of his age. He never had a proper job again.

One day, I was shocked to find empty bottles of brandy and whisky in the airing cupboard. When Bill subsequently threw a heavy leather shoe at me and nearly broke my chin, I knew I needed to make a difficult decision. Paul, who was now twenty-nine, advised me 'to get a life' and leave Bill. So one Saturday, in early 2006, when Bill was at the local pub watching rugby with his mates, I packed up my car and left him, never to go back.

Later that year, at a dinner party given by friends, I met Mark, and we fell in love. My divorce from Bill went through in October and I moved into Mark's home in Cornwall. In 2010 we went on holiday to a Greek island, where we were stranded by the Icelandic ash cloud and stayed for an extra week. We happened to see an advert on a shop noticeboard advertising a house for sale. We had no intention of buying a house in Greece, but we fell in love with the small stone home with dark green shutters and bought it! Mark and I married in 2017, and we are very happy, living in Greece for three to six months every year.

Although I do not go to church at the moment, I strongly believe that my faith and the power of prayer have helped me with the mental struggles I have experienced since 1964. As I look back on my life, it is all too easy to say, 'Why me?' I had no history or signs of mental illness before I was admitted to Holloway Sanatorium as a fifteen-year-old girl. A lot of questions remain unanswered. Why did the school arrange for me to go there and tell me that it was for a sinus operation? And why were my parents not informed that I would have ECT?

Over the years, I have been told by different NHS doctors' practices that I have manic depression – a label that seems to follow my medical notes and is always flagged up on the GP's screen. I keep asking myself: would I have had depression if I had not been admitted to Ward Five? If I'd never come under the care of Sargant and Pollitt?

Today, I still have a general feeling of shame that I was an in-patient on Ward Five and often wonder what my life might have been like if I had not been so mentally 'bruised' by the experience. On the plus side, I am blessed with a wonderful son, daughter-in-law and two gorgeous grandsons and an incredibly loving second husband. I am also very proud to have had a job for most of my working life.

Most importantly, I have not experienced any depression since I met Mark nineteen years ago. With all that I have gone through in my seventy-four years, I am very blessed, but my life from

1964 to the present could have been so very different. I'm finally happy and stable, but it's because of my own determination to lead a 'normal' life, and the support from loved ones, not because of Sargant and his Sleep Room. The only medical legacy is my six-monthly blood tests and repeat prescription of a low dose of lithium carbonate – first prescribed on Ward Five more than sixty years ago.

Some people find a way to forgive those that have wronged them. I struggle to forgive Sargant and Pollitt. I came across a YouTube video recently about Sargant. I had not heard him speak for more than thirty years and it sent a shiver down my spine. Such a strong, distinct voice. It reminded me that you never disagreed with him – he was so confident in what he was saying. He had convinced himself he was helping people, but in reality it was a very cruel experiment.

Ultimately, he and Pollitt were given the authority for their treatments by St Thomas' and the NHS. We patients and our families innocently put our trust in them, but they shattered our lives, which were never to be the same again. In my darker days, I take comfort from a quote by Paul F. Davis, which I share with friends when they are low: 'The sun always shines above the clouds.'

13

'There are all sorts of ways of spending a honeymoon'

Sargant's personal life took a dramatic turn in August 1940, when he married a young British woman called Peggy. It could so nearly have been an American woman called Alice, whom he had met the previous year while attending a medical meeting in St Louis. After wiring Alice to say that he was leaving for Britain, they had spent one last night together. He couldn't expect an American to risk the dangers of war in Europe.

Peggy, on the other hand, seems to have been made of sterner stuff. She was working for the local Red Cross Society in Sutton at the outbreak of war and Sargant had turned to the charity in search of suitable people to work in his laboratory at Belmont. During his year in Boston, he had noticed how many 'intelligent Boston ex debutantes' – he had an eye for debutantes – had volunteered to work at Massachusetts General Hospital. He duly sought out 'intelligent Sutton girls' who had enough money to volunteer as unpaid laboratory assistants.

We don't know a lot about Peggy (born Dorothy Glen),

because she 'did not want to be talked about too much' in Sargant's autobiography. 'I believe Peggy came from a wealthy family,' says Nita Mitchell-Heggs, who worked on Ward Five in 1968 as a post-registration house officer (a newly qualified junior doctor). 'William appeared proud of her background. She was tall, slim and strikingly good-looking, rather than beautiful. Softly spoken and dignified, with great taste too. She ran a wonderfully appointed, traditionally decorated town house in Hamilton Terrace and was an excellent hostess. I recall eating superb beef Wellington.'

She carried herself well, with swept-back hair and make-up perfectly applied. In a rare photo of her, taken when she accompanied Sargant on one of his many international trips, she is standing beside Samburu tribeswomen in northern Kenya, wearing trousers and a blouse. 'Peggy was immaculately and elegantly dressed, in a very classic, tailored way,' Mitchell-Heggs adds. 'The hand-sewn hems on her beautiful dresses were the clue to their being expensive and bespoke.' She was also very game. When the tribeswomen wanted her to dance with them in 'mixed dancing', Sargant recalled: 'After some difficulty in picking up the rhythm, she found that the only way to imitate the dancing was to imitate the movements of sexual intercourse.'

Lord Owen once went to a cocktail party at their house on Hamilton Terrace and remembers Peggy as 'beautiful, very attractive', but also 'expensive'. She was, he thought, 'high maintenance'. Several people have spoken of a quiet sadness about her too. 'I wonder, in retrospect, if this could be explained by the fact that she and William had no children,' Mitchell-Heggs says.

Sargant and Peggy married in the grand surrounds of the King's Chapel of the Savoy in London, and took a seven-day honeymoon near Warwick. It was just as Birmingham began to be bombed, forcing the couple to retreat to an air-raid shelter. Bombing raids were to become something of a feature of their early life together. On their return to Sutton, honeymoon cut short, they rented a top-floor flat opposite the hospital, but spent their nights in the communal shelter on the ground floor.

Sleep proved elusive. The Sargants were surrounded by snorers and everyone knew that they were newly-weds, much to his embarrassment. He and his fellow doctors at Belmont were also being blamed for the bombing, as the hospital was thought to be a target. It wasn't a great start to married life, but the only other option was living with his mother-in-law, which held even less appeal for Sargant. They soon found a small air-raid shelter in a nearby field, abandoned by its owner because he couldn't bear the sound of dropping bombs, which was amplified by the ventilator shaft. Sargant, on the other hand, seems to have derived a particular thrill from the noise. 'The sound of falling bombs eventually came to have certain pleasant associations for us. There are all sorts of ways of spending a honeymoon!'

Belmont was on the main railway line to London. A month after the marriage, the hospital took a direct hit. Three wards, one above the other, were destroyed. Sargant and his colleagues dug unconscious patients out of the wreckage, but sixteen were killed. The experience left Sargant traumatised, but it seems to have troubled his wife less. After rushing out into the street, where she was unable to establish if she was now a widow, Peggy had gone back to bed.

At the outbreak of war, Belmont had been designated a joint general and neuropsychiatric hospital within Britain's Emergency Medical Service. It was one of many neurosis centres set up to deal with an anticipated outbreak of mass civilian hysteria at the beginning of the war (eight hundred beds were prepared), but it never happened. The British upper lip remained defiantly stiff.

To relieve boredom among staff during the so-called Phoney War, the hospital admitted ordinary psychiatric patients, many of them from the Maudsley site at Camberwell. Military patients were few and far between, but Dunkirk changed everything.

Belmont soon started to receive hundreds of traumatised soldiers who arrived directly by train from Dover. 'I shall never forget the arrival of these Dunkirk soldiers in their "tin hats" and filthy uniforms, some of them wounded, many in states of total and abject neurotic collapse, slouching along, mixed with Belgian and French civilians who had scrambled aboard the boats at the last minute,' Sargant wrote movingly in *The Unquiet Mind* (with more than a little help, one suspects, from the pen of Robert Graves).

Here was an unprecedented opportunity for Sargant to test, at scale, the efficacy of the new wave of shock treatments that had been developed in Europe in the 1920s and 1930s. At his disposal was a seemingly endless supply of human guinea pigs. Out of the first thousand admissions at Belmont, 150 were men suffering from 'acute hysterical loss of memory' – a condition rarely seen in peacetime. 'Opportunities of treatment and research were showered upon us at Sutton.'

By 1944, ten thousand military casualties had passed through Belmont, most of them suffering from what Sargant called 'acute battle shock' (known today as post-traumatic stress disorder). He also treated a variety of other psychiatric symptoms that he knew could seldom be observed in such numbers except in wartime.

Much later, in an interview in 1967, Sargant talked about his war years at Belmont with barely concealed enthusiasm. 'War time was a tremendous experience, because here for the first time you saw so many normal people breaking down under very great stresses.' The horrors of the battlefield – and the numerous breakdowns that ensued – represented a unique career opportunity for an ambitious psychiatrist. Sargant couldn't believe his luck.

One of the earliest Dunkirk casualties Sargant saw was a soldier whose whole body was shaking uncontrollably. In addition to the tremors, he was also suffering from what would be known today as transient global amnesia – shock-induced memory loss.

He had no recollection of being taken off the beach at Dunkirk or of being brought back across the Channel. Sargant also noticed that there was total paralysis of the man's right hand.

Puzzled by the sight before him, Sargant injected the soldier with sodium amytal, a quick-acting sedative that he'd brought with him to Belmont for experimental use on air-raid casualties. The effect was as strange as it was disturbing. The soldier began to talk, describing, with dramatic gestures, how he had come across his own brother lying by the roadside with a severe abdominal wound. After his brother had pleaded with him to end his suffering, he had dragged him into a field and shot him.

Exhausted, the man's tremors ceased. More remarkably, he now had full use of his right arm again – it was his right hand that had fired the fatal shot. A few weeks later, Sargant and Dr Eliot Slater, his clinical director at Belmont, wrote an article for the *Lancet* about their new treatment for 'acute shell shock'. The article mentioned the case of the soldier with a paralysed hand and was intended to offer emergency advice for other psychiatrists dealing with returning war casualties. But Sargant's desire to rush into print once again had unfortunate consequences. On the day of publication in the *Lancet*, the *Daily Mail* ran a story with the headline 'Hypnotised Soldier Tells of Secret Grief – he shot brother'. Sargant sent for the solider at once, apologised and arranged for his immediate discharge from the Army.

The incident says much about Sargant's eagerness for wider recognition as a psychiatrist. He was determined to prove, once and for all, the shortcomings of psychotherapy, which had been used to treat shell shock victims in the First World War. It took too long – a particular issue in the fierce cauldron of war – and didn't work. Later, he used to joke that his predecessor at St Thomas', Dr William Stoddart, told medical students in 1916 that they feared the German's Zeppelins and bombs because they were phallic symbols that aroused homosexual feelings and fears.

Sargant had clearly forgotten that he'd formed his own 'pleasant associations' with falling bombs and Peggy in an air-raid shelter near Belmont.

Sodium amytal, developed by the Lilly Company in 1927, was one of a new type of short-acting barbiturates that soon became the most popular sedative on the market. Sargant was keen on it from the start. Extremely addictive, it replaced 'bromides' such as the foul-tasting 'mist pot brom' (potassium bromide), which had been used to sedate schizophrenics in asylums.

Sargant had used sodium amytal for the first time the previous week, on another patient suffering from acute battle neurosis. He couldn't speak and his bladder had swollen to the size of a beach ball – he had not been able to urinate for days. His hands also shook as if he had Parkinson's. Not sure what to do with him, Sargant administered an intravenous injection of sodium amytal. The effect was startling. The patient's bladder emptied all over the couch, his speech returned, the trembling stopped and, according to Sargant, he became intelligent, articulate and relatively normal. At least, he did until the effects of the injection had worn off – a coda that was so often overlooked by Sargant.

It was the beginning of what Sargant called 'front-line' sedation. Giving intravenous injections of sodium amytal, sodium pentothal and other barbiturates, he began to treat waves of troops returning from the war. Key to the treatment's success was the speed with which the barbiturates were administered after the trauma. The longer the delay, the more chance that neurotic patterns of behaviour would become fixed in the patient's brain. 'It was like the surgical rule which requires that a fractured leg must immediately be put into a splint.'

Sargant claimed many successes, but he also became highly selective about whom he treated – only patients who would respond well to his treatment. 'No psychiatrist can yet make a silk purse out of a sow's ear,' he wrote. It was a strategy that would serve him well throughout his career. People of 'good previous personality' became his mantra.

Intriguingly, it wasn't only the *Daily Mail* who had noticed Sargant's use of sodium amytal. Military intelligence was interested too. The ability to persuade someone to reveal something, seemingly against their will, had obvious implications for interrogating prisoners of war. Sodium amytal wasn't just a sedative. It was a truth serum too.

14

'This form of therapy remains dangerous'

Six days after his article had appeared in the *Lancet*, Sargant received a letter from Colonel John Rawlings Rees. Formerly the medical director of the Tavistock Clinic, Rees had been appointed in 1939 as consultant psychiatrist to the British Army, working in the Directorate of Army Psychiatry. 'Dear Sargant,' he began, 'My warmest congratulations to you and Slater on the admirable article in the *Lancet*. I hadn't time to read it until last night, but I think it is extremely useful and the beginning of what I hope will be a lot of first-class work.' We don't know whether Sargant replied, but he was now on Whitehall's radar. For the next thirty years various government agencies, including the intelligence services, would turn to him for advice and help.

What was it about Sargant's work at Belmont that had particularly piqued Rees' interest? Time and again, Sargant had noticed that soldiers, once sedated with sodium amytal, would start to recall gruesome details of their ordeal on the front line. There would be an outpouring of emotions, ranging from the horrors of the battlefield to anger at their commanding officers. A torpedoed merchant seaman recalled being in the sea next to his close friend, who had disappeared beneath the waves. When the emotions became too painful, Sargant would increase the dose of sodium amytal to dampen them down.

Ironically, Sargant was tapping into the 'cathartic method' pioneered by the founder of psychoanalysis, Sigmund Freud, and Freud's mentor Josef Breuer. In *Studies in Hysteria* (1895), they had explained how pent-up emotions associated with a particular psychic trauma could be discharged by talking about them. They had called their technique 'abreaction', a term that Sargant adopted for his own very different drug-induced treatment. (The German verb, *abreagieren*, linked to the noun *Abreaktion*, means to vent or let off steam.)

Sargant was also following in the footsteps of a physician called J. Stephen Horsley, the first to discover that barbiturates could loosen tongues. In 1931, when women in labour at the London Hospital had been given the barbiturate Nembutal, Horsley noticed that they began to reveal their intimate secrets. Later they had no recollection of what they'd said. After testing his theory on embarrassed nurses, Horsley realised Nembutal had a potential role in psychiatry, where it could speed up analysis. 'In an hour the physician obtains a quantity of relevant information which he would not have obtained in a month by ordinary methods.' He began to experiment with other barbiturates, including sodium amytal and sodium pentothal, and called the technique 'narcoanalysis'. Following a brief flurry of media interest in the 1930s, however, it was largely forgotten – until Sargant came along.

Sargant was keen to publicise what he was discovering at Belmont, particularly the use of sodium amytal as an abreactive sedative. He wrote about it again in the *Lancet* on 25 January 1941. The slow, intravenous administration of a suitable narcotic – literally keeping the patient on the needle – allowed him to explore 'deeper into obscure episodes' and lay bare 'amnesias previously unsuspected'. A few months later, in June 1941, he spoke at the Royal Society of Medicine about emotional abreaction. John Rawling Rees, now a brigadier, must have been increasingly concerned by all the publicity, as Sargant was about to discover.

On 1 February 1942, Sargant wrote to E. Clayton-Jones, assistant editor at the *Lancet*, about another article he'd penned on sedation and sodium amytal. Sargant was due to send it in for publication when he received an 'urgent call' from Rees, who was 'considering the desirability of not publishing it because of its possible value to the army in the near future, and the undesirability of this work getting into enemy hands'. As Sargant explained to Clayton-Jones, 'They have now definitely made up their minds that they do not want it published.' Sargant didn't seem too upset. 'I quite see their point of view . . . perhaps they are deciding to do something on these lines.'

Indeed they were. Concerned by reports of their use by the Nazis, British military psychiatrists were already exploring the potential of barbiturates in interrogations. But Rees had a particular interest in Sargant's revelations. A year after he'd first written to Sargant, he was one of two psychiatrists who helped the intelligence services debrief Rudolf Hess, Germany's deputy Führer, after Hess had flown on an apparent peace mission to Scotland. (Hess had parachuted out of a Messerschmitt Bf 110 fighter bomber that he'd piloted himself – Hitler thought he was insane and disowned him.) From June 1941 to Hess's appearance at the Nuremberg trials in 1946, Rees oversaw the mental health of Hitler's incarcerated deputy. At some point, he was given barbiturates, including Evipan, to discover the real reason for his trip.

Intriguingly, Sargant's private papers include a translation of a document written by Hess. Dated 1945, it's a long, rambling account of the German's experiences during his imprisonment in the UK, including detailed descriptions of his medical treatment and own state of mind. At Nuremberg, Hess's mental health was assessed by a number of international psychiatrists, including Ewen Cameron, who would soon become Sargant's friend.

Despite – or perhaps because of – the military's interest, Sargant continued to develop his own drug-induced version of hypnosis. After the war, some medical students remember Sargant playing tape recordings of abreaction. He also liked to give live demonstrations, including one patient who had been trapped in a sea of boiling oil at Dunkirk. According to Ann Dally, after being given sodium amytal to release his memories, he would scream and leap all over the place. The medical students apparently loved it. 'He'd bring him back week after week . . . Sargant thought he was omnipotent.' The fact that the patient was able to repeatedly relive his experiences to order suggests that they might not have been permanently purged.

Barbiturates also changed the landscape of sleep. Regardless of their inherent risks, they superseded alcohol, opium, ether, chloroform and bromide, all of which had been used as sedatives. In the 1920s, Jakob Klaesi, a Swiss psychiatrist, had given patients a shot of morphine, followed by Somnifaine, a barbiturate derivative, to induce a twilight sleep for ten to twelve days. Klaesi recommended that it was best carried out in a darkened room with careful observation of the pulse and other bodily functions. 'The treatment must be stopped if vomiting or cardiac failure occur, and during menstruation.'

The first treatment in Britain was given in 1924, when Somnifaine was used on thirteen patients at the Maudsley. It was promptly dismissed as carrying 'considerable risk' with 'no special advantages'. By 1925, deep sleep treatment using Somnifaine had a mortality rate of 5 per cent and was widely acknowledged as being highly dangerous. But despite its well-documented hazards, psychiatrists continued to use it in the 1930s.

In February 1936, Dr D. N. Parfitt, deputy medical superintendent of Warwickshire and Coventry Mental Hospital, reported in the *Lancet* on fifty-six female patients whose various psychoses had been treated with continuous sleep for ten to twelve days. Three patients died, including one suffering from acute mania, who developed a temperature of 38.9 degrees on Day 11. The treatment was stopped but the patient 'soon began screaming ceaselessly'. Profound exhaustion set in, and she died from a high fever on Day 13, with a temperature of 42.6 degrees. Parfitt concluded that prolonged narcosis often produced improvement, sometimes dramatic, but warned that 'this form of therapy remains dangerous'.

It was against this backdrop of high risk and hazard that Sargant used barbiturates to induce sleep at Belmont. He gave patients barbiturates to put them to sleep for a couple of days when they first arrived. Abreaction would then be given if, on waking, they showed signs of functional memory loss or limb paralysis. Patients who were still anxious would be put back to sleep.

Sargant believed that narcosis was best suited to the 'acutely ill anxiety neurotic', a much more common phenomenon in wartime than in peace. The aim of the treatment was to provide twenty hours' sleep out of twenty-four, for a period that varied from a few days in 'the acute anxiety state' up to three weeks in 'the deeply depressed or acutely excited patient'.

Sargant used Somnifaine as well as sodium amytal and paraldehyde (a sedative that gave patients foul-smelling breath) to 'provide the fine adjustment of the depth of the narcosis'. Somnifaine was extremely toxic and required too dangerous a dose to induce narcosis on its own. Sodium amytal alone provided a 'smoother narcosis' but it was hard to induce a deep sleep. Nurses were also given strict instructions to make sure patients drank lots of fluid to avoid risk of poisoning, just as they would later in the Sleep Room. And they had to monitor blood pressure and urine, and administer insulin to combat Somnifaine's extreme toxicity. An enema was given before sedation, which was repeated every second day 'if bowel action is unsatisfactory'.

The patient was effectively in mortal danger day and night, for an extended period of time, which wasn't the case with other shock treatments. Risks included broncho-pneumonia, respiratory depression, cardiovascular collapse, urine retention, dehydration fever, vitamin deficiencies, toxic confusional states and barbiturate withdrawal fits. As if all that wasn't enough, a 'wrongly placed injection in the buttock' could cause sciatic nerve damage.

Sargant seemed to relish these dangers. 'To get the best results, the depth of the narcosis, especially in disturbed psychotic patients, may have to be pushed to limits that demand the highest degree of skill and training,' he said in the first edition of *Physical Methods of Treatment in Psychiatry* (1944). As with insulin coma therapy, he felt the risk of death burnished his own credentials as a physician in general medicine at a time when psychiatry was not regarded as a high-ranking or academic specialty.

There were other reasons too why Sargant embraced narcosis. It was at Belmont that he first realised sleep allowed him to administer ECT to patients who were too frightened of the treatment to receive it while they were awake. (He himself dismissed ECT as a 'not very exciting ritual'.) It also enabled him to keep the 'agitated indecisive patient' in hospital on a voluntary basis, avoiding 'the blow to family and patient of certification'.

Narcosis, in other words, was a way of sectioning a patient without the paperwork.

15

'His wife is very well indeed but not quite perfect'

Much like a good night's sleep, putting the kettle on for a brew has long been seen in Britain as a way to relieve stress. But tea played a different role in another of Sargant's go-to treatments at Belmont and later Ward Five. Tea and boiled potatoes. Modified insulin treatment was a variation of the high-risk insulin coma therapy that he'd finally been allowed to administer at the Maudsley in 1938. Noticing that schizophrenics had put on weight during the coma treatment and depressives tended to gain weight before they improved, Sargant decided to see if it was possible to stimulate recovery by 'artificially fattening them up'.

Silas Weir Mitchell, a physician, scientist and poet, had done something similar in the American Civil War, curing patients by confining them to bed, where they would be fattened and reddened. Inspired by the Weir Mitchell rest cure, as it was called, Sargant gave his own patients large doses of insulin and, the moment they dropped into a coma, brought them around by feeding them huge quantities of sugar via a stomach tube.

Some put on weight but most remained depressed. Sargant was disappointed, even more so when Dr Louis Minski, Belmont's medical superintendent, told him that he was consuming precious amounts of the hospital's rationed sugar. Sargant tried liquidised potatoes instead – unlike sugar, potatoes were never rationed. Although it took longer for patients to process the potato starches into sugar and come out of their coma, the alternative seemed to work.

When the Germans began daylight bombing raids, patients expressed their fear of being trapped in a permanent coma if they were hit during treatment. Undeterred, Sargant decided to give the patients a plate of potatoes just *before* they slipped into unconsciousness. There was now no need for stomach tubes and no danger of being bombed into eternal unconsciousness. The happenstance of war had led to a new therapy.

At one point, fourteen patients at a time were being treated in one ward at Belmont, which must have been an eerie sight. Later, in 1944, when Sargant worked at Graylingwell Hospital in Chichester, he had thirty casualties from the Normandy landings in a large dimly lit hall, all being given a combination of modified insulin treatment and narcosis. Nurses ran the place, but Sargant was on hand if something went wrong. 'There is no need for flurry as it will be some time before the patient will be in any danger from the induced glycaemia,' he said. As for the treatment itself, the patient, who had fasted from 8 p.m. the night before, was given 20 units of insulin at 7 a.m., increasing by 10 units a day until a dose of 100 units was reached, provided that the patient was still capable of eating food at the end of three hours.

The room was kept in semi-darkness and the patient at complete rest, much like in the Sleep Room. Constant vigilance was also necessary. Insulin in such large doses had a sedative effect and the patient was given sugared tea the moment he showed signs of slipping into a coma. 'The aim is to stabilise the dose at one just short of producing sopor or early coma.' Three hours after the injection, the patient was roused and given sugared tea, 16 oz of mashed potatoes, bread and butter, vitamin B supplements and an egg. 'Further amounts of potatoes are urged on him if he will take them.' Afterwards, the patients were given a full lunch, tea and supper and encouraged to take strenuous exercise, while being monitored for aftershocks. No treatment was given on Sundays. 'Often a patient would gain a pound in weight a day and eat two plates of mashed boiled potatoes each morning, and before long had put on nearly thirty pounds.'

Sargant claimed the treatment worked for Dunkirk and Blitz casualties who were suffering from anxiety or acute hysteria and had lost a lot of weight before they'd broken down, but he admitted it was markedly less successful for those suffering from severe depression and long-standing neurotic traits. Again, despite falling out of fashion in the 1950s, Sargant would continue to use a modified insulin therapy on Ward Five until the 1970s, not just for anorexics but for narcosis patients while they were in the Sleep Room.*

Many of them were appalled at the weight they had gained. 'I put on three stone during a four-month stay – I was enormously fat,' says Susannah, who thinks she was given modified insulin treatment in 1973 on Ward Five. 'I used to be seven and a half stone. I was white as a sheet, because I'd been lying in the dark for two months, vastly fat and dazed. They used to take us out for walks on the embankment as exercise. The nurses had their distinctive gabardine coats and little brimless hats, but I couldn't shut my coat – it had to be held together with safety pins. People must have known exactly where we were from. There was no dignity in it at all. Afterwards, when I was an outpatient at Scutari,

* Narcosis patients who were also given modified insulin therapy while in the Sleep Room would not be given their morning dose of sedatives on the day of treatment.

they used to weigh you after every appointment. I said, "I can't get the weight off, it's terrible, I feel awful." And it mattered to me, suddenly putting on all that weight. I'll never forget what the doctor said to me: "Buy bigger clothes."'

What Susannah didn't realise at the time was that if she hadn't put on weight, or responded to the continuous narcosis she also thinks she was given in the Sleep Room, she would have been lobotomised.

Of all the so-called heroic treatments, a lobotomy was undoubtedly the most invasive. To remove part of the brain in a bid to cure mental illness was the ultimate expression of Sargant's belief in physical methods of treatment in psychiatry. And he was keen to bring lobotomy to Belmont, inspired by his meeting with Walter Freeman and his patients in America. Freeman was eager to support him too. In 1942, he would send three copies of his book, *Psychosurgery*, to Europe: one to Egas Moniz, one to a Swedish psychiatrist and one to Sargant.

The Ministry of Health and the LCC once again did all they could to thwart Sargant's ambitions. But in Eliot Slater, his clinical director at Belmont, he had a firm ally who didn't oppose Sargant's experimental treatments. Slater went on to be Sargant's lifelong friend, co-authored all five editions of *An Introduction to Physical Treatments in Psychiatry* and shared a house with him in St John's Wood after the war. Something of a Renaissance man, Slater has often been overlooked in the Sargant story. A painter and poet with a love of Schumann, he was awarded, aged seventy-seven, a PhD for trying to prove that Shakespeare wrote *Edward III*. He also had troubling links with Nazi Germany.

Slater had joined the Maudsley in 1931 and was an active member of the British Eugenics Society. Encouraged by Aubrey Lewis, he had won a Rockefeller fellowship in 1934 to Germany, where he studied under Bruno Schulz and Ernst Rüdin at the Psychiatric Research Institute in Munich. Rüdin spearheaded the Nazis' *Rassenhygiene*, a programme designed to encourage a 'pure' and 'healthy' Aryan race by avoiding miscegenation and procreation among mentally ill people. Enforced sterilisation, for example, had been introduced in 1933 to prevent interbreeding between the 'feeble-minded' and schizophrenics. During the war an estimated three hundred thousand psychiatric patients would be exterminated in Germany, Austria and occupied Poland as part of the related Aktion T4 programme.

Slater distanced himself in later life from his connection with Rüdin, as did the British and American eugenics movement, which sought to rebrand eugenics as the more palatable 'psychiatric genetics'. But British and American eugenicists in the early twentieth century undoubtedly had much in common with what would later become *Rassenhygiene*. Slater himself claimed that his marriage to Lydia Pasternak, a Jew and sister of the Russian author Boris Pasternak, was proof enough of his disdain for Nazi ideology. (He was later awarded a CBE and headed up the Medical Research Council's genetic research department.) But there's no denying one incontrovertible piece of evidence against Slater.

In April 1939, just five months before war broke out, Slater had contributed to Rüdin's sixty-fifth birthday celebrations, writing an article, in German, for Rüdin's Festschrift, a book celebrating his academic achievements. Hitler personally presented Rüdin with a Nazi medal as a 'pathfinder in the field of hereditary hygiene'. Slater always insisted that he could only remember meeting Rüdin once, at an annual departmental dinner hosted by the German's wife at their home in Munich. 'We all arrived by arrangement together, one of our number carrying a large bouquet of flowers to be presented with a "*Küss' die Hand, gnädige Frau*" to the Frau Professor when she graciously received us.'

Slater, who would be divorced from Lydia Pasternak by 1946, didn't object to Sargant sending patients to be lobotomised at

Belmont, provided that he could guarantee the necessary neurosurgical facilities. However, the LCC once again stepped in. And once again Sargant set about circumventing authority. He wrote to Frederick Golla at the Burden Neurological Institute in Bristol, asking him to introduce lobotomy. The precedent might help Sargant to change the LCC's mind.

Golla duly obliged. On 11 December 1940, a year after he had introduced ECT to Britain, Golla oversaw Britain's first lobotomy. A young neurosurgeon called Wilfred Willway carried out the operation. Cheerful, debonair and bright, he could play chess against four people simultaneously. He also knew that death was 'close upon' him – he had Hodgkin's disease and would be dead four years later, aged thirty-six. Without access to Moniz's leucotome, he severed the frontal lobes of his first patient using a paper knife. 'My feeling at the moment is that a fairly extensive mutilation is necessary,' he said.

Golla himself called it a 'brutal and bloody operation'. Willway carried out more than eighty lobotomies before he died. The first eight were written up in the *Lancet* in July 1941 and declared by Sargant to be 'most successful'. The results suggested otherwise. There were, in fact, nine initial operations, but the ninth patient, a twenty-seven-year-old woman, died after a blood vessel was accidentally severed and her case was excluded from the initial report. As for the remaining eight, one died two days after the operation (heart attack), four remained in hospital and three were discharged, two of them with double incontinence.

Sargant was eventually granted permission to carry out lobotomies at Belmont, but only occasionally and provided that every case had been vetted by his seniors. Sargant wasn't satisfied and turned to Slater, who had also been put temporarily in charge of the psychiatric department at St George's Hospital. As a teaching hospital, St George's wasn't subject to the same control by the LCC or the Ministry of Health. Sargant, with Slater's blessing, discharged from Belmont those patients he felt would benefit from a lobotomy and promptly re-registered them at St George's, where Wylie McKissock, a cigar-smoking neurosurgeon, was only too happy to oblige. He'd just set up a neurological unit at the Atkinson Morley Hospital in Wimbledon, St George's former convalescent wing.

'This was what the New Testament calls "doing good by stealth",' Sargant said. If McKissock couldn't help, Sargant had 'understanding friends' at other hospitals, including the West End Hospital for Nervous Diseases. Between 1942 and 1945, Sargant was able to operate on a number of patients – 'by one ruse or another'. At his own admission, however, the results were not great. 'Our earliest experiments were not as satisfactory as one would have desired.'

It's not clear how many soldiers Sargant sent to be lobotomised, but many of those he dispatched to McKissock were civilians of 'good previous personality' ('well preserved' neurotics) who were suffering from anxiety, hysteria and depressive and obsessive states. The operation would be repeated several times if necessary.

Despite his Scottish-sounding name, McKissock was from suburban Staines. Dressed all in white in the operating theatre, he worked at lightning-quick speed, stopping only to puff on a cigar between patients. The operation could take as little as six minutes. He would go on to be responsible for more lobotomies in Britain than any other surgeon, his enthusiasm for psychosurgery matched only by Sargant's.

Terry Gould, McKissock's anaesthetist in the 1960s, estimated that he carried out three thousand operations in total (a figure only surpassed by Walter Freeman's 3,500), travelling around in his motor car at weekends with his theatre sister to visit rural psychiatric hospitals in Northampton, Chichester and Abergavenny. 'He used to say, "If Dr X wants it done, you do it."' And 'Dr X' was more often than not Dr Sargant.

But even McKissock had his reservations. He regarded

lobotomy as an experimental procedure. Patients were left with 'amnesia, confusion, somnolence and lack of initiative', he wrote in 1943. A few patients subsided into a 'harmless vegetable existence'. One husband reported that his wife had been left 'very well indeed, but not quite perfect'. Later he modified the Freeman-Watts procedure and developed what he termed a 'rostral leucotomy' that involved cutting holes in the top of the skull rather than the side.

Between 1947 and 1948, Monica was a young nurse at the Atkinson Morley. Nineteen at the time and now ninety-five, she still has vivid memories of McKissock and his operating theatre. 'It was so intense. I remember him boring into the skull with a drill,' she says. 'The patient, a young man, was sitting upright, and McKissock was operating on the top of his head. We were all terrified of him. He was such an autocrat. And we were the theatre runners, the skivvies. I remember it was very hot. Once he said, "Mop, girl, mop." And this nurse ran out of the room to get the mop for the floor. And he meant his forehead, you see, because he was sweating. Of course, he turned around and said, "You stupid girl." She was quivering with fright.'

By 1954, twelve thousand lobotomies had been performed in England and Wales, many of them by McKissock, who was also a consulting neurosurgeon at Belmont. After his retirement in 1971, he was knighted for services to medicine, but glowing obituaries in *The Times* and *Independent* in 1994 made no mention of lobotomy, or of his close relationship with Sargant.

Interviewed in 1977, Sargant revealed that he had recommended 350 people for lobotomies in the past two years through his private work, but only two had had the operation. The number of patients who received the procedure declined in the 1980s, when the Mental Health Act 1983 introduced the need for much greater consent, but limbic lobotomies, a microscopic version of the operation, were still being performed in the 1990s. (Various targeted neurosurgical treatments continue to be carried out today, including cingulotomy for stubborn OCD and persistent pain.) Sargant himself remained committed to lobotomy throughout the 1970s, and to the belief that mental illnesses, including psychosis, had an organic cause. 'There is a tract within the brain and I think that neurosurgeons will find it,' he said in 1977.

Almost fifty years on, that quest to discover biomarkers – biological evidence – of mental health conditions continues. Although some progress has been made in the field of 'precision psychiatry', using functional magnetic resonance imaging (fMRI) brain scans to predict which treatments might work best for different mental health conditions, there remains no physical test for depression or evidence of any brain abnormality that is specific to depression. And the jury is out whether the brain of someone with schizophrenia is physically any different from 'normal' grey matter. Neither of which invalidates a patient's suffering, but points to ongoing limitations in diagnosis and treatment. As Professor David Kupfer, chair of the DSM-V task force, said on publication of the latest edition of the *Diagnostic Statistical Manual of Mental Disorders* (2013), often referred to as the bible of psychiatry, 'We've been telling patients for several decades that we are waiting for biomarkers. We're still waiting.'

16

'Every dog had its breaking point'

Towards the end of the war, Sargant's office at Belmont had become a lively place. It was here that he used sodium amytal to induce trances, coaxing patients to relive their horrific battlefield experiences in what he called an 'amytal hypnoid state'. 'I remember about the third or fourth patient almost chasing me around the room re-living his experiences,' he said. Sometimes, it was obvious they were reliving actual events, but patients would also enter the realms of hellish fantasy. For others, sodium amytal wasn't enough to release – or abreact – their emotions and Sargant would mix the barbiturate with Benzedrine, the amphetamine he had first taken at London Zoo. Later, he switched to using ether to produce a more extreme reaction.

In many ways, Sargant was doing nothing new. Hypnosis had been used in the First World War by the likes of William Brown, a neurologist, to induce shell-shocked patients to relive traumatic experiences. But Sargant began to experiment with fictitious scenarios and was soon dreaming up terrifying situations for his patients. He might, for example, tell a member of the Royal Tank Corps that he was trapped in his burning vehicle and needed to fight his way out. 'If we could raise the crescendo of a patient's outburst to a grand finale of rage or terror, a state of temporary emotional collapse might follow.' Afterwards the patient would soon come round, feeling much better about life.

Sargant found that these implanted false suggestions could stir up a far greater 'emotional discharge' than the memory of a real event, particularly when he pushed the patient to the point of exhaustion. The key to success, he said, was for traumatic events to be 'relived in the present tense'.

It was around this time that Sargant was given a book by Ivan Pavlov, the well-known Russian neurologist. *Conditioned Reflexes and Psychiatry* was presented to him by Dr Howard Fabing, an American military psychiatrist and friend. Fabing thought that Sargant would appreciate the Russian's analysis of animal behaviour under acute stress and how it might relate to acute neurosis in humans. Pavlov believed that every dog had its breaking point – something that could also be said of the thousands of traumatised soldiers returning from the front line.

Pavlov is perhaps best known for his laboratory experiments on animals and in particular his concept of the conditioned reflex. This was based on his observations that a dog would begin to salivate not just at the sight of food, but when he saw the laboratory technician who regularly came to feed him. If Pavlov sounded his famous bell (it was more likely to have been a tuning fork or whistle) before the dog was fed, the animal would come to associate the sound with food and salivate. Pavlov's emphasis on the nervous system, rather than Freud's interest in the subconscious mind, chimed with Sargant's mechanistic approach to psychiatry. Both canine and human behaviour could be explained in purely physiological terms. There was no need to psychoanalyse why a dog salivates at the sight of the technician: it was a simple biological response. Pavlov, in other words, was Sargant's kind of guy. 'An anti-Freud for the biopsychiatry vanguard', as the author Mike Jay has memorably called him.

Pavlov's book had become available in translation in 1941, but copies in Britain were few and far between. His work had also largely been ignored in the West because of reservations about animal testing. Dogs also weren't thought to possess that uniquely human component so beloved of Freud: a soul.

Sargant, however, lapped it up. He had fallen ill in September 1944 with a combination of pneumonia and infectious hepatitis and had plenty of time for reading during his convalescence. 'Pavlov's clinical descriptions of the "experimental neuroses" which he could induce in dogs proved, in fact, to have a close correspondence with those war-neuroses which we were investigating at the time.' And he was quick to use the Russian's theories as another stick with which to beat the Freudians – 'unless it be conceded that Pavlov's dogs had . . . super-egos, egos and ids'.

Pavlov had won the Nobel Prize in 1903 for his work on animal digestion and was becoming increasingly interested in what happened to dogs when they were put under duress – and, later, how their behaviour compared to mental breakdowns in humans. He was presented with a unique research opportunity in 1924, when the Neva River flooded his laboratory in Leningrad. As the waters rose, his conditioned dogs began to panic, swimming around at the top of their cages, barking hysterically. A lab technician arrived at the last moment, bringing the dogs out through the water to safety.

A number of the dogs collapsed and were in a stupor after their rescue. The stress of the situation had overloaded their nervous systems. This 'rupture in higher nervous activity' had caused them to enter what Pavlov called a protective state of 'transmarginal inhibition' – in effect, a complete and self-preserving shutdown. Pavlov identified three distinct phases in dogs, which Sargant saw paralleled in humans: 'equivalent' (a person in this state might display 'no more pleasure on receipt of a five-pound note than on that of a sixpence'); 'paradoxical' ('sixpence may give, as it were, greater pleasure than a thousand pounds'); and 'ultra-paradoxical', in which conditioned responses were spectacularly reversed ('small things often upset an exhausted man to the point of passion, though he may smile at an almost overwhelming disaster').

It was this last, ultra-paradoxical phase of transmarginal inhibition that most intrigued Pavlov. Following acute stress, the brain seemed to suffer from reverse polarity. In Pavlov's traumatised animals, the reaction to the flood was startling. A dog would attach itself to people it had once disliked, and attack those that it had loved. 'Its behaviour, in fact, becomes exactly opposed to all its previous conditioning.'

It was immediately obvious to Sargant that Pavlov's stress-induced ultra-paradoxical phase had dramatic implications for humans and, in particular, for totalitarian leaders eager to change a nation's political beliefs. Towards the end of his life, whether by choice or obligation, Pavlov turned his attention to studying humans rather than dogs, and by the 1950s, long after his death, his theories were being widely deployed by the Russian state for political conversion. Sargant professed his abhorrence of this practice, but he didn't blame Pavlov personally.

Others were more vocal in their criticism. The Dutch psychoanalyst Joost Meerloo, who was interrogated and tortured by the Gestapo in Holland, coined the term 'menticide' to describe the psychological destruction of an individual. He even compared Pavlov's 'perverted' conditioning to nuclear war, suggesting that it was 'worse than an atomic explosion'.

Sargant was aware that Pavlov's theories could equally be applied to religious conversion. Just before falling ill, he'd paid a brief visit to his parents in Highgate, where he had picked up the second volume of John Wesley's *Journal* in his father's library. He was surprised to read a description of an emotional collapse caused by Wesley's fiery pulpit preaching. Sargant had grown up in a Methodist household and it occurred to him that Wesley's threats of eternal damnation and the hot fires of hell were not so different from his own suggestions to soldiers of being trapped in burning tanks. In both cases, subjecting someone to intense emotional stress had changed patterns of behaviour, echoing the Russian's ultra-paradoxical phase. 'Pavlov has shown by repeated and repeatable experiment just how a dog, like a man, can be conditioned to hate what it previously loved, and love what it previously hated.'

Furthermore, Pavlov found that dogs were subject to 'abnormal suggestibility' after they had collapsed. This too had implications for psychiatrists wishing to establish healthier patterns of thought in broken patients, who would now believe whatever the psychiatrist told them. Politicians of more sinister intent could also exploit such heightened suggestibility for their own ends. 'It was as if the recently printed brain-slate had been suddenly wiped clean, and Pavlov was able to imprint on it new conditioned patterns of behaviour,' Sargant said. Later, Pavlov slipped a hosepipe into the laboratory and turned on the tap. The dogs once again panicked – and once again lost their conditioned responses. Their brains, it seemed, could be wiped at will.

Brainwashing was in the air at the end of the Second World War. It would only be a few years until the publication of George Orwell's *Nineteen Eighty-Four*, in which O'Brien famously says, 'Power is in tearing human minds to pieces and putting them together again in new shapes of your own choosing.' Aldous Huxley had also made mind control a theme of his writing, in particular in 1932's *Brave New World*. In his prescient novel, a fictitious recreational drug called 'soma' had heightened the suggestibility of users.

Sargant was convinced that Pavlov's notion of transmarginal inhibition had therapeutic possibilities. In his insulin coma therapy and ECT treatments, he saw Pavlovian theories at work, stressing the nervous system to a point of collapse. The consequences, however, were often disastrous. Sargant admitted that in the years immediately after his arrival at St Thomas' in 1948, he was forced to transfer some of his patients to psychiatric hospitals because they had responded so poorly to his treatments.

The arrival in Britain in 1953 of Largactil would change everything. The first generation antipsychotic enabled Sargant to induce a state of transmarginal inhibition within the confines of Ward Five. There, in the half light of the Sleep Room, he was free to disrupt unhealthy patterns of thought and behaviour until, like Pavlov's dogs, his patients had reached their breaking point.

17

'The upper eyelid of the patient is pinched between thumb and finger'

By the end of the war, Sargant had already become a controversial figure. Plans to reunite the Maudsley's two warring tribes – from Belmont and Mill Hill – at its original home in Camberwell only exacerbated his divisiveness. His extreme treatments might have been acceptable for soldiers returning from the front line, but they began to look inappropriate for civilians in peacetime. Accused of being 'soullessly one-sided', he seriously questioned whether he wanted to remain part of the teaching hospital. Mapother, Sargant's hero, was dead, and the more conservative Aubrey Lewis was in pole position to succeed him as head of the Maudsley.

On a visit to the London County Council, Sargant's brother, Tom, was appalled by what critics were saying about his sibling. They accused him of often being 'cruel and irresponsible', venting his own 'repressed and subconscious aggressions' on patients.

In the end, the LCC Selection Committee reappointed Sargant to the staff of the reunited Maudsley. Sargant, though, could see no future for the hospital. He continued on a part-time basis at the Maudsley and Belmont, while applying, unsuccessfully, for other posts at several well-known psychiatric hospitals. His reputation was more damaged than he thought. He was not even shortlisted for any of the jobs.

America called. In early 1947, he was granted two months' study leave and went with Peggy to New York. It was the first time he'd been to America since his departure in 1939, and he promptly ran into a crowd of old friends at a meeting of the American Psychiatric Association. The adulation that followed must have been a welcome tonic after the badmouthing he'd received in London. Finding himself 'suddenly famous', he went on a lecture tour, visiting Baltimore, Cincinnati, Topeka and Boston. He also visited Duke University in Durham, North Carolina, where he was invited to become visiting professor of psychiatry for a year. It didn't seem to matter that Sargant was not actually a professor, and he duly accepted the position.

Sargant felt quite at home at Duke. The buildings reminded him of the Second Court at St John's College, Cambridge. Tobacco fields and factories lay all around – heaven for a forty-a-day man. Sargant was covering for Professor Richard Lyman, who was on sabbatical. An eccentric and wealthy neurologist, Lyman ran the department of psychiatry at Duke Medical School and had chosen to spend a year working at Tuskegee Hospital in Alabama, an institution reserved for war veterans of colour. When Sargant went down to spend a few days with him at Tuskegee, he was horrified to discover patients held in crude restraining devices, an image that reminded him of George III. The experience appeared to trigger a flashback, recalling memories of his own breakdown at Hanwell and hinting, perhaps, at his own porphyria-induced psychosis. 'I morbidly imagined myself confined there as a result of a sudden mental attack.'

His first thought was to give these patients a lobotomy. As he reminded Lyman, his friend Walter Freeman was successfully carrying out the operation at the George Washington University School of Medicine. He also waxed lyrical about lobotomies in England, where thousands had already been performed. Lyman agreed to talk to the superintendent of the hospital.

The timing couldn't have been better for Freeman. Frustrated by the shortage of neurosurgeons, he had recently developed the 'transorbital lobotomy', a DIY version of the operation that could be performed by psychiatrists. Later dubbed an 'icepick lobotomy' by its critics, the procedure allowed psychiatrists to cut into the frontal lobe of the brain without the need for a surgeon or operating theatre. The only instruments required were a mallet and a steel leucotome. (This was later replaced by a stronger 'orbitoclast', a steel tool that resembled an icepick, after a leucotome had snapped and lacerated a patient's eyeball.) ECT was given beforehand to knock out the patient. Then, 'The upper eyelid of the patient is pinched between thumb and finger, bringing it away from the eyeball,' Freeman explained. The point of the leucotome was introduced parallel with the bridge of the nose and 'tapped lightly with a hammer to drive it through the orbital plate'. When the leucotome had been inserted 4 cm, it was pushed laterally to sever brain fibres and then 'gently driven' to a depth of 7 cm. After further sweeping cuts had been made (imagine the action of a windscreen wiper) it was withdrawn and a further electric shock given. The patient was awake and talking within an hour. Not surprisingly, a headache was 'usually present', the patient felt nauseous and his eyelids were swollen, but it tended to clear 'within a day or two'; penicillin was used to reduce the chance of infection.

Sargant suggested to Lyman that one hundred patients at Tuskegee should be selected for the procedure: fifty would be given Freeman's transorbital lobotomy, fifty would just be given ECT, but would also undergo the operation if the results were positive. It was a 'wonderful chance' to 'do a controlled experiment'.

Lyman took the bait. Permission was apparently sought from relatives and Freeman volunteered to perform all the operations himself for free. But then word reached Washington, where the Veterans' Administration (VA) ordered a ban on the operation. Dr Glen Spurling, national neurosurgeon to the VA, was adamant that the procedure would not be performed by someone who wasn't surgically qualified. 'Over my dead body,' he was said to have remarked. As Sargant lamented, 'The whole Negro-rescue plan had to be cancelled.'

To many, the proposed mass lobotomy at Tuskegee in 1948 had little to do with salvation. It was part of a wider pattern of experimenting on American war veterans, an estimated two thousand of whom were lobotomised between 1943 and 1955. (Tuskegee had been subject to another notorious experiment in 1932, when six hundred African Americans were denied treatment for syphilis for the next forty years, even after penicillin had become available, in order to study the progress of the disease.) It was also part of Freeman's decade-long 'head-hunting' odyssey, in which he travelled around America in search of people to lobotomise. He visited an estimated two hundred asylums and, during a twelve-day spree in 1952, lobotomised 228 patients in four state asylums in West Virginia – one of America's poorest states.

Sargant's year at Duke was to have one other profound influence on him, after his eye was caught by a lurid newspaper report of snake-handling at a service for white people in a small church in Durham. The town, in the heart of America's Bible Belt, had witnessed a great many Revival meetings in the nineteenth century – series of services held over many days at which new converts were recruited and sinners encouraged to repent.

Sargant attended one of the services with Peggy and a group of Duke students. After the pastor had whipped attendees into a trancelike state, helped by Sargant, who at one point led the clapping, poisonous snakes were removed from a box in front of the choir. Converts would handle them first, before they were passed around. Suddenly, someone handling a snake would be seized with frenzied hysteria before collapsing in a stupor – behaviour that was likened to 'wiping the slate clean for God'. Having used similar techniques on his Dunkirk and Normandy patients, Sargant recognised a kindred spirit in the pastor. He also saw parallels with the conversion techniques of John Wesley, and the indoctrination methods adopted by fascist and communist regimes.

One of Sargant's laboratory assistants had his own particular use for it. A regular at the snake-handling sessions, he had discovered that women became suggestible and receptive to his sexual advances when they had collapsed. According to Sargant, the assistant used to follow one of the female worshippers out of the church for sex. But he couldn't understand her indignance when he tried, later, to arrange another meeting: 'I am not that kind of girl,' she said.

Sargant didn't seem too concerned by the assistant's predatory behaviour. Later in life, he was determined to prove that sexual abandon induced the same sort of suggestibility as drug-induced abreaction, an obsession that he would write about in his last book, *The Mind Possessed* (1973) – and one that would cause further trauma to his patients.

PART 2

18

'The final one did it. The final one did it!'

Sargant's second stay in America was brought to a sudden end in 1948, when he was offered the post of Physician in Charge of the Department of Psychological Medicine at St Thomas'. Sargant was delighted. It was a plum job for someone who had been turned down for other posts before he'd left for America – and came as a surprise to everyone. Though it might have helped that his old Cambridge friend, John Harman, was on the hospital's new board of governors.

Alfred Loomis lent Sargant his flat in New York for one last week of luxury. Sargant's membership of the Savage Club in London allowed him to use the Lotos Club, a five-storey mansion at 5 East Sixty-sixth Street. 'We are having a good ending,' he wrote from the club to Leslie Hohman, Professor of Psychiatry at Duke University. Peggy would have preferred to stay on in America, but they sailed back to Britain on the *Mauretania*, arriving in Southampton on 18 August. Sargant, too, was sorry to leave and had been offered the job of running a large psychiatric hospital in Baltimore before taking the role at St Thomas'.

It was all change when he arrived back in London. Aneurin Bevan and the Labour government had just inaugurated the National Health Service and St Thomas' was no longer under the control of the London County Council or a medical superintendent, but the Ministry of Health. It now had its own medical and management committees, run by consultants, and a new sense of freedom and independence.

Sargant had remained on the staff of various London hospitals while he had been away in America, but now he needed to streamline his workload. Reluctantly, he dropped his post at the West End Hospital for Nervous Diseases, where he ran an ECT clinic for outpatients, but he was determined to stay on at the Maudsley. It had recently merged with Bethlem Royal Hospital ('Bedlam'), but it was now run by his nemesis, Professor Aubrey Lewis. Sargant had asked for clinical beds to be allotted to him on his return from America, but Lewis demurred, prompting Sargant to resign. As one colleague later remarked, quoting a Chinese proverb, 'Two tigers cannot live on one hill.' Sargant was left with five NHS sessions a week at St Thomas', two at Belmont – now a civilian psychiatric hospital again – and three sessions of private practice. (Each session was four hours.)

Sargant claimed that the main attraction of private work was not the fees but the opportunity it gave him for personal contact with patients. His hospital commitments, he said, were far more important. But he wasn't slow to set himself up in private practice. Within a few weeks of his arrival back in Britain, he was using Harman's consulting rooms in Harley Street, before sharing with a neurologist further down the street at number 23. Peggy also found them a house in north London – 'at the Lord's end of Hamilton Terrace', as he later described number 19 to Robert Graves.

Peggy had looked at no fewer than 150 properties before

settling on this one. They lived in the five-storey Regency house with Sargant's old Belmont colleague Eliot Slater. For eight years, the Sargants lived upstairs, the Slaters on the ground floor, but the house was never formally divided. The Sargants also shared a house in Cranborne, Dorset, with two other couples, retreating there at weekends.

Sargant's first job at St Thomas' was to sort out the dank basement where psychiatric outpatients were treated from 1949. It had been requisitioned as an air-raid shelter during the war and was nicknamed Scutari, after the grim barracks in Istanbul where Florence Nightingale had treated wounded soldiers during the Crimean War. She founded modern nursing at St Thomas', giving her name to the hospital's celebrated Nightingale nurses. Sargant seemed to find it darkly amusing that confused patients regaining consciousness after ECT might see rats running along the basement's water pipes and conclude that they had finally gone mad.

It was nothing that a lick of paint couldn't sort. Sargant tapped into the hospital's pecunious endowment funds, persuading the authorities to spruce the place up. No doubt he raised the matter in April 1949, when he was formally introduced to St Thomas' board of governors, which included both Harman and Robert Sainsbury, the supermarket businessman and philanthropist who would go on to be a generous benefactor of Sargant's work.

The basement was divided up into consulting and research rooms, a waiting room and a ten-bed ward where outpatients could recover after treatments that included drug abreaction, modified insulin treatment and methamphetamine injections. The only problem was a lack of beds for psychiatric inpatients – there were only two in the entire hospital. Fortunately for Sargant, if not for those who would end up in the Sleep Room, St Thomas' had merged with the nearby Royal Waterloo Hospital for Children and Women and his newly formed department was allotted the entire top floor, which had once been used for private patients.

Attendances shot up in the first few years as patients were sent to Scutari from all over the country. Sargant liked to claim that there were almost as many psychiatric patients attending St Thomas' as all other forms of illness combined. In 1948, 4,477 outpatients attended the Department for Psychological Medicine. By 1953, the figure had risen to 16,708. Scutari had become a Piccadilly Circus for the mind.

At the same time, Sargant was also establishing his new fiefdom at the Royal Waterloo, away from St Thomas'. As Peter Tyrer, his former house physician, remembers: 'It was a completely isolated unit on its own and it operated under its own rules, and you couldn't challenge them. It was a unit run by someone like Donald Trump, you know. Any time you challenged William Sargant you got shouted down, not quite so abusively as Trump, but not far off.'

One of Sargant's first tasks was securing the financial means to pursue his own particular therapeutic vision. Who exactly funded him has since become a source of much controversy. There are suggestions that his work, particularly the Sleep Room, was paid for either by the intelligence services, Big Pharma or a combination of both. Under the National Health Service Act 1946, teaching hospitals such as St Thomas' were permitted to manage their own endowment funds, overseen by the hospital's board of governors.

The Royal Waterloo, now part of St Thomas', was allowed to keep its own endowment funds too and the St Thomas' Hospital – Royal Waterloo Endowment Account was duly set up in 1948 at the Westminster Bank. The account comprised money transferred from the Royal Waterloo's Building Fund Deposit Account and the Royal Waterloo Special Amenities Fund, both of which were closed after the merger. Sargant would prove especially adept at applying for a slice of these funds, which were traditionally used for research and amenities for staff and patients. The Royal Waterloo boasted no fewer than twenty-nine special funds, eight of which did not pass into the ownership of St Thomas' board of governors. Others, such as Matron's Christmas Chocolate and Crackers Fund, and the Fund for Endowment of Nightingale Medals for Nurses, were transferred to the governors, who merged them into the general endowments of St Thomas' Hospital.

In the early days of Ward Five, Sargant was given permission to approach the Mrs Smith Fund for £300 towards furnishing the patients' day room. A 'charitable source' would be tapped up for a further £400. He was also good at extracting money from St Thomas' Endowment Sub-Committee to pay for study leave, both in the UK and abroad, and for research staff. Between 1950 and 1953, sixteen sessions a week were allocated to research, compared to fifteen for consultants. In the following years, he would also turn to other anonymous sources to pay for his researchers.

Sargant himself was initially allotted five sessions a week at St Thomas', which was increased to six in 1953, at an additional cost of £300 per annum. His NHS salary in 1953, including two sessions per week at Belmont, was £2,400 – equivalent to £85,000 in 2025. Private income from his Harley Street sessions would have almost doubled his salary and Sargant often complained of paying too much tax.

Some time in the mid 1950s, a dedicated Ward Five account was set up, using money donated by former patients evidently happy with their treatment. The minutes of St Thomas' Finance Committee began to include small entries referring, in different ways, to the fund. New furniture was bought 'from the monies which have been donated for Ward Five'. Five divan beds and mattresses were purchased 'from Ward Five fund'. A telephone outside the day room was paid for with 'funds received for the benefit of Ward Five'. A consulting room in the attic of the building's hexagonal turret, reached by a staircase, was paid for with 'donations specifically given to Ward Five'. One record cabinet 'to hold 50 LP records' would be paid for from 'funds that have accrued for the benefit of Ward Five'. And so on.

There's nothing to suggest that contributions came from anything other than grateful patients and supporters, of whom there were many. In 1957, for example, the minutes record the donation of a TV to the day room. Another typical entry reveals that a relative of a former patient in Ward Five presented the ward with 'a cinemagraph projector'.

Initially, Ward Five had twelve inpatient beds. By 1952, it had twenty, mostly in single or double rooms. It soon boasted a dining room too, and a new communal space in the turret (below the consulting room). It had been furnished by the same City of London charity that had provided Sargant with the money to buy his first shock box in 1940.

Sargant, to his credit, did all he could to integrate psychiatric patients with general medical cases, often arranging for neurological or psychiatric registrars to visit them on ordinary medical wards. As he said, patients under his care were 'not being treated as lunatics'. The only people he couldn't accommodate were psychopaths, whose 'compulsive suicidal gestures and general irresponsibility can completely disrupt the work of such a unit'.

Two hundred and seventy people were admitted as inpatients to Ward Five between 1950 and 1953. They were given a range of Sargant's favourite physical treatments: deep insulin coma (31); lobotomy (28); ECT (68); modified insulin treatment (99); aversion treatment (22); Cardiazol in insulin sopor (6); abreactive treatments (27); acetylcholine shock therapy (44), endocrine (hormone) therapies (54) and narcosis (3).

The development of anti-psychotic drugs was a watershed moment in post-war psychiatry. The compound chlorpromazine had first been synthesised in 1951, in the laboratories of Rhône-Poulenc, a French pharmaceutical company. It subsequently sold the drug to Smith, Kline & French (now part of GSK, formerly GlaxoSmithKline), who marketed it under the brand name Largactil in Britain and Thorazine in America. Initially it had been used during surgery as a '*stabilisateur végétatif*' to induce an artificial state of hibernation and prevent shock. Patients would lose all interest in their surroundings but remain conscious, if drowsy. Psychiatrists soon realised its potential to quieten agitated patients, and it became available on prescription in France from November 1952. Chlorpromazine blocked dopamine receptors in the brain, which seemed to relieve psychotic symptoms such as hallucinations and delusions. A psychopharmacological revolution had begun.

The popular press in Britain dubbed Largactil a 'wonder drug', a soubriquet Sargant felt was fully deserved. It allowed him, for example, to treat acute schizophrenics in a general hospital setting rather than dispatching them to mental hospitals to languish for years. They could now be sent home on 'maintenance doses' after an average of six weeks' treatment on Ward Five.

Today there is a greater awareness of the serious side effects of first-generation antipsychotics, particularly when the patient takes them for a long time. Sargant, though, was more concerned by GPs who took their patients off the drug too soon. 'We must provisionally accept the view that some patients will need to take chlorpromazine for the rest of their lives.' He also gave the drug in huge quantities, claiming that, unlike bromides, the new generation of tranquilisers could be taken 'in massive doses without clouding the patient's consciousness, without any danger to health'. He also argued that they were 'not addictive'.

For Sargant, side effects were an acceptable trade-off, but for the patients, they were horrific: 'extra pyramidal' symptoms that triggered tremors in the arms and legs similar to those with Parkinson's disease; tardive dyskinesia, including facial twitching, grimacing, smacking the lips, sticking out the tongue;

weight gain; dry mouth; restlessness; and significant falls in blood pressure when standing.

The sedative effects of the drug so dulled the senses that it was soon being dubbed a 'liquid cosh' or 'chemical straitjacket'. One trial, carried out in 1954, concluded that Largactil's principal effect was 'psychic indifference'. Sargant was unmoved. What mattered was that formerly troublesome patients were now manageable, either in general hospitals or in the community. By 1967, he predicted that within twenty-five years 'nearly all psychiatric patients will be readily cured with simple drugs mostly prescribed by general physicians'.

Largactil would go on to play a central role in the Sleep Room, but in the 1950s and early 1960s, narcosis was still perceived as a highly risky treatment. In the past, Sargant had put people to sleep using barbiturates, combined with paraldehyde, a process he had described in 1944 as one of the two 'most problematic' treatments (injecting patients with malaria to treat general paralysis of the insane was the other). Largactil opened up new possibilities. Mixed with barbiturates, it enabled Sargant to induce a lighter – and apparently safer – sleep. But he still wasn't keen on the treatment. 'Continuous narcosis is ... very seldom required nowadays when we have so many other possibilities at our disposal,' he wrote in the fourth edition of *An Introduction to Physical Methods of Treatment in Psychiatry* (1964). It prolonged depression in many patients and only dealt with the 'superficial symptomatology' of schizophrenia, while 'leaving the deeper process untouched'. Dismissive words from someone whose name would soon be synonymous with continuous sleep treatment. (Sargant later revealed that he had given narcosis treatment to 123 patients between 1962 and 1964, but the average duration was only 3.3 weeks.) There still remained one good reason to use it: sleep allowed him to do whatever else he wanted to patients who weren't in a position to protest.

By contrast, the number of lobotomies soared in the early

1950s. Between 1948 and 1955, more than a thousand patients a year had the operation in England and Wales. Numerous cases were sent from all over the UK for Sargant's second opinion. After an assessment, he would dispatch them to Wylie McKissock or Harvey Jackson, St Thomas' resident neurosurgeon, often more than once. By 1955, 462 patients had had more than one lobotomy.

Peter Tyrer treated a patient for thirty years whom Sargant had subjected to no fewer than four lobotomies. 'She worshipped him,' Tyrer says, 'insisting that "The final one did it. The final one did it!"' And Ann Dally said she was aware of Sargant sending one patient with a severe obsessive disorder for five lobotomies, in a bid to stop him building fences throughout his house. After each operation, he'd dismantle the fences, only for his obsessive disorder – and the fences – to return.

19

'Somehow they took his soul apart'

In the early 1950s, one subject was beginning to occupy Sargant's mind more than any other: brainwashing. It would haunt former patients too, some of whom felt that they had been victims of brainwashing experiments in the Sleep Room. Sargant had taken an interest in the subject as early as 1944, when he'd first read Pavlov. When relations between the West and Russia later froze over, Sargant found himself ahead of the curve – and an obvious person for Western governments and their intelligence agencies to consult. How were the communists apparently able to brainwash people at will?

Sargant established his credentials as a global authority in 1951, when he wrote a controversial paper for the *British Medical Journal*. In 'The Mechanism of "Conversion"', a lecture he had first presented in Spain, he argued that religion, politics and psychiatry faced a common problem: how to seek 'the most effective means of bringing about rapid changes in an individual's beliefs and actions'.

The paper built on Sargant's wartime interest in abreaction, religious conversion and Pavlov's theory of transmarginal inhibition – that point of a stress-induced breakdown when beliefs are reversed and suggestibility is at its greatest. Drug-assisted abreaction could break up patterns of recently implanted behaviour in the same way that the Leningrad flood had so dramatically changed the behaviour of Pavlov's lab dogs. Sargant argued that the therapeutic goals of a psychiatrist were, therefore, essentially the same as those of the political brainwasher (and the religious leader such as John Wesley): to turn a patient's unhelpful patterns of behaviour and thought into diametrically opposite ones.

Such an approach was particularly appealing to Western intelligence services, who were playing catch-up with the communists and keen to harness any technique that could alter people's minds. If abreaction didn't do the trick, Sargant had a lockerful of other shock treatments – including ECT. 'Substituting an electrically induced convulsion for a psychologically induced abreaction, and giving a series of these, can produce truly dramatic results,' he wrote. 'Thought rumination is dispersed; recently formed attitudes lose their hold on the patient, and older-established patterns of thinking are restored.'

Insulin coma therapy and the inhalation of high-CO_2 mixtures, both of which led to coma, were also recommended. Reflecting on past shock treatments, Sargant wrote: 'Older methods, such as ducking- and swinging-stools, the firing off of guns, and other methods of producing terror states in the mentally deranged, would hardly have been used by psychiatrists of the past if good results had not sometimes occurred.'

On a purely physiological level, Sargant was right. Shock treatments operated on the principle that a tremendous blow to the central nervous system could somehow reset it. The American evolutionary biologist Richard Lewontin once compared the process to a 'mental enema'. In that sense, such treatments had much in common with the medieval ducking stool, which was used primarily as a form of punishment for witches and misbehaving women ('scolds'), some of whom might have been manic, disinhibited or psychotic. As with waterboarding, the victim thought they were about to drown (and sometimes did). The prospect of death was enough to shock them back to their senses.

If all those treatments failed, there was one other to change unhealthy patterns of thought: lobotomy. There were certain cases in which ideas and 'abnormal emotion' became so deeply fixed in the brain that relief was only finally obtained 'by sectioning certain brain tracts'.

Not surprisingly, 'The Mechanism of "Conversion"' caused uproar in the letters pages of the *BMJ*. 'Can it be right that any person should be placed so completely under the power of another?' asked E. Weatherhead from Folkestone. A more metaphysical broadside was launched by R. D. Laing. A rising star in the anti-psychiatry movement, Laing argued that Sargant regarded man as a machine and that, when it went wrong, he used methods that were similar to giving a radio a smack. 'The justification of this procedure, with man as with the wireless set, is that "it works", as indeed it does ... but has the paradoxical result of regression to barbarism.'

The letter marked the beginning of a long and simmering rivalry between the two stars of post-war psychiatry. Known variously as the 'acid Marxist' and the 'Mick Jagger of psychiatry', the Glasgow-born Laing couldn't have been more different from the pinstripe-suited Sargant. Laing argued that insanity was a perfectly rational adjustment to a mad and dangerous world. He sought to blur the boundaries between the professional and the patient, the psychotic and the sane, hugging his patients rather than electrocuting them. Mental breakdowns, he argued, could also be seen as mental breakthroughs and the 'schizoid' experience was another valid way of being human.

The rivalry between Laing and Sargant would come to a head in 1967 when the BBC broadcast a controversial TV docudrama,

In Two Minds. Directed by Ken Loach, it featured a young woman, Kate Winter (played by Anna Cropper), who suffered from schizophrenia. The play, based on *Sanity, Madness and the Family*, co-authored by Laing and fellow psychiatrist Aaron Esterson, was a direct challenge to Sargant and, in particular, *The Hurt Mind*, a BBC documentary series on mental health in which Sargant had waxed lyrical about lobotomy, ECT, abreaction and insulin coma therapy.

After *In Two Minds* was broadcast, Joan Bakewell moderated a lively debate between Laing and Sargant in a special edition of BBC2's *Late Night Line-Up*. Bakewell remembers Sargant as being 'severe and on the defensive – not a warm figure at all'. The debate over, the men retreated to the green room, where, according to Laing, Sargant addressed him 'the way a General addresses a Major, a junior officer', saying: '"Ronald, we are both on the same side, you shouldn't talk like that in front of the children" . . . His argument at that time was, well, we completely disagree and my whole approach was a load of shit, while his was the scientific one . . . You know, I'll vouch for him as a member of the club, but I shouldn't make the criticisms of psychiatry that I do.'

In the gospel according to Sargant, however, the shock tactics of terror and anger, rather than empathy and hugs, were the best emotions to arouse in order to disrupt unhelpful patterns of thought – and to allow new ones to be implanted.

'Brainwash' had first entered the public consciousness in September 1950, when the journalist and CIA propagandist Edward Hunter coined the word in an article for the *Miami Daily News*. In the first of many anti-communist tracts, Hunter described how Chinese leaders used force to persuade people to convert to communism in a process known as '*xi-nao*' – literally translated as 'mind cleanse'. Subsequent articles by Hunter linked Pavlov's theories, which were being popularised by Sargant at the time, with plans to convert the Russian man to socialism, citing the Moscow show trials of 1936–8 as evidence.

Western observers had undoubtedly been baffled by the trials, at which members of the Bolshevik old guard, showing no signs of physical torture, admitted freely to their guilt and pleaded to receive the harshest possible punishments. 'The proletarian court must not, and cannot, spare my life,' urged Alexei Shestov, a Bolshevik party member and trade unionist. In America, the Dewey Commission agreed that the trials were 'frame-ups'. And in Britain, the *Daily Mail* concluded: 'No mystery in history matches what is going on in Moscow.'

Ten years later, Western observers were equally confused by the apparent confession of Cardinal József Mindszenty, head of the Catholic Church in Hungary and a potential future pope. After being arrested on Boxing Day 1948, he admitted in court to plotting to overthrow Hungary's communist government, trigger a third world war and take over the country once America had defeated Russia. According to witnesses, his speech in court was slurred, his eyes glazed. The British Foreign Office concluded that his demeanour was 'wholly unlike what we know of the cardinal's real personality'. The Americans were similarly perplexed. Mindszenty was being controlled by 'some unknown force', according to a CIA security memorandum, which speculated that he had been hypnotised. Paul Linebarger, a US Army intelligence adviser, drew a simpler conclusion: 'Somehow they took his soul apart.'

And then, in July 1951, two Soviet agents were seized in Germany, along with suspicious cylinders containing liquid and syringes. According to a declassified CIA document, the men were carrying an injectable substance that would make the victim 'amenable to the will of the captor for an indefinite length of time'. The victim could walk and stand erect, and would show 'no evidence of narcosis'. Despite extensive laboratory analysis, the substance was never identified, only adding to the West's paranoia – and interest in drug-induced sleep.

Such events served to convince the American intelligence

community that the Soviets had discovered the secret of brainwashing. And they were prepared to go to any lengths to find out how they were doing it. Parallel with a build-up of nuclear weapons in the 1950s, a different global battle had been joined, prompting a psychopharmacological arms race to unlock the human mind.

Western fears were compounded by the apparent confessions of American pilots captured during the Korean War. Early on in the conflict, in May 1951, the North Koreans accused America of attacking their country with smallpox biological bombs, and dispersing germ-infected insects from aircraft. In May 1952, two captured US pilots confessed to the charges, reading out signed confessions that were broadcast on Peking Radio. A further thirty-six pilots made similar confessions, sparking worldwide indignation.

America's use of biological weapons in the Korean War has never been proved or disproved. But one thing is clear: true-blue American pilots were unlikely candidates to reveal operational details to the enemy. As far as the West was concerned, they had been brainwashed. 'The words were mine, but the thoughts were theirs,' as one pilot said on his eventual return to America.

Western intelligence was now convinced that the Russians had a deadly new weapon in their Cold War arsenal. Brainwashing could not only be used to persuade the masses of the merits of communism; it could also be deployed during interrogation to extract information from individual prisoners, to plant new thoughts – and possibly commands – in their minds, turning people into programmable assassins. It might have subsequently become the stuff of movies, but in the early 1950s the perceived threat was very real.

Sargant was intrigued. Brainwashing had much in common with his own psychiatric approach to traumatised soldiers. There was, after all, a fine line between the therapeutic benefits of healing a sick mind and the dangers of corrupting a healthy one. The point was not lost on Sargant, who was once again keen to make links between Pavlov, Wesleyan conversions and abreaction. 'I began to wonder whether the same principles must also hold good for political techniques of brainwashing.'

Sargant was also interested in why prisoners often made false confessions to the police. During the war, inmates from Brixton prison were sent, under armed escort, to Belmont, where Sargant would give them brain wave tests to check for possible epilepsy. Some of the prisoners had been forced to confess to serious crimes that were punishable by hanging. (Later they asked to withdraw these confessions.) Sargant examined police interrogation methods, looking for parallels between Pavlov's ultra-paradoxical state and prisoners' brain reactions during stressful questioning. 'Wesley, Pavlov, battle-shocked soldiers, the police, MI5, or the Russian OGPU [secret service] – here was material for an over-all physiological thesis,' he wrote.

It would take another mental breakdown and a chance meeting in Majorca with Robert Graves to turn that thesis into *Battle for the Mind*, Sargant's bestselling book on brainwashing. The media, meanwhile, was already intrigued. The very first episode of *Panorama*, the BBC's flagship current affairs TV programme, was aired on 11 November 1953, with a guest appearance by Sargant. He wasn't named – under the rules of the new NHS, doctors weren't allowed to advertise themselves. Instead, he was billed as a physician and expert on brainwashing. More than seventy years later, *Panorama* is still going – it's reportedly the longest-running TV news programme in the world – but its debut was such a disaster that the show very nearly got cancelled after one episode.

Patrick Murphy, the presenter, was an accomplished *Daily Mail* journalist, but it was his first time in a TV studio. The editor, Dennis Bardens, had tapped up his wartime contacts to secure an interview with British businessman Edgar 'Ted' Sanders, who had been released three months earlier from jail in Hungary. Hungary's secret police had arrested Sanders in November 1949. When he was put on trial in February 1950, he was found guilty of espionage and other charges, and sentenced to thirteen years. Only the previous year, Cardinal Mindszenty had made his strange confessions at a similar show trial, fuelling fears in the West that brainwashing techniques were thriving behind the Iron Curtain.

It was just the sort of scoop needed to launch a new programme. Bardens had even managed to find a recording of Sanders' confession in court, which had been broadcast on Budapest radio. The plan was to play the recording at the top of the programme. Murphy would then interview Sanders and Sargant would explain how brainwashing worked. Unfortunately, Murphy managed to play the recording backwards, filling the studio with a screeching sound. The programme was pulled for a month, while senior management decided whether to axe it. Murphy was replaced.*

Sadly, no recording of the disastrous programme exists, but we know what Sargant said. Among his personal papers is an unmarked document that's never been published: his scripted conversation with Murphy and Sanders. 'Here is a physician specially interested in some of the methods that may have been used,' Murphy began, cueing up Sargant to elaborate on his Pavlovian theories of conditioned behaviour. 'It may sound odd to talk about the mechanics of the mind, but in some ways our brains are machines,' Sargant said, before turning to Pavlov's lab dogs and the Leningrad flood. 'There is a close resemblance between such findings and the "brain washing" practised by the communists. Early in the breakdown of the normal mind under

---

* To be fair to Murphy, he had to operate a huge and unwieldy tape recorder called a Sound Mirror that had two seven-inch reels and a joystick that moved in four directions. 'When the moment came to play the tape,' Bardens recalled, 'Murphy got into a technical panic and didn't know whether to turn the joystick north, south, east or west.'

stress, the most fantastic suggestions may start to seem more sensible. What we call a state of increased suggestibility may occur ... during the "brain washing" itself, previously implanted habits can not only be wiped out, but exactly opposite ones can take their place.'

Sargant proceeded to show photographs of a young woman at a Revivalist meeting in America. She had just handled a rattlesnake and was entering a final state of collapse. 'The methods adopted in the case of Edgar Sanders were basically very simple when these principles are understood,' he said. 'We in British medicine are now learning all we can about these terrible and effective methods of changing man's beliefs and habits of thought on a large scale. It is vitally important to do so, because ultimately the fate of the world will depend on the conversion of the masses to one ideal of life or another.'

It was a strange choice of words. The fate of the world lay not in the hands of its politicians, spies and military leaders, but with British medicine. Sargant then interviewed Sanders, who admitted that after a long interrogation he almost 'began to believe' what the Hungarian authorities had been trying to get him to admit. 'Do you bear any ill will against the people who did these terrible things to you?' Sargant asked. 'Curiously not,' Sanders replied. Sargant was fascinated. Sanders should have hated his captors, but his views had been reversed, if only briefly, like the dogs in Pavlov's flooded laboratory.

From the moment Sanders had been released in Vienna, the Foreign Office had carefully briefed him on what he could and couldn't say to the press. Lord Reading, Under-Secretary of State for Foreign Affairs, personally met Sanders when he arrived back in the UK in August 1953 and was concerned by his constant talking and chain smoking. At Lord Reading's request, the Foreign Office's News Department contacted the *Daily Herald*, which had signed Sanders up for a series of exclusive interviews, asking the paper 'to consult us if he includes anything in his draft which is objectionable on personal or security grounds'. The News Department also liaised closely with the BBC about Sanders' possible appearance on another show in August.

Given the degree to which the Foreign Office micromanaged Sanders' media engagements, it seems highly likely that his appearance on *Panorama* was handled with equal care. Bardens claimed to have arranged the interview through his contacts with the 'murkier side of the Foreign Office', which suggests MI6. The intelligence service would have certainly not objected to the BBC's presentation of Sanders as a victim of brainwashing, as it helped to undermine his embarrassing confession that he was a spy.

Sargant also had his own intelligence connections at the time. His old Cambridge Union contact, Selwyn Lloyd, was Minister of State for Foreign Affairs from 1951 to 1954, becoming Foreign Secretary in 1955, a role that gave him ultimate responsibility for MI6. The fact that the exchange with Sanders had been so carefully scripted beforehand only adds to the suggestion that Sargant's involvement had been sanctioned – and possibly choreographed – by MI6.

As it happened, the Hungarians were right to suspect Sanders. While in Budapest, he was working for an American communications company, International Telephone and Telegraph Corporation, with known CIA connections at the time. He was also still on the Army List while in Hungary. During the war he had served as a captain in field security and in the Army Intelligence Corps and, it seems, acted as a courier for MI6. He was, in many ways, an ideal intelligence asset for operations behind the Iron Curtain. And Sargant, now an expert on brainwashing, was the ideal person to interview him.

20

'Such sudden social degradation can prove most effective'

In 1954, Sargant suffered a second breakdown. He was on a six-week visit to the US, to attend meetings of the American Academy of Neurology, catch up with the latest research on lobotomies and go to the annual meeting of the American Psychiatric Association in St Louis. (St Thomas' Endowment Fund had paid £300 towards the cost of the trip.) At one particular session, Sargant heard a speaker talking about modified insulin treatment and how it was based not on Sargant's own pioneering time at Belmont but on the work of Sigmund Freud. It was all too much and he felt shooting pains in his chest. His worst fears had been confirmed. America's psychiatrists were in thrall to Freud.*

---

* In July 1964, Sargant would write a coruscating article for the *Atlantic* ('Psychiatric Treatment: Here and in England'), in which he expressed bewilderment at American psychiatry's continuing obsession with psychoanalysis at the expense of biological treatments. 'The soul of man is becoming as easily treatable as the body in many instances, and by simpler and more effective measures than the long years of psychotherapy which we once had to use.'

At another meeting the next day, Sargant was gripped wih the same sense of anger, which caused more shooting pains, followed by flu and a temperature. His chest continued to hurt back home in London, not helped by competing in the tug-of-war at St Thomas' student sports day. The following morning, 8 July 1954, he couldn't even get out of bed. Peggy summoned his old friend John Harman, who listened to Sargant's chest and immediately diagnosed tuberculosis.

Harman put him on a course of three antibiotics. Sargant didn't ask to see his X-ray confirming Harman's diagnosis, nor was he shown it. He had already begun to feel overburdened by his work before his trip to America, suspecting lung cancer because of his chain-smoking habit. But, like many doctors, he had not got it checked. Was it tuberculosis or another bout of depression? It could have been both – comorbidity of TB and depression is common. Sargant once again attributed his poor mental state to an underlying biological issue that could be treated organically. 'What a difference it makes when the cause of a near-breakdown is recognized as a curable physical disease,' he said.

Harman formally signed Sargant off as 'incapable of work'. It was a year before Sargant returned to St Thomas' and another two and a half years before he stopped taking the antibiotics. Peggy looked after him at home, where he received a steady stream of visitors. Friends corresponded with him too, urging him to cut down on his work when he was better. His younger brother, Norman, who had been consecrated as Bishop of Mysore in 1951, wrote from the Nilgiri Hills in southern India about how fat they were both becoming. 'I show every promise of obtaining father's figure before I reach fifty.' Cassocks and other ecclesiastical outfits, along with tropical clothing, had been kind to his waistline – unlike English suits, which were less forgiving. And a female friend wrote from Lexington, Massachusetts, hoping that they could get a nurse to help Peggy. 'I should suggest a beautiful blonde of great intelligence, strength and wit – someone just like Peggy, in fact,' she said. 'But they are hard to come by.'

While convalescing, Sargant had time to transform his thoughts on Pavlov, religious conversion and brainwashing into a book. After six months of bedridden life, during which he spoke chapters into a Dictaphone, he had completed a first draft of what would become *Battle for the Mind*.

Sargant was, however, worried that the book would cause religious offence by linking Wesley to Pavlov's experiments on dogs, snake-handling in the Deep South and lobotomy. Perhaps he also knew that he wasn't a gifted writer. His syntax was often clumsy, his sentences convoluted. 'William couldn't put two words together coherently,' remembers Peter Tyrer. So it was a stroke of luck that he bumped into Robert Graves while he was recuperating in Majorca at the end of his year off, between March and June 1955.

Sargant and Peggy spent three very happy months on the island, renting a house near Deià, where Graves lived. He would return many times over the following years, staying around Palma and Peguera. On this first trip, the weather was good and his health improved. He also seemed to have spent a lot of time lying 'godlike' on the beach, observing the local 'mortals' as they courted young girls from England and France.

After a day of what he called 'social psychology', Sargant and Peggy would meet up with the local expats. Ever the psychiatrist, he described them as psychopaths and alcholics. At 6 p.m., they would all drink the local brandy, tongues were loosened and couples began to row. It was then that the wife-swapping began. 'Spouses would easily get switched, and not always in the same way.'

It's an interesting aspect of his life in Majorca for Sargant to include in his autobiography, given the stories that would later circulate about his own drinks parties at Hamilton Terrace, which were rumoured to go with a swing. Ann Dally's daughter

Emma remembers her mother talking about the notorious events. 'My parents didn't go for drinks at Hamilton Terrace very often, but she said there were two types of guests: those that left at normal times, and those who stayed, waiting for the fun to begin. It was the 1960s, you know. My mother certainly wasn't interested in that. You do wonder who was the enthusiastic person wanting those parties. Was Sargant's wife as keen on them as he was?'

Sargant would shed more light on his liberal attitude to sexual relationships in his article about pornography for *The Times* in 1976. Alluding, perhaps, to his own marital arrangements, he suggested that there would be fewer prostitutes and broken marriages 'if activities slightly off the normal path were more widely accepted, provided nobody was in any way harmed or mentally hurt by them'.

He was quick to point out in his autobiography that Graves, who worked hard and drank little, was 'an outstanding exception' in Majorca, although the author famously had many mistresses and muses, eight children, and once lived with his first wife and another woman in a relationship he called 'The Trinity'. In the late 1950s and 1960s, Deià also became a bohemian hub for beatniks, artists, musicians and hippies, drawn in part by the poet's presence on the island.

Graves had first moved to Deià in 1929, on the recommendation of his friend Gertrude Stein, who reportedly told him that 'Majorca was paradise – if you can stand it'. His autobiography, *Goodbye to All That*, had just been published and *I, Claudius*, a historical novel, would cement his reputation four years later. In the early 1950s, he spent a couple of years in Palma (where his children were at school), before moving back to Deià. *The White Goddess*, his seminal book on poetic inspiration, had been published in 1948, and he was working on *The Greek Myths*, which would have wide appeal when it appeared in 1955. Graves' friend George Simon, a radiologist at St Bart's, advised him not to help

Sargant with his book, dismissing the psychiatrist as 'a charming man known for his eccentric views on lobotomy and hallucinogenic drugs', but at the time Graves desperately needed the cash and was effectively hired as a ghostwriter.

Sargant and Graves didn't get off to the most auspicious start. On his return to London in June 1955, Sargant wrote to Graves to thank him 'for all your kindness to us when we were in Majorca'. He also sent him a revised introduction to *Battle for the Mind* that Graves had polished. Unfortunately, he began the letter 'Dear Charles', a subliminal reference, perhaps, to Graves' younger brother, also an author, who was earning more money than Robert.

'Dear Will,' Graves replied. 'Your psychologists are always making the most pitiful Freudian slips: imagine identifying me with my evil brother Charles!' Graves added that he'd recently experienced something similar, when his publisher had addressed him as 'Rupert' – a reference, presumably, to his fellow war poet Rupert Brooke.

Graves agreed to re-write (or 're-English', as he described it to his friend Spike Milligan) the entire manuscript by November 1955, but not before the two men had argued over financial terms and who paid more tax. Graves also suggested that he should be paid before publication, at the hourly rate he charged for writing book reviews for London journals. 'I will devote my leisure time to ... keeping a steady saliva flow, which will double the appeal among the non-technical public.' In the end, they agreed that Graves should receive a third of the royalties, 'which should butter a few carrots,' the poet wrote, predicting correctly that the book would be 'a great hit'.

Graves' revised draft was sprinkled with classical allusions, including a reference to his own recent translation of Apuleius' *The Golden Ass*. He also wrote a chapter under his own byline, 'Brainwashing in Ancient Times'. Otherwise his name does not appear in the book, apart from an acknowledgement in Sargant's foreword. Graves was more than happy to maintain a low profile, for both their sakes. Two years earlier, in *The Nazarene Gospel Restored*, he had revisited the gospels to tell the 'true' story of Jesus, upsetting Protestants and Catholics alike. 'I am Public Enemy No. 1 to the churches.'

Sargant, however, was delighted by the literary connection and was soon showing Graves off to friends at his drinks parties at Hamilton Terrace.*

Battle for the Mind proved an instant success when it was published in the UK and America in 1957, helped in no small part by Aldous Huxley, who mentioned the book on TV. 'This had the immediate result of selling over 1,000 copies that week,' Sargant wrote excitedly to Graves. Perhaps Huxley's plug was a thank-you for Sargant's glowing review, a few years earlier, of *Doors of Perception*, his paean to the psychedelic drug mescaline. Bertrand Russell also wrote to Sargant to say that he'd found his advance copy of the book 'absorbingly interesting'. Sargant had replied: 'We shall find out how many are still terrified by the thought that they may be ruled by their brains rather than their souls!'

Sargant, with Graves' considerable help, had set out his stall in the introduction, spinning the book as a survivor's guide – a manual to educate the Western world about the dangers of being brainwashed by communists. He was keen, however, to present

---

* In 1967, Graves would turn to Sargant for help when his twenty-three-year-old son Juan had a psychotic episode in Majorca. Initially, Sargant sent a large jar of pills to Graves, who passed the medication on to Juan. His condition seemed to improve but then he had a complete breakdown. His brother William believes it was caused either by taking too many of Sargant's pills, strong medication that should have been overseen by a doctor, or Juan's drink had been laced with LSD at a party, or a combination of both. Either way, William arranged for a sedated Juan to be flown in early July to London. He was received by his mother, Beryl, and Sargant oversaw his admission to the Royal Waterloo. William doesn't know if Juan was admitted to the Sleep Room, but he was treated by Sargant for three months, eventually returning to Majorca in October.

himself as an impartial observer, unaligned with any ethical or political system. His sole concern was to show 'how beliefs, whether good or bad, false or true, can be forcibly implanted in the human brain'.

In the early chapters, Sargant revisited his interest in Pavlov, comparing men's suggestibility to dogs' and how it was possible to diametrically switch the behaviour of both ('box the compass') if they were subjected to extreme stress. John Wesley and his methods of conversion also featured prominently. Sargant must have been particularly gratified to discover that he and Wesley shared a love of giving people electric shocks. In one of the book's footnotes, he pointed out that the preacher had a Leyden jar – a primitive battery that stored and dispensed static electricity – and was an early advocate of electrotherapy. With barely concealed delight, he quoted Wesley in words that could have been his own: 'When I hear any talk of the danger of being electrified (especially if they are medical men who talk so), I cannot but impute it to great want either of sense or honesty . . . we know it is a thousand medicines in one; in particular, that it is the most efficacious medicine in nervous disorders of every kind, which has ever yet been discovered.'

Ultimately, Sargant felt that Wesley had been a successful preacher because he launched an assault on his congregation's feelings rather than its intellect, creating 'high emotional tension' in potential converts. 'Fear of everlasting hell' affected the nervous system of his followers just as 'fear of death by drowning' had traumatised Pavlov's dogs.

Later chapters looked in depth at the mass brainwashing techniques used by politicians, including Mao Zedong and the People's Republic of China in the early 1950s. Sargant had a word of warning for the Ministry of Defence, who seemed to be quite satisfied that, of the forty British prisoners of war in Korea who had been brainwashed, none were officers. 'It seems very difficult to believe that the holding of a senior non-commissioned or officer rank in the British Army renders one so immune to methods which can result in at least the temporary breakdown of a Cardinal Mindszenty.'

Perhaps the most disturbing chapter is on 'The Eliciting of Confessions', in which Sargant moved away from a position of impartiality to offering advice on how to interrogate someone – and, crucially, how to resist interrogation. Some suggestions were attributed to well-known sources, such as *Nineteen Eighty-Four*, which 'seems to be based on factual accounts filtering from Eastern into Western Europe', but he also referenced a secret report by Drs Harold Wolff and Lawrence Hinkle, consultants to the United States Defense Department.

Wolff was ostensibly a global expert on migraines and headaches at the New York Hospital-Cornell Medical Center, but he was also a leading adviser to the CIA, helping to channel funds and conducting his own uncompromising research that involved 'potential harm of the subject'. The report, 'Communist Interrogation and Indoctrination of Enemies of the State', was only published in a declassified version in August 1956, a few months before *Battle for the Mind* was released. Mindful of publisher deadlines, might he have had access to an earlier, classified version that appeared at the beginning of April that year? Either way, the report's basic message was that neither the Chinese nor the Russians had a secret weapon. They were just using traditional brutal police methods such as solitary confinement, humiliation, long periods of standing, sleep deprivation and bright lights. When the prisoner finally broke down, he was ready to be interrogated. Sargant was keen to cast this approach in Pavlovian terms. He was also overly careful not to suggest that he had inside information. 'There should be no mystery made about the details of these police techniques. They are in the public domain.'

Other parts of the chapter, however, were unattributed, including a section on how to disorientate a person of 'authority or consequence' by putting them in old and ill-fitting prison clothes, including trousers that he must hold up with his hands. 'Such sudden social degradation can prove most effective.' It's a curious switch of style, from reportage to recommendation. 'For the phlegmatic and unyielding,' Sargant continued, 'many extra stresses are found that may still keep within the law against the use of torture or physical violence.' One was solitary confinement, followed by placing a prisoner in a cell with two or three other inmates who were in on the game, under instructions to persuade him to confess. 'The influence they exert is that of the tamed elephant on the newly captured one.'

Elsewhere, Sargant urged an interrogator to go through a prisoner's past life in great detail to find sensitive subjects. Having found a 'sore spot', the examiner should keep touching on any experience which was 'tremblingly alive' in the prisoner's mind. He should sometimes be made to fill in long questionnaires to fatigue him further. Finally, 'unless some accident brings the examination to a premature end', the prisoner's brain would be too disorganised to respond normally. 'It can become transmarginally inhibited, vulnerable to suggestions, paradoxical and ultra-paradoxical phases may supervene, and the fortress finally surrenders unconditionally.'

Such techniques bear an uncanny similarity to Sargant's own insistence that a patient's history should be taken in great detail before breaking down patterns of behaviour with drugs, ECT and narcosis. (One of his house officers recalled taking nine hours to conduct an admission history for an OCD patient admitted to the Sleep Room.) The book also lends credence to the claim that Sargant once worked at Maresfield Camp in Sussex, when it was the headquarters of the British Army Intelligence Corps. A year after *Battle for the Mind* was published, in September 1958, a new Psychological Warfare Centre was set up at the camp to train elite troops in how to resist communist interrogations.

The Americans were obsessed with interrogations too. In 1963, the CIA compiled *KUBARK Counterintelligence Interrogation*, a 128-page secret manual detailing the most effective ways to interrogate 'resistant sources'. It drew on MKULTRA, the CIA's mind control project, and its research into heightened suggestibility, hypnosis, isolation, narcosis and reactions to pain and fear. 'This work [KUBARK] is of sufficient importance and relevance that it is no longer possible to discuss interrogation significantly without reference to the psychological research conducted in the past decade,' the manual stated.

Alfred McCoy and Naomi Klein have both argued that KUBARK's central approach to coercive interrogation – a prisoner needs to be regressed to a state of total dependence if he is to yield up his secrets – owes more than a little to Ewen Cameron and Donald Hebb's work on sensory isolation at McGill University. Sargant's theories about interrogation, however, are very much part of the KUBARK playbook too. 'All of the techniques employed to break through an interrogation roadblock, the entire spectrum from simple isolation to hypnosis and narcosis, are essentially ways of speeding up the process of regression,' the KUBARK authors wrote.

In 1977, Sargant said that he regretted that *Battle for the Mind* had become 'a sort of policeman's guide to breaking people down'. Three years earlier, however, he'd expressed pride in Pavlov's ideas in a letter to *The Times*. Writing about fourteen Irish Republicans, known as the 'Hooded Men', who had been interned and tortured without trial, he said: 'Recent Ulster revelations – including the use of induced mental fatigue, fasting, hooding, persistent disturbing noises, on and off interrogation and so on – show how well Pavlov's teaching has been absorbed and refined by modern political and police medicine. When any difficulty arises, one simply adds drugs, such as LSD, which make intelligent resistance even more difficult when used with what is now called "sensory isolation".'

The tone is more knowing than rueful. Sargant must have

realised that enhanced interrogation and NHS psychiatry made for uncomfortable bedfellows, and that it was unusual for a former consultant at St Thomas' to be so familiar with the 'Five Techniques', as the British interrogation methods were called. But it didn't stop him finishing his book with some practical advice. Victims of attempted brainwashing or the eliciting of a confession should not lose weight by worrying and must learn to snatch sleep wherever possible. 'Though men are not dogs, they should humbly try to remember how much they resemble dogs in their brain functions, and not boast themselves demigods.'

The nation had been warned.

21

Linda Keith

It was Jimi Hendrix who sent the money for my air ticket back to London. I was a twenty-three-year-old *Vogue* model into sex, drugs and rock 'n' roll, and he was a huge star. Nobody knew I was back in London, and I wanted to keep it that way. I would only leave my parents' home in West Hampstead to score dope, to keep myself under control.

My parents always referred to me as 'being ill' rather than the more accurate description of me: a pleasure-seeking, music-obsessed drug addict. What they wanted was a tame, house-trained lapdog. They couldn't face my real afflictions, which is why, in early 1969, they sought out completely the wrong person to cure me: Dr William Sargant, champion of the lobotomy, deep sleep treatment and electro-convulsive therapy. What on earth were they thinking?

My parents drove me past his house on Hamilton Terrace in St John's Wood to persuade me what a great man he was. They were full of him, thought he was going to help me so much. They even gave me his book, *Battle for the Mind*, as if, by reading it, I'd consented to his treatments. I couldn't read a page and refused to see him. No way was I going to be violated by his brutal methods, but my parents had already contacted him, describing me as being ill with depression.

I was a wild child of the sixties and wanted to sort myself out in my own way, but I knew it would take a great deal of soul-searching. Going cold turkey at some point was also inevitable. I didn't want to do it just yet, so I went out to score – one more time. When I returned, I headed straight up to my bedroom and got myself high. Everything was fine and then the peculiar sensations began. My head felt enormous, full of fluid, red and bloated, my eyes seemingly popping out of their sockets. Then I had a fuzzy feeling, like pins and needles, and my tongue started to feel too large for my mouth. I opened my mouth and it seemed to fall out, big and floppy. My tongue got bigger and longer, way past my chin now, and was still lengthening. And there was nothing I could do about it. I tried to stuff it back in but that didn't work. And then I realised that I was struggling to breathe. I phoned 999 but couldn't talk, so I had to find my parents for help. I put a towel over my ridiculously elongated tongue and grunted at my parents as I handed over the phone. The paramedics gave me a shot of something, and the facial paralysis weakened. My tongue went back to its normal size in my mouth too. I agreed, in my terrified state, to see Sargant.

My parents arranged for me to be admitted to Ward Five under his care. I have no memory of getting there or of being put to sleep in his Sleep Room. All I know is that I didn't wake up for six weeks. My memories are necessarily patchy, dim recollections from when I was woken up to be fed, washed or be given ECT. The room was in almost complete darkness, except for a small pool of light from a dim lamp. It was eerie. Silence apart from the moan of sleeping patients, as many as eight of us crammed close together. I was in the first bed on the right, behind the door.

I am told that my mother came in frequently to see me, but that might have been later. We were woken every few hours to go to the loo and be fed. It was a twilight world and I have a tinge of fear even now as I force myself to think about it – the enormous amount of ECT that I was given.

I have no idea how they dealt with my withdrawal from drugs. I'm guessing that the cocktail of medication that they gave to put me to sleep tempered my physical withdrawal symptoms. I had no understanding of what was going on or being done to me. Time didn't exist. Nothing existed! I was without a mind. I had been rendered completely helpless, but I was strangely aware of my helplessness at some unconscious level.

After my narcosis treatment, I was taken from the Sleep Room to a small room on Ward Five overlooking Waterloo Bridge. My memory of these few months is also limited – just vague impressions remain. But I do remember being taken in a van with other patients over to St Thomas' to have ECT twice a week. It was the same anaesthetist every time: a good-looking man, tall and kindly, who would always say, 'Small prick coming.' I don't know whether he meant he was a small prick, but it made me laugh every time. I would try to savour the momentary high that I experienced as the drugs entered my system. I remember a block of rubber being placed in my mouth and the contact jelly rubbed into my temples. Then I was off. I never recalled anything of the shock itself and would come to in the recovery room shortly afterwards.

The nurses there were fabulous. I remember their kindness. It was a pleasure coming round to a cup of tea and chatting with them. There were so many patients being treated with ECT – it was like a conveyor belt. I must have had almost fifty ECTs in total during my entire stay on Ward Five. I count myself lucky, blessed even, to have a full complement of faculties today, in my mid-seventies, but I have few memories of that horrific time. The ECT has destroyed most of them, which is just as well.

Only once was there a glimpse of the old me. My mother told me later that I had managed to manipulate her into bringing in my passport for some practical administrative reason. Somehow,

I managed to get myself to New York and the Salvation Club for a private gig that Jimi wanted me to attend. Once I had my passport the rest was a breeze.

A car was waiting for me outside the hospital, arranged by Jimi, and I was whisked off to Heathrow and onto a flight to New York. I arrived just in time to go to the club. I have little recollection of the gig or the rest of the night, but I do remember telling everyone that I was in a psychiatric hospital in London. I also took some drugs. Of all things, I took Tuinal, a sleeping pill. It's what people took in clubs before Mandrax.

The next morning, I found myself on a plane bound for London. I dutifully rolled up to the Royal Waterloo and rang the bell. I'd become so institutionalised that I wanted to return to hospital. I suppose nobody believed where I'd been – they must have assumed I was delusional, like a lot of Sargant's patients: 'Been hanging out with Jimi Hendrix in New York, have you? Of course you have.' But, amazingly, that's exactly what I had just been doing.

I remained in the care of Sargant as an outpatient when I went home to my parents to recuperate. Twice a week I took a direct bus to St Thomas', where I had my ECT treatment in the Scutari outpatients' ward. I don't think I could have managed a more complex journey.

My time in the Sleep Room left me hugely mentally incapacitated. I couldn't make any decisions on my own. I needed help to choose what clothes to put on in the morning, what to order in a restaurant, and what to do with myself during the day. Most shockingly of all, I could no longer read. I recognised letters and words, but they made no sense to me, so I gave up. I watched television instead and sat with my parents like the dutiful lapdog they had always wanted me to be. I wasn't happy or unhappy – I wasn't there. It was as if my brain and personality were dead. I have no idea if my parents were satisfied with the new me, or whether they regretted Sargant's brutal annihilation of my character.

Once, after my release, I had an outpatient appointment with

Sargant at his private practice at 23 Harley Street. He was a huge man, tall with an ugly mouth. My parents called him dapper. I asked him when I might read again, and he said that he didn't know. No one had had as much ECT as me, so he had no frame of reference. I found this horrifying, but not as much as what happened next – he actually came on to me. Tried to hug me and kiss me on the mouth. I wasn't as docile as he expected and lashed out. I ducked and ran, hitting him sideways, and he went over onto an ottoman pouffe in the middle of the room. He was lying sprawled on the floor as I made my exit.

My parents loved me, but they didn't like me very much. My father, Alan Keith, was a well-known radio presenter, who had long-running shows on the BBC including *Your Hundred Best Tunes*. He often used to say to me, 'You must live within the narrow confines of middle-class society.' It became a bit of a mantra in our north London Jewish family – and maybe it was why I rebelled so hard against him and my mother.

I grew up in Cholmley Gardens, a 1920s mansion block in West Hampstead. At school, I always felt that I was behind in classwork. I hated it. I used to bring cigarettes into school to smoke in the toilets, or play truant, wandering down Tin Pan Alley, where I'd frequent the guitar shops and ask questions. What sort of guitar did Chuck Berry use? Could you show me one?

From a ridiculously young age, I'd had this passion for black, rhythm and blues music. And thanks to my father, I had extraordinary access to the BBC Gramophone Record Library. At my request, he'd bring home 78s, 45s and LPs – recently released imports such *Best of Muddy Waters* and *Best of Little Walter*.

My parents just couldn't understand their young daughter's obsession with these old black men. Why didn't I want to hang out at the telephone boxes in Golders Green with my girlfriends and a bouffant hairdo? It was then, I think, that they started to worry and publicly call me 'a bit odd'.

I was only fourteen, but I was already going once a week to the Sunset Club on Carnaby Street and developed a love of Caribbean music, bluebeat and ska. I was also sent to Geneva to visit my uncle, where something awful happened to me at a teenage party that haunts me to this day. It involved a man in his twenties and was frightening and foul, but no one would tell me afterwards exactly what had happened. Any memory of the incident was later completely wiped by the ECT Sargant gave me.

Back in England, I was allowed to leave school just a few months short of fifteen. After a while, however, my parents couldn't take any more of my lifestyle and my father found me a job at *Vogue* through a member of our synagogue. I made the coffee, dealt with the mail and loved it. *Vogue* was a prestigious magazine to work for, but it never occurred to me to pursue a career as a model. Then, aged sixteen, I was asked to go up to the top floor to be photographed, simply because the model hadn't turned up. My first photo session at Vogue Studios, on 20 May 1963, was published on Katharine Whitehorn's page in the *Observer*.

I registered with Lucie Clayton's, Britain's top modelling agency at the time (Jean Shrimpton and Joanna Lumley were on their books) and picked up lots of work. Nothing big, just a regular modelling job doing advertising and knitting patterns. It was then that I started to use my diet pills. In those days they were amphetamines, and I began to take them to get me going in the morning. It was the start of what was to become a life of destructive, merry-go-round drug abuse that would eventually lead me, six years later, to the Sleep Room.

I was still only seventeen the night I first met Keith Richards. He was nineteen. It was a Friday night at a launch party for a new Beatles record at the Town and Country Club on Haverstock Hill. At last, here it was, that throbbing warmth that creeps up your body and lands bright red in your cheeks. Keith was talking to my best friend, Sheila, so that was easy. I walked over to them, face aglow. 'Hi, I'm Linda.' I made a comment about the Rolling Stones' single 'Come On', referenced Chuck Berry and Johnnie Johnson, and we were away, lost in conversation about rhythm and blues. As Keith later wrote in his autobiography, 'She made a straight line for me. And I was absolutely, totally in love.'

Keith was such a shy guy, but I would ask him question after question, and he kept chatting to me. We discussed Muddy Waters, Howlin' Wolf, Lead Belly and Little Walter. All my old friends. All the old black men. Later that night, he stayed over in the tiny guest bedroom at my parents' flat. My mother met him the next morning and thought he was 'a nice enough boy'. We didn't stay for breakfast. We went to his place in Kilburn. One bedroom for Mick, one for Keith. Overflowing ashtrays and old teacups littered Keith's room, which had a mattress on the floor and clothes strewn around, but it didn't take us long to get our kit off.

Keith was very attentive throughout our relationship, putting up with my no-time-to-lose approach to life. 'When you change with every new day', as the lyrics go in 'Ruby Tuesday', the song Keith wrote about me after we'd split up. For the next two years, I lived with Keith as the Rolling Stones exploded onto the music scene. They were exciting times. We left Kilburn to live in Hampstead, my old stamping ground. Keith and I were in the basement, Mick and Chrissie [Shrimpton] had the first floor.

It was then that disaster struck. In June 1964, while Keith was on the Stones' first USA tour, I headed to Stonehenge for Midsummer's Eve. On the way back to London, I was in the front passenger seat of a stranger's Mini Minor when it collided with a roundabout. I was flung through the windscreen – I wasn't wearing a seatbelt – and the car ended up upside down. I don't remember the accident itself, but an ambulance took me to hospital.

When I woke up the next morning, I was terrified. I couldn't speak or move. I had fractured my skull, severed my olfactory nerve and lost my front teeth. Later I was transferred to a private room at University College Hospital in London, where I stayed for two months. They'd covered the mirror with a sheet, which freaked me out. As a model, my face was my livelihood. The whole thing was traumatic, but Keith was very loving and paid for the skin grafts on my face, which healed.

I moved into Keith's flat in St John's Wood after I'd recovered and went back into modelling, working with all the great fashion photographers of the time, including David Bailey. One night in 1966, when I was in America during the Stones' tour, I decided to go to a new club in midtown Manhattan. A group called Curtis Knight and the Squires was playing rhythm and blues, with someone called Jimmy James on lead guitar. I couldn't take my eyes off him – the astonishing moods he could bring to the music, his charisma, skill and stage presence.

Jimmy noticed me and played it up, shooting his guitar at me like a machine gun. We laughed. And then he performed his bag of tricks – just for me – and started to play with his teeth, behind his head, exaggerating his very sensual moves. I was thunderstruck.

Jimmy came back to my friends' apartment after the gig, and we talked about music. We took some acid too – the first time Jimmy had tried it. Jimmy and I fell in love that night. It was tender, romantic and devastatingly sensual – but also platonic. I kept leaping up to play him music, delving into my own box of 45s to impress him. From then on, we were joined at the hip. The next day, we went up to the room Keith and I had at the Americana Hotel. Jimmy thought it was a treasure trove of guitars and artefacts. I told him to pick a guitar to borrow while Keith was away – his own guitar was in a pawnshop. Still on his first acid trip, he chose Keith's white Fender Stratocaster.

I was still with Keith, just having a good time with Jimmy while he was on tour. In truth, I was starting to yearn for Jimmy's touch. There was a broken-heart melancholia about him, which was part of his charm. I was also loving the drugs too much. I had started to use a needle and was constantly running to the bathroom in the clubs to keep the high going. Sadly drugs had now become a big part of my life.

I was relieved when Keith went back to England – I didn't want him to see me so spaced out. What I didn't realise was that Keith had gone to hatch a plan with my father to 'rescue' me from America. A few nights later, I was sitting at the Café au Go Go with a friend, tripping, and said to her, 'My God, that bloke over there could be my father.' This figure continued walking towards me – it was my father! He'd come to take me home.

The flight back to London was like a silent movie. My father was all grey: grey face, grey hair, grey overcoat. And I was all black to reflect my state of mind. Shades and a Moroccan *burnous*, hood up, craving all sorts of drugs, adamant that I didn't need rescuing. We both smoked furiously. I could see his strained face, his sunken cheeks. It was agonising and I felt for him, but we didn't exchange a word the whole way home – *plus ça change*.

We arrived back at Cholmley Gardens, where Keith was waiting for me. His plan to get me home had worked. I was furious that people were making decisions on my behalf, and I ordered him out of my room. I lost my way after Keith and I broke up, slid further down the slippery slope of drugs. I also had this idea that I was now free to start a relationship with Jimmy. But Jimmy had other plans, as I found out when he came over to England and immediately formed a relationship with someone else. He'd also changed his name from Jimmy James to Jimi Hendrix.

By 1967, I had become a detached and elusive spectre. I was still working, but it was becoming increasingly difficult to get to jobs on time. I would party every night, desperately trying to avoid Jimi and his new crowd, but we occasionally came across each other. We'd have sex, followed by a crashing argument about monogamy, and then part bitterly. My modelling career was now all but over and I was getting myself into deeper and deeper water with drugs. By 1968, I was back home with my parents, trying to work again, but I'd become disenchanted with the swinging sixties. Peace and love had been replaced by agitation and conflict, and I ran away again, as I always did. To America. Of course, I was really running away from myself. I was soon flat out of money, stranded on the west coast. My drug use was completely out of hand, and I was looking terrible, so I made plans to head home to London, but I only had enough money to get to my friend Suzy's apartment in New York.

When I arrived, I found Suzy strung out on heroin and turning tricks to maintain her habit. Like her, I was at rock bottom, and it was an easy step to take drugs too. Whenever she had a male caller, I'd step out onto the fire escape and sit there until her business had finished, swinging my legs as I stared at the overflowing trash bins below.

Did Sargant and his Sleep Room help me? It temporarily broke the cycle of drug addiction, got me through withdrawal, but nothing else. I still craved drugs afterwards. Even after all the treatments, the deep narcosis and the ECT, I could never accept that I was loved for anything other than my looks.

I think I owe my ultimate recovery to the people I met after I left Ward Five, like my first husband, Lawrence, who helped me to re-learn the daily rituals of getting dressed, going to the shops, and even getting a shopping list together. With his care, I overcame my mental defects caused by the ECT. I had nightmares about my treatment for a long time. I don't any more. When I was anxious, I'd rub my forehead, try to get the gel off my temples. It's transferred into a hair gesture now, sweeping back my hair behind my ears. An anxiety tic, I suppose.

My recovery also had a lot to do with me. Ultimately, I found the inner strength to enjoy life without substances. I even managed to teach myself how to read again, beginning with picture books for three-year-olds that I borrowed from our local library. After five years of hard work, I completed a one-year Open University science foundation course. I also taught myself how to remember again, devising a system in which I 'pushed in' information, visualising the memory carving channels into my grey matter.

I had to come off all the meds that had been prescribed by Sargant when I stayed in a drug-free therapeutic community in a squat in Finsbury Park. It was a fantastic relief to be free of the anti-depressants, which had stultified my personality and enjoyment of life. I ended up living with the man who ran the commune. We moved to Wales, helped set up the first drug-free therapeutic community in Holland and got married, but it didn't last.

Later, I worked for an advertising agency and stayed off the drugs, except for the occasional joint. It was only when I met John Porter, my husband of forty years, and had two daughters with him, that I found real happiness, in Britain and in America, where he worked as a successful record producer. I still had bouts of depression, but I thought it was just a way of life that everyone experienced. I could feel it coming on, like a thunderstorm brewing on the horizon of my life.

My moods were certainly easier to manage once I'd had children. Later I discovered Jung and learnt a lot about myself and my relationship with my parents. I also confronted the trauma of the Sleep Room and whatever had happened to me in Geneva. Being prescribed Prozac in the 1990s had an immediate and positive effect on me too. I could have been a poster girl for Prozac!

I also had a rapprochement with my mother, shortly after my father died. I'm so pleased I can think of her now in a loving, positive way. Later, when I had grandchildren, a psychiatrist diagnosed me as bipolar and I was put on different medication (aripiprazole). I also went in for some mild psychotherapy, the talking kind that Sargant hated so much. In addition to being bipolar, I have an addictive personality disorder. Marijuana has helped me to curb my more wayward impulses. And, late in life, I've found Zen meditation, the traditional Buddhist discipline, which has brought me tranquillity and insight.

Today, I describe myself as a contented grandma living in Wiltshire. I sometimes wonder what I would say to Sargant if I saw him again. Probably what I said when I saw him on Bond Street, a few years after he'd stopped treating me. He thought he was being very friendly and that I'd be thrilled to see him, but I called him a monster – to his face. I said it to the person walking past me too. 'This man is a monster.'

And then I walked on.*

* This chapter is based on author interviews with Linda Keith. It also draws on her own forthcoming autobiography, *Whatever Happened to Ruby Tuesday?*

PART 3

22

'Ewen was being fished by the CIA'

Sargant's interest in brainwashing inevitably drew him into the murky waters of espionage, both in the UK and in America, leading to further speculation that the Sleep Room was funded by Western intelligence services. But official references are few and far between. The only mention of Sargant in declassified CIA papers appears in '"Truth" Drugs in Interrogation', an Agency document written in spring 1961 and declassified in 1993. In it, the author George Bimmerle writes about the importance of 'subject-interrogator rapport', adding that 'the British narcoanalyst William Sargant recommends that the therapist deliberately distort the facts of the patient's life-experience to achieve heightened emotional response and abreaction'. The same wording, except for a misspelling of Sargant's name ('Sargent'), was repeated at a hearing of the Senate Select Committee on Intelligence, convened to investigate MKULTRA in 1977.

The link between Sargant and the spooks was first made by the late Gordon Thomas, a former war reporter and investigative journalist who encountered him while working as a TV producer in the BBC Science Department in the 1960s. Thomas wrote more than forty books that sold forty-five million copies, including *Gideon's Spies: The Secret History of the Mossad*. His father-in-law was Joachim Kreamer, an MI6 officer who ran a network of spies in East Germany. Conspiracy theorists have lapped up Thomas' various accounts of Sargant's intelligence work, while other authors, including Hank Albarelli (in *A Terrible Mistake*) and Anthony Frewin (in *Lobster* magazine), have questioned their veracity.

The fact remains, however, that Thomas knew Sargant better than any other journalist or author, living or dead. Thomas had apparently met Sargant up to twenty times and had personal access to his private diary and correspondence. *Journey into Madness*, written by Thomas in 1988, is the origin story of all subsequent narratives that connect Sargant with the spooks. It was one of the earliest books to investigate the CIA-sponsored mind control experiments conducted by Sargant's friend Ewen Cameron at McGill University. In it, Thomas also claimed that Allen Dulles, Director of the CIA between 1953 and 1961, invited Sargant to his parties because he regarded him as 'Britain's leading medical expert on communist methods of eliciting confessions'. And he revealed the close professional relationship between Sargant and Cameron, who sought Sargant's advice on how to 'strip patients of their selfhood and introduce into their minds what he wanted them to believe'. On one occasion, Sargant scribbled a note to Cameron about brainwashing: 'Whatever you manage in this field, I thought of it first!'

Journey into Madness was well received, even prompting an editorial in the *Lancet* about the abuse of medical science. The references to Sargant were, by and large, measured and had an old-school journalistic authenticity about them, based on fireside conversations and off-the-record briefings, rather than hard documentary evidence. Thomas' real target was Cameron, and Sargant was clearly an important source whom he was keen to protect from similar charges. When Sargant heard about Cameron's idea of giving patients intensive ECT while they were kept asleep for weeks at a time, Thomas quoted him dismissing the treatment as 'medical madness' – a response we now know to be disingenuous at best. And in a chapter about a Washington cocktail party thrown by Dulles in 1954, Cameron was allegedly ushered into the director's study at the end of the evening with various senior CIA officers, including Sidney Gottlieb and Harold Wolff, while Sargant was driven back to his hotel. Again, Thomas appeared to be protecting his source from accusations of CIA collusion. At times, however, Thomas let slip Sargant's knowledge of American intelligence. The British psychiatrist was 'understanding of how such matters worked' and had concluded that 'Ewen was being fished for by the CIA'.

It's fair to say that *Secrets & Lies*, also by Thomas, was less scrupulously researched. Published twenty years later, in 2008, the book repurposed much of the same material that had appeared in *Journey into Madness*. It also included some more outlandish claims about Sargant, particularly in the epilogue, written after he'd heard about one of Sargant's Sleep Room patients. When Thomas contacted Anne White, she described to him her narcosis treatment on Ward Five. In those days the Sleep Room in London was not widely known about – it was one of medicine's dirty secrets. Thomas felt duped by Sargant. The psychiatrist appeared to have subjected his patients to the very same 'medical madness' – narcosis, ECT – that Cameron had administered in Montreal. It was a personal and professional slap in the face for Thomas, who had been keen to protect Sargant. But once he realised that Sargant had misled him, Thomas was keen to set the record straight.

'To discover all this was shocking for me,' Thomas wrote. 'Not just for what he did, but because I had counted on Dr Sargant as a friend. To learn he was a monster, who managed to hide the truth about his work even after MKULTRA had been exposed, was indeed painful.'

There is, however, another explanation. Sargant had told Thomas that he could only publish the more sensitive intelligence material that he'd shared with the author after he'd died. (Sargant happened to die two months before *Journey into Madness* was published, but it would have been too late for any additions to be made.) So in *Secrets & Lies*, he was free to write what he'd known all along about Sargant but hadn't been able to reveal, a volte-face prompted by hearing Anne White's story. (Later he would grossly exaggerate her experience in various newspaper articles, much to her understandable dismay, claiming that Sargant had weaponised her as a *Manchurian Candidate*-style assassin.)

Thomas once again described the cocktail party in Washington, only this time, instead of being driven back to his hotel, Sargant joined the gathering in Dulles' study. There was no protecting his source any more. Sargant was now portrayed as a close friend of Gottlieb and Dulles, whose wife, Clover, had been given a proof copy of *Battle for the Mind* by Sargant, signed and inscribed with the words 'Clover Dulles, a gracious lady'. Sargant was someone who conducted experiments on military volunteers at Porton Down and Maresfield, and was a 'willing tutor' on communist brainwashing techniques. 'Once he agreed to work for Britain's intelligence services, money was no longer a problem and through the US drugs companies, he met like-minded psychiatrists.'

Thomas also aimed a punch below the belt. Sargant had a 'voracious sexual appetite that could not be satisfied in normal relationships' and attended 'swinger parties' in English country mansions, where he found 'physical relief for his fantasies'. Later, Thomas wrote an article about Sargant's sexual peccadilloes for *Freedom* magazine, which is published by the Scientologists, sworn enemies of psychiatry.

Thomas provided no documentary evidence for any of these claims – the source for most of his allegations about Sargant was 'interviews with the author'. There is also the vexed question of why Thomas didn't include Sargant's closest secrets in the paperback edition of *Journey into Madness*, which came out in May 1989, almost a year after Sargant's death. (Thomas had apparently lobbied his publisher for a new edition, but 'this was not to be'.)

Thomas' contribution to the Sargant story cannot, however, be ignored. In among the chaff, there's a lot of wheat. Sargant did work, in some capacity, for various British intelligence services. He also had connections with US intelligence, as well as Big Pharma. And colleagues have confirmed the swinger claims, which wouldn't be relevant to this story if it weren't for subsequent sexual abuse allegations made by his patients.

Ultimately, only Sargant knew the true extent of his own involvement with the intelligence community. He used to make a big play of refusing to sign the Official Secrets Act (OSA), arguing that it would have hog-tied his lecturing and journalism. He once told Peggy that she was 'potty' to have signed the OSA when she worked with young offenders in prison. But his stance was ultimately meaningless. 'We didn't in those days sign the OSA,' according to Peter Dally, who worked for MI6. 'We gave advice.' As Nigel West, historian of the intelligence services, points out: 'Regardless of whether someone has signed the OSA, he or she is still liable to prosecution if they breach the Act. Any of us are. All it means, if you have signed it, is that you will get an extra five years when it comes to sentencing.'

During his research for *Journey into Madness*, Thomas said that he'd met Sargant for dinner at his home, presumably in the hamlet of East Woodyates, near Salisbury. Sargant, who was unwell and close to the end of his life, provided 'hitherto unsuspected insights into his fellow-psychiatrist' Ewen Cameron. It is entirely possible that Sargant also revealed more about his own career that night, on the understanding that Thomas could only publish his secrets after his death. In a tantalising passage in *The Unquiet Mind*, Sargant himself suggested that he might not have wanted to take his own secrets to the grave: 'On one or two occasions I confess to having been so scared by information given me that I have preferred to burn the records without delay, but now I sometimes regret it. Perhaps it should be the duty of those who possess explosive secret information to ensure at least that the record does not die with them.'

Was Sargant referring to his own role in one of the most controversial deaths in the history of the CIA?

23

'A Manhattan Project of the mind'

The problem with proving Sargant's links to the intelligence services is that any work he undertook, by its very nature, was secret and appears destined to remain so. The British authorities – Porton Down (now run by the Defence, Science and Technology Laboratory, or DSTL) and MI6 in particular – are reluctant to open any files that might shed light on Sargant's role, much to the dismay of his former Sleep Room patients. They would like to know either way if their harrowing experiences were part of a wider covert programme of experiments.

The earliest documentary evidence of Sargant's intelligence connections comes from a classified report in October 1951 by an American, Henry K. Beecher, Dorr Professor of Anaesthesiology at Harvard. Beecher's name would later become synonymous with upholding medical ethics, thanks to 'Ethics and Clinical Research', a paper he published in the *New England Journal of Medicine* in 1966. In a coruscating indictment of America's research establishment, he called out twenty-two (unnamed) experiments on human guinea pigs who hadn't given their consent, including one that involved injecting live cancer cells into senile patients without explaining that the cells were cancerous. The paper radically altered the way human experiments were conducted.

For ten years of his otherwise distinguished Harvard career, however, Beecher was engaged in clandestine work for US military intelligence and the CIA that not only contravened his own high standards for human research, but violated the recent Nuremberg Code and its enshrinement of the voluntary consent of human subjects in medical experiments. Beecher's report in 1951 was written for the US Surgeon General and summarised a trip he made to Europe in September that year. It identified and recommended various civilian doctors, psychiatrists and academics with whom the US intelligence community could safely 'join forces' on a top-secret project to control and influence human behaviour. One of those psychiatrists was Sargant.

The project, which had its scientific roots in Nazi Germany, was initially given the codename Bluebird (April 1950). By the time it was renamed Artichoke (August 1951) and then MKULTRA (April 1953), it had switched from being defensive to an unashamedly offensive CIA project that would go on to consume $25 million of US taxpayers' money over the next twenty years. And at its heart was an unethical programme to manipulate and control human behaviour and consciousness – 'a Manhattan Project of the mind', as it became known. It was the stuff of a thousand online conspiracy theories, driving the plots of films and TV shows such as *The Ipcress File*, *The Parallax View*, *Jacob's Ladder*, the Jason Bourne franchise, *The X-Files* and, most recently, *Stranger Things*.

MKULTRA is undoubtedly why Sargant's name has become inextricably linked to the intelligence services. And why it is so hard to disentangle conspiracy theory from fact. But despite its dystopian-sounding goals, MKULTRA was a real programme.

('MK' designated which CIA department would run it, in this case the Technical Services Staff; 'ULTRA' referred to the most secret classification of intelligence during the Second World War.) Between 1953 and 1973, the CIA covertly funded at least eighty American institutions – including forty-four colleges and universities, fifteen research foundations, pharmaceutical and chemical companies, twelve hospitals and three penal institutions – as well as 185 'non-government researchers and assistants'.

Payments to 149 subprojects were made through intermediate 'cut-out' organisations, such as the Society for the Investigation of Human Ecology (later renamed the Human Ecology Fund) in New York; the Geschickter Fund for Medical Research in Washington DC; and, briefly, the Josiah Macy Jr. Foundation. Many prominent psychiatrists, psychologists, neurologists and pharmacologists thought they were receiving grants to advance the cause of science rather than shore up national security. Others might have suspected who was funding them. One thing is certain: psychiatrists such as Sargant lay at the heart of the CIA's mind control programme.

Unfortunately, the majority of MKULTRA files were destroyed in 1973 on the orders of the Director of Central Intelligence, Richard Helms, who was spooked by the unfolding Watergate scandal. There are, however, a few remaining Project Bluebird documents that give a flavour of the original programme – and confirm how much it sat in Sargant's wheelhouse, particularly given his groundbreaking work with abreactive drugs. Like its successor Project Artichoke, Bluebird sought to improve interrogation techniques (and to encourage subjects to sing like a bluebird, hence the name) in order to obtain control of an individual. Some of the questions it hoped to answer included: 'Can a man be made to commit acts useful to us under post-hypnotic suggestion?' Another memorandum asked simply: 'Can a person under hypnosis be forced to commit murder?'

It was this suggestion, perhaps, that inspired Richard Condon's

1959 novel, *The Manchurian Candidate*, in which a captured American soldier is brainwashed to become a remote-controlled assassin programmed to kill the US president. Condon talked to many CIA insiders, and, as outlandish as his plot might sound today, nothing was off limits in the early years of MKULTRA. A list of mind control methods from 1950 included the use of drugs such as heroin and morphine, electro-shock therapy, lobotomy, hypnotism, sensory deprivation and torture. Another document stated that the CIA would consider 'special or unorthodox methods such as brain damage, sensory stimulation, hypnosis, so-called "black psychiatry", Pavlovian conditioning, "Brainwashing" or any other methods having pertinence for such procedures as interrogation, subversion or seduction'.

The intelligence community's quest to take control of someone's thoughts – either to reveal them against the individual's will, or to destroy and replace them with others – dovetailed with the work of a psychiatrist such as Sargant, who was also trying to destroy patterns of existing thought and replace them with new ones – ostensibly for therapeutic purposes. Indeed, he was already using a lot of these 'unorthodox methods' in his newly established fiefdom on the top floor of the Royal Waterloo. And many of his private patients might argue that 'black psychiatry' would have been a fitting brass plaque to hang outside 23 Harley Street.

Once Bluebird had been authorised by the CIA director on 20 April 1950, the search was on for civilian psychiatrists. In 1951, Morse Allen, the mastermind behind the project, approached a psychiatrist 'of considerable note' who was a professor at a medical school and had been cleared to work as a consultant for the CIA. (As John Marks, who first told this story, points out, the psychiatrist's name, like many other civilian consultants, was redacted in the CIA file.) The psychiatrist had reported that it was not only possible to elicit information from a patient in the aftermath of an ECT session, but that the patient would have no recollection of what they'd said.

It sounded too good to be true: revelations followed by amnesia – ideal for the interrogation of an enemy agent. The psychiatrist also confided that the machine, if turned down a notch or two, could deliver 'excruciating pain', as if the 'whole head was on fire', that might also be useful during interrogation: 'it had the effect of making a man talk'. Continuous shocks, however, would reduce the patient to the 'vegetable level'. One advantage for Allen was that ECT was undetectable, unless the subject was given a brain (EEG) scan within two weeks. Even better, Allen noted that portable ECT machines – the shock boxes so beloved by Sargant – were becoming widely available.

The CIA's Office of Scientific Intelligence, one of the many warring departments that briefly oversaw MKULTRA, duly gave the psychiatrist a $100,000 grant to develop 'electric shock and hypnosis techniques'. A year later, another psychiatrist was given $100,000 to explore 'neurosurgical techniques'. As Marks has said, this presumably meant lobotomy.

Sargant was a frequent visitor to America at the time. He was also an adept hypnotist.* It is unlikely, however, that he was one of the beneficiaries of the CIA grants. But the two payments illustrate just how blurred the lines had become between civilian psychiatry and military intelligence.

Beecher chose to focus on interrogation and truth serum drugs on his trip to Europe in 1951. Operating under the broad umbrella of Operation Artichoke, he was initially interested in mescaline but later switched his attention to LSD. (He had been well briefed by the Pentagon on its hallucinogenic properties.) He began with a visit to the Ministry of Defence in London, before embarking on a grand tour of academics in Oxford,

* Sue, a student nurse on Ward Five, remembers Sargant giving a talk on the value of hypnosis to a small group of junior housemen and nurses. Hypnosis, he said, made it easier for patients to talk more freely about their problems. 'And then he asked if anyone fancied a small trial,' Sue says. 'I said I didn't mind – I found it fascinating.' The next moment she was hypnotised.

Edinburgh and Cambridge, where on 13 September 1951 he met Sir Henry Dale, former President of the Royal Society and the Royal Society of Medicine, and a Nobel Prize-winner.

Back home, Beecher was a pillar of Boston society, a fan of ballroom dancing, lobster and tweeds. He was clearly well connected in Britain too. Dale, a distinguished physiologist and pharmacologist, was 'an acquaintance of longstanding'. He had no experience of truth serums but was 'non-committal as to the hazards involved'. But he did know people who might be able to help Beecher, including one person in particular. 'He suggested that I see William W. Sargant, London, a sound, progressive psychiatrist.'

Sargant's star was certainly in the ascendant. Recently installed as Physician in Charge at St Thomas', he was familiar to Dale. In September 1949, Sargant had personally briefed him on the guests attending a special symposium of American psychiatrists, including Walter Freeman, which was hosted by the Section of Psychiatry of the Royal Society of Medicine in Wimpole Street, followed by dinner at the Hyde Park Hotel (where *poulet poëlée polonaise* was served). Sargant was also well known for having pushed the boundaries at Belmont in the Second World War, when he had subjected thousands of soldiers to abreaction. It was, in effect, a method of interrogation that combined drugs with a form of hypnosis – what the Americans called narcoanalysis.

Sargant's work in this area had, of course, already attracted the attention of British military intelligence. In 1942, Colonel Rees, who would later oversee Rudolf Hess's incarceration, had asked him to desist from publishing anything further about abreaction for security reasons. (Interestingly, Rees chaired the first day of the London Symposium of American Psychiatrists in 1949 and had reassured Dale that 'Young Sargant' would brief him on the American psychiatrists in attendance.)

After Beecher had met everyone he wanted to see in Britain,

he continued on his quest to Belgium and then Germany, where he visited the European Command Intelligence Center at Oberursel, the former home of the Nazis' notorious Dulag Luft. Many downed RAF crews were taken there for interrogation before being sent on to permanent POW camps. After the war, the Americans renamed it Camp King.

A number of erstwhile Nazi scientists and doctors went on to work at Camp King for the Americans, including Dr Kurt Blome, the former director of the Nazis' biological warfare programme (he had tested sarin on inmates at Auschwitz in 1944), and Brigadier General Walter Schreiber, who was linked to gangrene trials on young Polish women at Ravensbrück. Blome's work at Camp King has never been declassified, but it appears that he was hired as part of Project Bluebird, most probably because of his knowledge of hallucinogens and poisons. Schreiber was described to Beecher as 'intelligent and helpful' and 'a good man to see'.

Beecher's wish list of candidates was growing and in his report, which was subsequently classified top secret, Sargant now found himself in the company of former Nazis.

24

'We must always remember to thank the CIA and the Army for LSD'

Beecher's trip to Europe seems to have had a galvanising effect on the West's intelligence community, which was beginning to realise the possibility of using drugs in interrogation. The wake-up call had been a secret tripartite gathering in Montreal earlier in the year. On 1 June 1951, a British delegation, including Henry Tizard ('Tizard the Wizard', who had met Alfred Loomis during the war), head of the Defence Research and Policy Committee at the Ministry of Defence, and someone from MI6 listed in the minutes simply as 'Dancy', had attended a meeting at the Ritz-Carlton Hotel. Also present were members of the Canadian Defence Research Board and the CIA. The discussion ranged from confessions, menticide, 'intervention in the human mind' and 'psychological coercion', to the Moscow show trials and Cardinal Mindszenty's later drugged appearance in a court in

Budapest.* The agenda then moved on to sensory isolation and how to implant new ideas.

In the years following this clandestine meeting, the CIA embarked on a wide range of LSD experiments as part of MKULTRA. The now notorious trials on students, prisoners and hospital patients soon involved American citizens being given LSD unwittingly, and were overseen by Sidney Gottlieb, head of the CIA's recently created Chemical Division of the Technical Services Staff.

If Gottlieb hadn't existed, Hollywood would have invented him. A brilliant chemist with a PhD and a stutter, he was on a quest to explore the dark frontiers of the human mind, using his bewitching intellect to charm or chill. He was fan of folk music and drank milk from his own goats. He was also utterly devoid of morals, ordering devious assassinations and Jacobean tragedy poisonings that picked up where the Nazis had left off.

MKULTRA experiments included subjecting seven inmates at the Federal Drug Hospital in Lexington, Kentucky to LSD for seventy-two consecutive days. Their remarkable drug tolerance led to another experiment, this time on an Indian bull elephant. Tusko was injected with 1,500 times the normal human dose of LSD at Lincoln Park Zoo, Oklahoma City, apparently to see if the drug might induce musth, a state of heightened aggression. It proved a cruel and fatal miscalculation.

Gottlieb's most notorious signing was George White, a hard-living narcotics detective who had once shot his initials into a hotel ceiling with a pistol. In Operation Midnight, White paid prostitutes to slip LSD into their clients' drinks, hoping that the age-old combination of drugs and sex would loosen the tongues of those in sensitive jobs. Two-way mirrors were fitted in a safe house in San Francisco, where White drank chilled Martinis

---

* Mindszenty's sister lived in Halifax, Nova Scotia and it was thought she might have been able to shed further light on her brother's weird behaviour.

in the monitoring room, sitting on a $25 portable lavatory, for which he later billed the CIA. As he wrote in his diary, 'Where else could a red-blooded American boy lie, cheat, rape and pillage with the sanction and blessing of the All Highest?'

White's lawless experiments leached across the city in a textbook demonstration of mission creep. LSD was soon being slipped into people's drinks in public bars, restaurants and house parties. Word spread and students started to volunteer for research experiments at hospitals and universities, unaware that they were being covertly financed by the CIA. Ken Kesey, author of *One Flew Over the Cuckoo's Nest*, and Robert Hunter of the Grateful Dead both took LSD for the first time as part of these trials. It wasn't long before Timothy Leary, the American psychologist, was telling the world to 'turn on, tune in, drop out'. It seemed to many that the CIA's desire to weaponise LSD had inadvertently helped to fuel America's counterculture. As John Lennon later told *Playboy* magazine, 'We must always remember to thank the CIA and the Army for LSD.'

LSD trials on unwitting subjects proceeded at a more reserved, though no less sinister, pace in Britain in the early 1950s. Many believe Sargant was involved. After Tizard and Dancy had returned from Montreal, work soon began at the Chemical Defence Experimental Establishment at Porton Down to research and develop potential truth serums. A rumour that Sandoz Pharmaceuticals in Switzerland was about to put one hundred million doses of LSD – 10kg – up for sale on the open market must have focused minds. It was enough (at the time) to keep the entire population of Britain high as kites for at least twenty-four hours. The rumour proved unfounded – the US military attaché in Switzerland had confused his milligrams with kilograms – but Sandoz agreed to keep the Americans informed of any interest from Eastern Europe.

A considerable amount of information has been released in recent years about trials at Porton Down in the 1960s that investigated LSD's properties as an incapacitating agent – a non-lethal, so-called 'humane weapon' that would disable rather than kill. Since its release, video footage of volunteers from 41 Royal Marine Commando being given the drug on exercise (in a 1964 trial called Moneybags) has gone viral, largely because of the posh, straight-faced commentary on soldiers rolling about in hysterics: 'Seventy minutes after the administration of the drug, with one man climbing a tree, the troop commander gives up.'

Unfortunately, very few official documents on the earlier, more secretive truth serum trials have been released, despite repeated requests for greater transparency. As the historian Professor Ulf Schmidt says: 'The stakes are simply too high for Western governments to allow greater insight into their psychochemical weapons arsenals.' The question is: was Sargant, the 'sound, progressive' psychiatrist, as recommended by Dale to Beecher, and head of psychiatry at St Thomas', an NHS teaching hospital, present at those non-consensual military experiments?

Schmidt believes that LSD trials at Porton Down in the early 1950s were conducted by MI6 at the request of the CIA's Office of Scientific Intelligence. If MI6, the most secretive of Britain's intelligence agencies, did carry them out as part of MKULTRA, it might explain the intelligence service's ongoing refusal to release details. All the more surprising, then, that it paid out modest compensation in 2006 to three servicemen for being given LSD without their knowledge. As Schmidt says, it was a rare admission of guilt – and a PR disaster. Anything to do with MKULTRA remains pure clickbait, and the internet suddenly found itself mainlining MI6, after the intelligence service had effectively admitted to committing criminal acts against its own citizens.

To be fair, Porton scientists tested LSD on themselves too, but presumably with better knowledge of what they were doing. Intelligence officers also volunteered. Writing in *Spycatcher*, Peter Wright, MI5's former principal scientific officer, revealed that he had volunteered in the 1950s as a guinea pig in 'extensive trials' at Porton Down, cooperating with MI6 on 'a joint programme' to investigate LSD's use in interrogations.

But what did Wright mean by a 'joint programme'? Cooperation between MI6 and MI5, the domestic security agency? Or between the UK and the US? The British government has never acknowledged any US involvement in the trials, but we know that relations between Porton Down staff and their American counterparts at Fort Detrick, a military research facility in Maryland, were close during the Cold War, particularly when it came to the West's biological weapons programme. They were 'all the same family', according to one American official.

Was Sargant part of that family? Repeated freedom of information requests to the Defence Science and Technology Laboratory, the government organisation that now runs Porton Down, have yielded nothing more than the standard brush-off: 'No information in scope of your request is held.' If the CIA had put pressure on the UK to run its own trials, it seems to have made the British authorities particularly nervous of upsetting their transatlantic allies – even seventy years later. A psychiatrist, possibly several, would have been needed to record the subjects' mental state. After all, the trials were designed to discover if it was possible to take control of someone's mind during interrogation. And it was common to bring in civilian scientists and medical staff as consultants.

One key player was Dr Harry Cullumbine, the scientist responsible for human experiments at Porton Down during the 1950s. Although records suggest he was travelling a lot at the time, he had also been in overall charge of the nerve gas tests, in which Ronald Maddison, a twenty-year-old airman, had died of sarin poisoning in May 1953. His tragic death sent shockwaves through Whitehall and very nearly led to human trials being banned.

When MI6 came along in the same year, asking for LSD to be tested on unwitting subjects, Cullumbine and his staff would have been particularly mindful of the risks. In his unpublished, hitherto unseen autobiography, he hinted at the tension that existed between the two organisations when he wrote of a clandestine 'truth drug' interrogation in Düsseldorf in 1955. MI6 had asked Cullumbine to fly out to Germany to 'open up' a 'short, stocky, swarthy' Russian with LSD. Cullumbine's air ticket would be found inside a copy of the *Evening Standard* 'on a settee' near the Germany desk at London airport. 'It sounded too much like a James Bond story to me,' he wrote. 'What was I supposed to do with the LSD?' Cullumbine felt sufficiently concerned by the nature of the interrogation to bring along, as insurance, 'a doctor working in our division . . . who had been involved in the LSD trials'. MI6 was not amused. 'I had upset their plans.'

Sargant wasn't on that particular trip, but he would have been ideally suited to screen volunteers at Porton Down, given his work at Belmont during the war. He was also very familiar with LSD. In a letter to Gordon Wasson, an American banker and amateur mycologist who discovered psilocybin, the psychoactive ingredient in magic mushrooms, Sargant wrote: 'Quite a lot of interesting work is going on over here with regard to lysergic acid.' And, although Sargant included only one mention of LSD in the third edition of *An Introduction to Physical Methods of Treatment in Psychiatry* (1954), the drug featured prominently in the fourth edition ten years later. Sargant advocated its use in drug abreaction, recommending 25μg in 5cc of water at 9 a.m. on the first day, increasing gradually to as much as 150μg on subsequent days. 'Distortion of body image, disturbance of time sense and drowsiness are common,' he wrote. Sargant's colleague Peter Dally confirmed that LSD was used 'on everything' at St Thomas' in the 1950s. 'We were experimenting with it . . . using it in a very indiscriminating way because we wanted to know what its value was.'

Part of the drug's appeal to psychiatrists was that it seemed to mimic a form of psychosis (a 'psychosis in miniature', according to Beecher), offering unique insights into schizophrenia. The profound changes in consciousness that the drug induced were also thought to have therapeutic potential, a line of research that has become newly fashionable in the UK and the US. (The world's first formal centre for psychedelic research was opened at Imperial College London in 2019.) Ronald Sandison was doing a lot of research at Powick Hospital in Worcestershire in the 1950s on the use of LSD for treating mental illness. He was supported by Professor Joel Elkes, head of the Department of Experimental Psychiatry at the University of Birmingham, who was already doing 'humdrum' work for Porton Down on anti-cholinesterases and German chemical warfare agents. Elkes went on to help with a second wave of LSD trials at Porton in the mid 1950s, but it's unclear whether he, or Sandison, was involved in the initial MI6 trials. Basil Clarke, Porton's consultant psychologist, was also present in 1953, and Cyril Cunningham, an occupational psychologist and expert on brainwashing and interrogation, was probably there too.

Was Sargant there as well? Eric Gow, for one, believes that he was. And he should know. One of the three former servicemen who received compensation in 2006, he was given LSD at Porton Down in January 1954, when he was an eighteen-year-old radio operator in the Royal Navy. Gow was eighty-nine when we spoke on the phone, but his recall of events more than seventy years earlier was still razor-sharp. And after being sent a photo on WhatsApp of Sargant, taken at about the same time (1954), he said: 'The more I look at him, the more familiar he gets.' Five months later, he messaged again, reiterating how recognisable Sargant looked. 'Must admit your guy seems to get familiar as I see him.'

If he didn't recognise Sargant immediately, it's perhaps not surprising. For all but fifteen minutes of their possible encounter, Gow was tripping on acid.

25

'The big radiator in front of us . . . began to play like a concertina'

It was quite common for young servicemen to volunteer for trials at Porton Down in return for some beer money and a trip to the Wiltshire countryside – more than twenty thousand military volunteers have passed through its secretive doors since it was founded in 1916 – and Eric Gow thought he was taking part in an innocent test to find a cure for the common cold. He was on shore leave at the time, in Nissen hut barracks just outside Plymouth. A message was posted on the noticeboard, asking for volunteers. 'Ten shillings, weekend leave and a travel warrant,' Eric remembers. 'Four of us volunteered.'

When they arrived at an army base close to Porton Down, they were put in a dormitory with fourteen other naval volunteers from all over the country. The next day, with a foot of snow on the ground, they were picked up in an open truck and driven over to Porton Down, where everyone was told to sign the Official Secrets Act. 'We were asked if we'd suffered from any illnesses and I put down pneumonia. But at no point was there any mention of what was going to happen.' They weren't given any psychiatric screening or mental health checks before the experiment either.

Eric and his Welsh friend John were suddenly separated from the rest of the group and taken to an office in a different part of the building, where a man was sitting behind a desk. 'He didn't tell us his name. He wasn't looking like a doctor. He was wearing a darkish suit. I took him to be a doctor. A southerner. Many years later, I was to learn that he was part of MI6 and looking for a truth drug. He explained that we were going to do some simple tests, drink something, and then attempt the tests again, which we might find more difficult. I remember thinking, with all the bravado of an eighteen-year-old, That's what you think.'

The three simple tests involved Eric and John writing down their names and addresses on a sheet of paper, remembering how chairs had been laid out in a pattern in an adjoining room, and adding three numbers together. They managed all three tests without any problem. The man then presented them with a sherry glass each of clear liquid.

'They were cut glass,' Eric remembers. 'He pushed them across the desk and said, "Bottoms up." This guy had a genial attitude. Quite friendly. He put you at your ease. You weren't worried when you picked up the glass and drank it. But the liquid had a funny taste to it.'

The effect was almost instantaneous, and Eric soon began to suspect that the trial had nothing to do with the common cold. 'The big radiator in front of us, one of those old-fashioned cast-iron fluted ones, began to play like a concertina, squeezing in and out. And the floor, it was brown plastic and had heel marks on it from the snow outside. They were all spinning like Catherine wheels going off. You didn't know what was going on.

We assumed it was the drink. He'd said it might make us feel a bit weird.' Eric failed to add up the numbers or write down his address – his handwriting was huge. 'We were laughing our heads off, had no idea what was happening. In the end, the psychiatrist gave up the idea of us arranging the chairs.'

At this point, there is the first of several blanks in Eric's memory. The next thing he remembers is riding a bike down the corridors of Porton Down, laughing and screaming. 'I was pedalling, John was on the crossbar. A woman in a white coat came out of a lab and told us to stop cycling. She took us back into her lab, sat us down and made us a cup of tea.'

Another blank, followed by being in the NAAFI canteen, early evening. 'John is talking about this packet of Daz powder dancing along the shelf behind the bar.' And then they are in a phone box outside Porton Down, having decided to go to a dance in Salisbury, despite a warning from the woman in the laboratory not to leave the base. 'Every window of the phone box was a beautiful technicoloured picture of Indians, with cowboys chasing them. The old kaleidoscope-type pictures. We ended up going dancing, still wearing our wellies. I don't think we got a date that night.'

They didn't get back to Porton Down either. Eric remembers waking up in a cell with John. They had been picked up by the police while wandering through the countryside, throwing snowballs at road signs, and were taken to a small RAF base at Old Sarum. 'The next morning, they gave us a large breakfast, treated us like kings, and took us back to Porton, where nobody asked any questions and we weren't told off for anything.'

Gow took part in two more trials, which involved mustard gas being dripped onto his bare arms. He had an inch-square patch of dark skin for fifty years afterwards. His memory of the LSD trials is significant. He went on to be a Justice of the Peace for twenty-nine years and gave crucial evidence to Operation Antler, an inquiry by Wiltshire Police from 1999 to 2003 that investigated human experiments at Porton Down, including the death of Ronald Maddison. The circumstances of his death had been covered up for half a century, as well as the subsequent use of his body parts for military research. A second inquiry, held as a result of Operation Antler's findings, concluded in November 2004 that Maddison had been unlawfully killed. His family finally received compensation.

For historians of the secretive research centre, 1953 has undoubtedly gone down as Porton Down's *annus horribilis*. Not only was it the year when Maddison tragically died, it was also when the non-consensual trials of LSD began. Gow believes that the doctors in attendance at his own experiment – who might have included Sargant – behaved irresponsibly, as he and John were not kept under close supervision. Later, a senior member of staff at Porton would describe the early LSD trials as 'inadequately controlled'. It was pure luck that Gow didn't experience a bad trip. As he says, 'To use your own as guinea pigs and put them in any harm's way at all is not really on, is it?'

The late Don Webb was another volunteer at Porton who recognised Sargant's face. He took part in LSD trials in 1953, when he was a nineteen-year-old corporal in the Royal Air Force. A friend had recommended that he attend, after he'd received an extra week's pay for being subjected to the common cold. It was a skive, his friend said. But it turned out to be anything but. The experience left him deeply traumatised, and he suffered flashbacks for ten years afterwards.

Like Gow, Webb and one other volunteer were separated from the main group of guinea pigs and taken to a laboratory, where they were presented with glasses of clear liquid by two men in civilian clothes and white coats. 'They told us there's something in [the water],' Webb recalled to Dominic Streatfeild for his acclaimed book *Brainwash: The Secret History of Mind Control* (2006). 'They told us, "We're going to see how you react to this stuff."' Webb initially felt nothing but then began to laugh uncontrollably, all the time being quizzed by the doctors. 'How are you feeling now?'

The next day, he was taken back to the laboratory on his own and given another glass of clear liquid. 'Really weird things started happening in the walls and the floor. Everything looked as if it was covered with about six inches of clear fluid ... then people's faces started to peel open. That was weird! The faces, the flesh would peel open, and there was a skull looking at you ... it was horrible.'

Webb has also talked of 'walls melting, cracks appearing in people's faces ... eyes would run down cheeks, Salvador Dalí-type faces ... a flower would turn into a slug'. (In 1981 he would write a play, *Mindrape*, about his experiences.) As he tried to calm down from what was clearly a very bad trip, he was subjected to psychological tests, including Rorschach inkblots, and neurological equipment was used to check his reaction speed. A week after his trial, he returned to Porton to complain of lurid flashbacks, but was sent away with sleeping pills.

In 2009, Webb was interviewed for a BBC Radio 4 programme about Sargant. In *Revealing the Mind Bender General*, the presenter James Maw asked him about one of the men who had run the trial. He had talked to Webb, when he was hallucinating, in a very 'interested, authoritative manner', saying: 'This was quite normal, it's not going to hurt you, it's just some effects we're trying to find out about. Don't worry about it, you're quite safe.' Webb said, 'At the same time he was saying this to me, he looks like something out of a nightmare.'

Maw then showed Webb video footage of Sargant to see if he recognised the psychiatrist. 'It could well have been him,' Webb said. 'The way he held himself. It could very easily have been the same man. Very easily.' He added: 'The person who I was engaged with mostly was ... so far as I could see, the psychiatrist. He was in charge of the entire thing. I would blame him if it was the same man. He was in charge of it, he was running the whole thing.'

A spokesperson for DSTL was careful in her choice of words when Maw asked if Sargant had taken part in any of its LSD trials. 'We can only say that he definitely wasn't directly employed by us.' As Maw observed in the radio programme, 'directly' was the important word here. The LSD trials were MI6's shout, not Porton Down's. Read between the lines of the official statements and there's a real sense that Porton resented MI6 for asking it to carry out the trials for them.

Further evidence of departmental differences is found in Cullumbine's unpublished autobiography. 'People from MI6 would occasionally visit Porton,' he wrote.

> They would call on —— the chief superintendent ... One time they wanted a quicker, more certain-acting drug than the cyanide capsules their agents swallowed after being captured. On another visit, they wanted something that would cause a tree to slowly die. It was a particular tree, one planted near Stalin's grave in Moscow. They thought it would cause consternation, and some soul-searching, if it were to wither away. An injection of mercuric nitrate into the trunk was thought to be a possibility.
>
> We had received a small sample of LSD just after it had been synthesized at Sandoz. We tested it on volunteers, giving tiny doses by mouth, which is how its properties had been discovered. It had psychological and hallucinogenic effects; some people were not affected at all, some became disorientated. It was suggested that during the disorientations, a person might forget to lie and might tell the truth under questioning. We stopped our trials with LSD when it was reported that, in a few people, it might produce suicidal tendencies. But MI6 was eager to try it as a 'truth drug'.

We'll never know for certain whether Sargant did work on the LSD trials at Porton Down, given MI6's reluctance to declassify any further files. (Porton's hands would appear tied. The Foreign and Commonwealth Office, which oversees MI6, also declined to respond to a Freedom of Information request, citing the involvement of the intelligence services, who are exempt from FOIs.) All we can say is that two of the guinea pigs, Eric Gow and Don Webb, were pretty sure that Sargant was the psychiatrist who conducted their own trials.

If Sargant was working at Porton Down while also working as an NHS consultant at St Thomas', the collaboration between the two establishments was not as unusual as it sounds. A few years after the initial LSD trials, in 1960, terminally ill cancer patients, including those suffering from leukaemia and lung cancer, began to be given two experimental viruses. Two doctors from St Thomas' (a consultant neurologist and a professor of haematology) and two scientists from Porton Down worked together, publishing a joint paper six years later in the *British Medical Journal*. None of the thirty-three patients survived. One died of respiratory failure three hours after inoculation.

The viruses in question were Kyasanur Forest disease and the related Langat virus, both of which were thought to attack cancer cells and tumours. The Kyasanur Forest disease virus also happens to be a biosafety Level 4 pathogen, which ranks it as deadly as the Ebola and Marburg viruses. The US military at Fort Detrick once considered using it as a biological weapon and looked into ways of using infected migrating birds to attack an enemy.

The experimental treatment, conducted with family consent, might have had the potential to help very ill patients. In the end, though, it failed. 'Transient therapeutic benefit was observed in only four patients.' But it did provide an opportunity for scientists at Porton Down to investigate possible immunities and develop live vaccines against biological weapons.

According to Gordon Thomas, Sargant played a role in the experiment, staying at an 'old coaching inn' close to Porton Down with Bill Buckley, who went on to be the CIA's station chief in Beirut in the 1980s (and was Thomas' main source within the CIA). Sargant apparently collected the paperwork on the autopsies, which had been carried out at Porton Down.

He was unquestionably the sort of psychiatrist whom Porton Down – and MI6 – might have turned to, following his work with abreactive drugs in the war and his burgeoning knowledge of brainwashing. Comparing Sargant to Ewen Cameron, the *Lancet* said in 1988, shortly after his death: 'Sargant's work with drugs and physical treatments likewise attracted the interest of the intelligence men.'

Lord Owen, Sargant's former registrar who later became Foreign Secretary, said in 2009: 'I wouldn't be a bit surprised if he was speaking to people who had been on the fringe of brainwashing.' Owen's views haven't changed. 'I'm sure he was linked,' he says. 'MI6 and MI5 take some of the best of the London top consultants in all their areas of specialty and St Thomas' gets probably more than most.'

One reason, perhaps, why a CIA expert in biological warfare called Frank Olson turned to Sargant in his hour of need. But, as Sargant's patients in the Sleep Room would also discover, it would prove a disastrous decision to trust him.

26

‘He said, “Norm, did you ever see a man die?”’

The death of Frank Olson, a CIA biochemist, lies at the heart of every article, blog, book and conspiracy theory that links Sargant to Western intelligence services. Olson worked for the Special Operations Division at Fort Detrick, home of the US Army’s biological warfare laboratories. His defenestration from the thirteenth floor* of a New York hotel remains one of the great unsolved mysteries of the Cold War. So too is the part played by Sargant. ‘He’s a very significant person in this story,’ Olson’s son Eric says.

The exact circumstances of Olson’s death have been subject to rigorous analysis, thanks to the lifelong work of Eric and many investigative journalists, including Seymour Hersh and Hank Albarelli, all of whom believe that Olson was murdered. Similar allegations were made in *Deckname Artischocke*, a 2002 German

---

* It is often reported that Olson fell from the tenth floor, because of the number of his room (1018A), but it was in fact the thirteenth.

TV documentary, many of which were repeated in *Wormwood*, a 2017 Netflix series.

On 18 November 1953, Olson attended a work retreat on Deep Creek Lake in Maryland. He had been invited by Sidney Gottlieb, who had also asked along three other people from Fort Detrick's Special Operations Division and four agents from the CIA's Technical Services Staff. On the second night, Gottlieb's deputy, Robert Lashbrook, handed around glasses of Cointreau to the assembled group, including Olson, who knocked his back with gusto. Twenty minutes later, Gottlieb asked if everyone was OK. When several people said they felt strange, he announced that the Cointreau had been laced with LSD.

Olson wasn't amused. Earlier, Gottlieb had talked about the necessity of testing substances such as LSD on unwitting volunteers, but Olson never assumed that Gottlieb had his own personnel in mind. He soon became 'quite agitated', unable to separate fantasy from reality. Olson returned home the next day, where his wife said that he 'was uncharacteristically moody and depressed'. He told her that he'd made 'a terrible mistake', but didn't elaborate. Had he revealed something under the influence of LSD? And if so, what?

After a subdued weekend at home, Olson returned to work, where he confided in his boss that he had 'messed up'. Gottlieb sent him to New York for treatment, but Olson felt increasingly paranoid and agreed to be hospitalised at a sanatorium in Maryland. It wasn't to be. At 2.25 a.m. on 28 November he died in a pool of blood on the pavement outside the Hotel Statler (later the Hotel Pennsylvania), a curtain billowing from a broken window thirteen floors above.

Olson was born to Swedish immigrants in Wisconsin and had begun working at Fort Detrick during the Second World War. Armed with a PhD in chemistry from the University of Wisconsin, where he had studied aerosol delivery systems, he was well suited to Cold War experiments, including a simulated anthrax attack on San Francisco.* He left the army in 1944 but stayed on at Fort Detrick as a civilian and was soon signed up to its newly formed Special Operations Division, which he would later go on to run. Some time in 1950, he joined the CIA. He remained within the Special Operations Division, however, and continued to specialise in bioweapons, devising delivery methods that would have made Ian Fleming's Q proud. Gadgets included shaving cream and insect repellents that contained anthrax, deadly lipstick, lethal cigarette lighters and an asthma spray that induced pneumonia.

The first signs that Olson didn't have the stomach for this sort of work came when he began to experiment on animals at Fort Detrick. According to Eric, his father didn't like it when they died in his laboratory. 'He'd come to work in the morning and see piles of dead monkeys. That messes with you. He wasn't the right guy for that.'

Norman Cournoyer, a close friend and former colleague, remembered that Olson's CIA career took him down a 'new path' that was focused on 'information retrieval' as part of Projects Bluebird, Artichoke and MKULTRA. His work involved psychoactive drugs and from 1950, according to Cournoyer, Olson began to visit black sites in Germany to work on special interrogations and truth serums. He was soon reporting directly to Gottlieb, who had joined the CIA in July 1951.

Olson's travel documents confirm that Olson visited Germany in the early 1950s. According to his diplomatic passport, issued on 26 April 1950, he was 'proceeding to the British Isles on official business for the Department of the Army'. Stamps reveal that he travelled to France, Germany, England and Sweden between 1950 and 1953. His itinerary bore all the hallmarks of a spy, using small

---

* Similar operations would soon be undertaken at Porton Down, including widespread airborne dispersal trials using zinc cadmium sulphide, which was used to simulate a germ warfare attack.

airfields such as Bovingdon, Northolt and Hendon to enter and leave the UK. Eric has also found evidence in his father's slides and home movies that Olson visited the CIA's West Germany offices in Frankfurt in 1952, and the US Army's headquarters in Berlin in August 1953.

It's clear, then, that Olson visited Germany, but what exactly did he witness when he was there? Cournoyer remembered Olson was troubled after one of his early trips. 'He came back and he told me … "Norm, you would be stunned by the techniques that they used. They made people talk. They brainwashed people. They used all kinds of drugs. They used all kinds of torture. They were using Nazis, they were using prisoners, they were using Soviets. And they didn't care if they came out of it or not."'

Olson visited Germany for a second time in June 1952, when he could have witnessed the interrogation of 'Patient Number Two', a suspected Soviet double agent. CIA documents reveal that this 'medium height, friendly individual who spoke no English' and who was 'somewhat apprehensive', was subjected to an intense interrogation in Villa Schuster, a safe house near Oberursel, on 13 June – the day after Olson had landed in Germany. A CIA memorandum confirms that between 4 and 18 June 1952, 'Artichoke techniques' were applied to 'two operational cases in a safe house'.

John Marks shed more light on the nature of these interrogations in *The Search for the 'Manchurian Candidate'*. When one of those present, Dr Samuel Thompson, a psychiatrist and naval commander, asked what would happen if something went wrong, a CIA officer turned to him and said, 'Disposal of the body would be no problem.' There were no limits, in other words, something that Eric says came to increasingly haunt his father.

For his final trip to Europe, in 1953, Olson spent time in London between 27 July (when he flew in to Northolt) and 2

August, and from 5 to 8 August. He also visited Sweden, France and Germany. He shot a lot of ciné film that summer, just like any regular tourist. Eric found footage of Big Ben and the Eiffel Tower.

Eric is adamant that his father also visited Porton Down while he was passing through Britain in the early 1950s. At an Artichoke conference in mid February 1953, Gottlieb reported that Porton Down scientists, 'in consultation with SOD researchers', were testing LSD and other hallucinogenic drugs on 'volunteer enlisted personnel'.* Olson was head of the Special Operations Division (SOD) until spring 1953.

According to Gordon Thomas, it was in Wiltshire that Olson had got to know Sargant. Given the Englishman had the right security clearance, Olson felt he could confide in him. 'And he came to London and made the mistake of thinking that, since Sargant was an MI6 psychiatrist, he could tell him what he was struggling with,' says Eric.

Thomas said that Sargant had described Olson as the 'quintessential' American abroad – 'the typical apple-pie-and-salute-the-flag man'. He had an 'endearing innocence', but his behaviour was different when they met for dinner in London. Sargant later told Thomas that Olson seemed a little excited and perhaps even apprehensive about his forthcoming trip to Germany.

Sargant suggested to Olson that they should meet up again when he was passing through London on his way home. The next time they met, the changes in Olson's personality were even more marked. According to Sargant, the biochemist had 'come face to face with his own reality' in Germany. He made no secret

---

* According to Eric Gow, who was shown US documents during the inquest into Ronald Maddison's death, the CIA marvelled at the number of volunteers the British had managed to recruit for its LSD trials. 'What are you telling them?' a CIA officer asked. 'Nothing,' came the British reply.

that he had 'witnessed murder being committed' by the CIA on 'expendables' in 'terminal trials'.

Cournoyer also recalled a marked change in his friend when he returned from his final trip to Europe. 'He sounded different,' Cournoyer remembered. 'He said, "Norm, did you ever see a man die?" And I said, "No." He said, "Well, I did. They did die. Some of the people that were interrogated died."'

Sargant also detected a strong sense of 'soul-searching' and 'seeking reassurance' in Olson at their final meeting. The American felt it would be the right thing for him, as a patriot, to report what he had seen. He couldn't believe his own country would do such things.

Thomas claimed that Sargant was sufficiently concerned by Olson's state of mind to contact MI6, who duly passed on the information to the CIA. The American had become 'someone who could go to the media and reveal what was going on'. Cournoyer was also aware of Olson's tendency to say what he thought, telling Jon Ronson, for his book *The Men Who Stare at Goats* (2004), that Olson had been about to confide in a journalist. 'He came so close it wasn't even funny.'

For Sargant, there was 'no question' of not tipping off MI6. 'I don't know what he said exactly, that he was "not on the programme",' Eric says. According to Thomas, Sargant recommended to MI6 that Olson should no longer have access to Porton Down. The British and the Americans were 'joined at the hip' and there were 'common interests to protect'.

Six months later, Olson was dead. Sargant heard the news after receiving a 'priority message' from the British embassy in Washington. He concluded that Olson 'could only have been murdered'. Had he known the fatal consequences of his tip-off? He appeared to have felt remorse about the 'bad business', later confiding in the CIA's Bill Buckley that he regretted his own involvement.

The CIA swung into cover-up mode the moment Olson's

body was found on the New York sidewalk. They spun a story that he had either fallen or jumped to his death after becoming depressed. There was no mention of LSD. Olson was largely forgotten until June 1975, when the Rockefeller Commission published a report about the death of an unnamed man who had been given LSD without his knowledge. When the *Washington Post* picked up on the story, Eric realised that it was his father. The Olson family duly filed a lawsuit against the American government for wrongful death, prompting President Ford to apologise personally to them at a meeting in the White House. He also agreed to pay them $750,000, in exchange for dropping all legal proceedings.*

But the exact circumstances of how he died remained a mystery. In a dramatic development in 1994, Eric had his father's body exhumed. A second autopsy revealed a haematoma under the front of the skull that suggested Olson had 'been rendered unable to defend himself so that he could be tossed out the window'.

In November 2008, Gordon Thomas sent Eric a 2,000-word memorandum confirming the details of Sargant's meeting with his father. Sargant, he reiterated, felt that Olson was a patriotic man who had been 'locked up in his lab mentality'. Whether he was subsequently murdered or committed suicide, Olson died after the CIA had given him LSD without his knowledge. And according to his son, Sargant had played a central role: 'It's what led to his death.'

* The deal was brokered by Donald Rumsfeld, President Ford's Chief of Staff, and his deputy, Dick Cheney, two individuals who would go on to play a central role in America's War on Terror after 9/11.

27

'Massive electroshock seemed promising'

The Canadian author Anne Collins was the first to point out that the work of Scottish-born psychiatrist Ewen Cameron in Montreal was inspired by and paralleled what Sargant was doing in London. There were some remarkable similarities between the two men's approaches to psychiatry. So many, in fact, that it's impossible to understand Sargant without understanding Cameron. Both men had little time for talking therapies, preferring instead the intensive use of ECT and drugs. More importantly, both had a Sleep Room. According to Gordon Thomas, the two psychiatrists also moved in US intelligence circles in the early 1950s.

Oddly, there is no mention of Cameron in Sargant's personal papers at the Wellcome Collection. You wouldn't know that that they had ever met, let alone become friends. Given the large number of letters that Sargant wrote, the absence of any correspondence smacks of redaction. There is, however, plenty of evidence in the medical literature that the two men shared the same platform at conferences and were on the same medical page.

Take, for example, talks that they gave in London. Both were high-profile Maudsley Bequest Lectures about schizophrenia. Cameron presented the first in 1962. The second, by Sargant the following year, was a riposte of sorts, suggesting that there was an element of rivalry in their friendship.

In his paper, Cameron summarised what he'd been doing at the Allan Memorial Institute for Psychiatry over the previous seven years to treat schizophrenia. His use of ECT was even more intensive than Sargant's. 'A survey of the existing literature showed that of the multiplicity of methods of treatment, massive electroshock seemed promising,' he wrote.

As John Marks has pointed out, the details of Cameron's controversial work were hiding in plain sight. They were recorded by Cameron himself in talks and articles in medical journals which he thought (ironically as it turned out) would shore up his reputation. He was, after all, one of North America's most well-known psychiatrists: a former president of the American Psychiatric Association (1952–3) and the Canadian Psychiatric Association (1958–9), and co-founder and president of the World Psychiatric Association (1961–6).

ECT was initially thought to cure schizophrenia because multiple electric shocks caused such complete confusion, disorientation and amnesia in a patient that schizophrenic symptoms would disappear along with the loss of memory and bladder and bowel control. Everything would be erased – the good and the bad. This process, which Cameron called 'depatterning', would wipe the slate clean. As a patient slowly regained her senses, however, schizophrenic symptoms would often return. So Cameron decided to maximise the initial confusion by using an approach known as the Page-Russell technique: administering electric shocks that were up to 50 per cent stronger than normal and with much more frequency. His goal? The human soul a *tabula rasa*. A young British psychiatrist, Robert Russell, and his colleague Lewis Page, had developed a device in the late 1940s that gave a series of up to fifteen shocks – 150 volts rather than the usual 90–110 volts – in rapid-fire bursts, usually once a day. Cameron used the machine twice a day, sometimes even three times, giving six electric shocks in quick succession.* Significantly, he also decided to administer the treatment while his patients were asleep.

'We had already found that prolonged sleep causes confusion,' he wrote. 'Thus we decided to administer intensive electric shock therapy to our patients in continuous sleep ... as a means of controlling excitement and anxiety.' Sargant would go on to say exactly the same about his own Sleep Room: 'Many patients, unable to tolerate a long course of ECT, can do so when anxiety is relieved by narcosis.'

Cameron, like Sargant, also used a combination of barbiturates and an antipsychotic (Largactil) to put the patient to sleep. After three days, he would begin to administer his own variation of the Page-Russell technique. Ugo Cerletti, inventor of ECT, called it 'annihilation therapy'.

Patients would be woken three times a day for food and to be helped to the bathroom. ECT would be given at different times. As the sound of screams echoed across the hospital, other patients at McGill avoided walking past the Sleep Room.

The first stage of depatterning was reached after five days of twice-daily treatments (60 shocks). 'There are marked memory deficits but it is possible for the individual to maintain a space-time image,' Cameron wrote. 'In other words, he knows where he is, how long he has been there and how he got there.' Things took a turn for the worse in stage two, after twenty days (240 shocks), when he lost all sense of time and space. 'He feels anxious and concerned because he cannot tell where he is and how he got there.' In the final, third stage, reached after as many

* According to John Marks, the doctor who actually administered the shocks confirmed that patients would often get three treatments a day in the early stages.

as thirty days (360 shocks), all feeling had gone, as well as any knowledge of time, space, second languages and marital status. He would be doubly incontinent, unable to feed himself or walk unassisted, and suck his thumb like an infant. Crucially for Cameron, though, 'all schizophrenic symptomatology is absent . . . he is completely free from all emotional disturbance save for a customary mild euphoria. He lives, as it were, in a very narrow segment of time and space.' Ironically, the patient was 'living in the moment', void of all thought and feeling.

Once the treatment was over, the patient was meant to pass back through the three stages in reverse. This period of 'reorganisation' was often 'turbulent' and a patient's anxiety was treated with more chlorpromazine, barbiturates and an antidepressant (a monoamine oxidase inhibitor, or MAOI). If the patient showed signs of a relapse, he was subjected to three more days of intense ECT treatment. At no point did Cameron engage in any psychotherapy: he found the talking cure to be 'positively calamitous'.

Sargant's use of ECT was arguably more restrained, but he shared Cameron's disdain for psychotherapy and his belief in the need to 'depattern' the brain, even if he didn't use exactly the same word. 'What we're doing is breaking up long, set patterns of behaviour,' he wrote in his autobiography.

In his own Maudsley Bequest paper, Sargant outlined his approach to treating schizophrenia. He was keener than Cameron on the use of insulin therapy, but ECT and chlorpromazine were central to both men's approaches. Nearly all cases of schizophrenia admitted to St Thomas' and Belmont were being given 'fairly intensive ECT', combined with chlorpromazine and modified insulin treatment. The result was rapid weight gain, the swift break-up of 'abnormal behaviour patterns' and better 'stabilisation' afterwards.

Although he wasn't using the intensive Page-Russell technique, Sargant was prepared to give prolonged treatment, particularly if the patient later relapsed into depression. He was not concerned about making 'set rules' about 'the exact number of ECT to be given'. A crossed-out paragraph of the speech typescript offered a further glimpse into the large amounts of shocks that he was prepared to give schizophrenic patients, whose nervous system 'seems generally far more tolerant of ECT'. Patients who had just been lobotomised were also fair game.

'I have recently advised a modified leucotomy on the nephew of one of the great rulers of the Near East, whose schizophrenia had failed to respond, except temporarily, to all other treatments,' Sargant wrote, unable to resist a name-drop, without quite breaching patient confidentiality. 'He did not even do well with this modified leucotomy, but made a dramatic further improvement when ECT was again given.'

Sargant's admirers often praised him for never giving up on a patient. His critics, like Cameron's, argued that he never knew when to stop, that he was possessed of a *furor therapeuticus** – a rage to heal – that was more in his own interest than his patients' and brooked no alternative treatments.

* *Furor therapeuticus* was most probably brought into usage by Sigmund Freud during meetings of the Vienna Psychoanalytic Society. He initially talked pejoratively of *furor sanandi*, which means much the same thing, when he accused fellow member Sándor Ferenczi of being too fanatical in his desire to cure patients.

28

'The voice seems to scream at me all the time'

Donald Ewen Cameron, the son of a Presbyterian minister, was born on Christmas Eve in 1901, in Bridge of Allan, Scotland. He would die, aged sixty-five, of a heart attack while climbing in the Adirondack Mountains in America. After studying psychological medicine at the University of Glasgow, he worked in Switzerland, Canada and America. In 1943, he was invited to McGill University in Montreal to become the first director of its Allan Memorial Institute for Psychiatry, housed in Ravenscrag, an imposing nineteenth-century mansion.

By all accounts, Cameron was a cold colleague, distant and enigmatic. Dr Elliot Emanuel, who worked with him, remembered an 'authoritarian' and 'ruthless' man – 'not very nice'. A tall figure, he retained his Glaswegian burr when he addressed female patients and staff as 'lassie' or 'girlie'. His trademark attire was an old suit, pockets stuffed with index cards, and he was known to nibble on the end of his tie. He read science fiction novels last thing at night, loved new cars and technology, and was driven by a burning desire to win the Nobel Prize. 'Girlie, we're going to cure schizophrenia,' he once told the head nurse in his Sleep Room.

Two events stand out in his early career. In 1931, two years after he had arrived at Brandon, a provincial mental hospital in Canada, he conducted an experiment that studied the effect of dehydration on twelve epileptics. The patients became increasingly desperate, eating snow from windowsills, drinking water from vases and stealing food and drink. One died. It was a cruel experiment that proved nothing more than Cameron's own tendency to put experimental research before patient welfare.

The second event was in November 1945, when Cameron was invited to assess the mental state of Rudolf Hess at the Nuremberg trials. He was there along with other psychiatrists from Russia, France, America and Britain, including Lord Moran (Sargant's former dean at St Mary's Hospital) and John Rawling Rees (who had asked Sargant to stop publishing papers on abreaction). Cameron concluded that Hess was 'not insane at the present time' and had been consciously exaggerating his amnesia during his captivity 'to exploit it to protect himself against examination'. Human memory was something that Cameron prized highly – it was the 'bastion' of man's being, he once said – which was ironic, given the lengths to which he would later go to destroy it. Exposure to the horrors of Nazi Germany might have made Cameron more determined to remain principled in his own work, but in fact it seemed to have had the opposite effect. 'Nuremberg was that moment when Cameron changed and became darker,' according to Stephen Bennett, who made a TV documentary, *Eminent Monsters*, about him in 2019.

Nine years later, in 1954, the Agency took an interest in Dr James Hebb, Cameron's colleague at the Allan Memorial, and his investigations into sensory deprivation. Hebb paid students to be blindfolded, wear earplugs and have their feet and hands bound in foam mittens. They would then be placed in a small soundproof chamber for as long as they could bear. (He would let them out as soon as they wished.)

The CIA, which saw the potential of isolation to break the human spirit, soon turned its attention to Cameron. He was pushing things far further than Hebb, not just with his intensive ECT treatments but with something even more disturbing. In 1956, Cameron had written a paper called 'Psychic Driving' for the *Journal of Psychiatry*. He described a new technique – 'an adaptation of Hebb's psychological isolation' – that involved bombarding patients with recorded audio messages, repeated thousands of times, either when they were in a drug-induced sleep or on LSD. Patients would resist, Cameron acknowledged, but 'if they are continuously overloaded their breakdown is to be expected'. He then added something that caught the eye of John Gittinger, the CIA's resident psychologist. 'Analogous to this is the breakdown of the individual under continuous interrogation.'

Psychic driving was arguably the most devastating of all of Cameron's treatments in his Sleep Room. He had begun to develop it in 1953, when he recorded a forty-year-old French Canadian patient talking about how her mother had threatened to abandon her as a child. Cutting her mother's words down to a single phrase – 'If you don't keep quiet, I'm going to leave you behind' – he played the recording back to her again and again, continually flicking the tape recorder switch, much to the woman's distress.

'Does it go on all the time?' she asked after nineteen repetitions. 'I hate to hear that. It upsets me; look at me shaking!' According to Cameron, the patient became red and restless, and began to breathe heavily. 'I hate everything!' she cried after thirty repetitions. Nine repeats later, she threatened him with her hands. 'Stop it! Stop it!' By the time Cameron had forced her to listen to the recording forty-five times, she begged him to turn the machine off and duly opened up about childhood traumas.

Cameron felt he was on to something – 'a gateway to a new field of psychotherapeutic methods' – not least because tape recordings offered a means to avoid long hours of tedious psychotherapy. Recordings, or verbal cues, as he called them, were initially of the patient herself ('autopsychic driving'), but were later provided by others ('heteropsychic driving'). He turned the cues into looped recordings. In the early days, they were on a single topic, no more than twenty seconds, and not played for very long: 'ten to thirty minutes' driving – repeated, if necessary, once a week.' And they were played through headphones, adapted from stenographers' headsets, a method that mimicked the auditory hallucinations experienced by schizophrenic patients in particular. 'This causes the patient to experience the driving with much greater impact . . . he frequently describes it as being like a voice within his head,' he wrote, adding that one patient reported: 'It's too close; it's horrible.'

To keep the patient listening, Cameron varied the volume and pitch of the repeated phrases, and even introduced an 'echo-back', which must have been particularly disconcerting. 'The voice seems to scream at me all the time,' one patient told Cameron. 'It is like the voice of a stranger, though I know it is my own.' Sometimes, patients misheard the message. One woman, who was struggling to enjoy sex with her husband, was played a short message: 'You are at ease with your husband.' But she misheard it as 'You are a tease to your husband', much to the staff's amusement.

Understandably, patients did all they could to escape the repetitive recordings and sought to 'move out of the area of exposure' – a euphemism for fleeing down the Allan Memorial's corridors. It was then that Cameron tried continuous narcosis treatment as a way to keep patients listening. Sleep was an interesting choice. Back in 1948, Cameron had seen an advert for a Cerebrophone, a device that played Linguaphone language-lesson records at night while the user slept, a learning technique called Dormiphonics. It was also used to cure people of bad habits, such as biting their nails. Although Cameron had tried and given up on the concept, the technology still appealed. He consulted his British lab technician, Leonard Rubenstein, who duly built a tape recorder that could relay multiple looped recordings through speakers in the ceiling or under the pillow in the Sleep Room on South 2 ward, where Cameron administered his most extreme treatments. 'A special mechanism has been built at the Allan Memorial Institute which enables us to co-ordinate delivery of eight separate sets of signals simultaneously,' he later boasted.

Cameron liked his gadgets and continued to modify his technique, varying the length of the recordings and experimenting with the methods of sedation, sometimes using LSD, as well as stimulating patients with Desoxyn (methamphetamine). But the biggest change was the ever-increasing duration and intensity of the psychic driving. 'If this thing worked after thirty repetitions, it was only common sense to see what would happen if the repetition was increased tenfold, a hundredfold or even more,' he wrote. He was soon subjecting patients to up to half a million repetitions over '20–30 days, 16 hours a day', which required much more restrictive methods to ensure they listened.

One tactic was the use of American football helmets that had been wired with speakers, but patients managed to rip them off, hurling them across the ward. Cameron revisited sleep treatment again, which was undergoing something of a renaissance thanks to the advent of chlorpromazine in 1953. Mixed with barbiturates, the tranquilising antipsychotic now made it much easier to keep someone in a pattern of relatively normal sleep for up to twenty hours a day. (Previous sleep treatments that only used barbiturates had put people into a state of deep unconsciousness, which was not good for psychic driving.)

In Cameron's Sleep Room, nurses woke the patients three times a day (8 a.m., 2 p.m. and 8 p.m.) to wash and feed them and check their vital signs. One patient was kept asleep for 65 days. Enemas were given if there had been no bowel movement for three days, and they were catheterised if they hadn't urinated in 12 hours. Medication was a mix of Largactil and barbiturates and milk of magnesia was given with night sedation. Some patients even had Sernyl, also known as angel dust, a recreational hallucinogen, to ensure 'heightened awareness of the verbal signals'.

Once the patient was sufficiently sedated, the tapes would begin. Messages, which he now called 'dynamic implants', would last for between twenty and thirty seconds. For the first ten days, for up to twenty hours a day, a patient would be subjected to looped recordings of negative messages. ('You let your mother check you up sexually after every date you had with a boy', for example.) She would then be subjected to ten days of positive messages about her relationship with her mother. ('Begin to assert yourself first in little things and soon you will be able to meet her on an equal basis.')

The CIA's appetite had been whetted. On the advice of Gittinger, who had read Cameron's article on psychic driving in 1956, the Agency decided to make Cameron an offer. Lt Col James Monroe, former head of the US Air Force's psychological warfare division, went to the Allan Memorial Institute and encouraged Cameron to apply to the Society for the Investigation of Human Ecology, of which he was executive director, for funds to develop his work.

Some people have given Cameron the benefit of the doubt and believe that he was unaware that the CIA was behind the society. The British psychiatrist Peter Roper, who worked with Cameron at the Allan Memorial, said in 2006 that 'almost all departments' benefited from military grants. 'I don't think [Cameron] ever knew the CIA was behind his funding.' Indeed, when the grant was approved, the authorisation memo stated that Cameron and his staff would remain 'completely unwitting' of its real source.

Cameron would already have been known to the intelligence services, thanks to his work with Hess in Nuremberg. He might even have personally known Allen Dulles before he became Director of the CIA in 1953. According to Gordon Thomas, it was Dulles who had personally asked for Cameron to be on the panel of international psychiatrists to examine Hess. As the author Anne Collins said: 'In 1957 a close inspection of the gift horse would easily have revealed the enemy lurking inside.'

Either way, Cameron put in a grant application, dated 21 January 1957, to 'study the effects upon human behaviour of the repetition of verbal signals'. Psychic driving, in other words, but this time used in conjunction with depatterning and other techniques he'd been working on, including sensory isolation, continuous sleep, LSD 'as a means of breaking down the ongoing patterns of behaviour', and four paralysing drugs, including curare, as a way of 'inactivating the patient during the period of driving' to ensure they listened.

Depatterning and psychic driving: Cameron was given carte blanche to dismantle the human psyche until nothing was left, and then reprogram it according to his paymasters' wishes. The CIA couldn't believe its luck, either. Here was an American citizen (Cameron had become one in 1942) working overseas (in Canada), allowing the Agency to notionally adhere to its principle of not operating domestically.

MKULTRA Subproject 68, signed off by Sidney Gottlieb on 26 February 1957, began on 18 March, when Cameron was awarded $38,180 to cover the first two years (payments were made every quarter). The funds paid for half the salary of Rubenstein ($2,500) as well as Leonard Levy, a research psychiatrist ($7,000), 'Concert Master continuous tape players' ($1,810) and 'message repeating mechanisms' ($320). A third annual payment of $19,090 was approved on 27 March 1959, followed by a final payment of $4,775, to cover a final extension to the project from 31 March to 1 July 1960. In total, Cameron was paid $62,045 by the CIA between 1957 and 1960, through the Society for the Investigation of Human Ecology. He wrote in April 1960 to thank the society for its 'invaluable' help, at the same time as applying for funding beyond 1 July. He was not successful.

Gittinger had apparently believed that a psychiatrist of Cameron's international standing would give the front organisation 'good cover' and a certain air of respectability, but he and the CIA regretted their investment. 'That was a foolish mistake,' he said, twenty-six years later. 'We shouldn't have done it ... I'm sorry we did because it turned out to be a terrible mistake.' Cameron's programme was 'of no interest' to the CIA and an Agency general counsel would characterise the experiments as 'repugnant'.

Ironically, Cameron would probably have continued on the same 'therapeutic' trajectory with or without CIA backing. By the start of the project, he had already given LSD to a thirty-nine-year-old alcoholic during twenty-five hours of psychic driving. And, in his 'adaptation of Hebb's psychological isolation', he had placed a patient in a dark room, covered his eyes with goggles and prevented him from touching his body. Both cases were written up in 1956, a year before the CIA funding started.

But the money clearly helped, paying for salaries, drugs and electronic devices. It also enabled Cameron to push sensory isolation to the limit. While subjecting a patient to negative looped recordings, Cameron would reinforce the message by 'applying galvanic stimulation to the leg' at the end of each repetition – an electric shock, in other words. Using $3,500 of the funds, he also built a box, or cubicle, in Ravenscrag's converted stable block, where he left one patient, Mary C, for thirty-five days of sensory deprivation. She'd already been subjected to other unimaginably intense treatments, including 'repeated depatterning' (ECT) and 101 days of 'positive' psychic driving, but 'no favourable results were obtained'. Her condition? She was a menopausal hypochondriac.

In 1960, Cameron addressed a meeting of the Canadian Psychiatric Association in Banff. In order for psychic driving to be most effective, Cameron stressed the importance of breaking up the existing 'personality pattern' and reducing critical awareness. Sleep (up to sixty days) was now his preferred form of depatterning, combined with ECT (up to thirty Page-Russell treatments). Depatterning and psychic driving had been combined in Cameron's Sleep Room into one hideous form of treatment, funded by the CIA.

29

'It was terrifying . . . you become very small'

In 1988, the CIA was forced to pay $750,000 in compensation to nine of Cameron's patients – the largest payment ever made by the Agency. The Canadian federal government, which also funded Cameron's work, paid out $100,000 each to seventy-seven patients in 1992, but 250 claims were turned down on the grounds that the individuals weren't 'tortured enough'. Lawsuits still rumble on, however, and the most recent compensation was made in 2017. A class action against the American government stalled in October 2023, but continues against the Canadian government, the Royal Victoria Hospital and McGill University.

Sargant would have realised as early as August 1977, when the *New York Times* published the source of Cameron's funding, that his relationship with his Scottish friend in the 1950s and 1960s could do irreparable damage to his own legacy. By the time the CIA had agreed to pay out compensation, he had had plenty of opportunity to expunge Cameron from his personal papers and to brief journalists like Gordon Thomas that he had always disapproved of him. In 1998, a decade after Sargant had died, Phillip Knightley wrote an article about the mysterious death of Frank Olson for the *Mail on Sunday*. Sargant had apparently told Thomas that what Cameron and the CIA were up to was as bad as anything in the Soviet Gulags. 'Sargant told me that he had urged the British government to distance this country from it. He said it was blacker than black.' Ten years later, in *Secrets & Lies*, Sargant was saying something similar to Bill Buckley, Thomas' main source within the CIA. 'What was being done to Cameron's patients was wrong, wrong, wrong.' If the quotes are genuine, either Sargant had been truly appalled by Cameron's work, which seems unlikely given how much their treatments had in common, or, more likely, he was desperate to distance himself from Cameron and the CIA.

Some things, however, can't be covered up. In the 1950s, Cameron and Sargant both emerged on the global stage as prominent players in psychiatry. They shared a desire to treat psychiatric patients in general hospitals and a passion for physical treatments such as ECT. Psychiatry, they both believed, deserved to be recognised as a proper medical science. They became good friends, as well as professional colleagues, who saw each other regularly at conferences. One onlooker remembers seeing them greeting each other in the early 1960s like 'long-lost friends'.

On 10 September 1957, nine months after Cameron had initially applied for funding from the CIA's cover organisation, Sargant invited him to give a talk in London at an Anglo-American symposium at the Royal Society of Medicine. The symposium, held at Wimpole Street, was hosted jointly by the Section of Psychiatry of the RSM (Sargant was Section president) and the Royal Medico-Psychological Association, which would later become the Royal College of Psychiatrists (Sargant was its registrar). Cameron opened proceedings with a talk about teaching psychiatry and Sargant chaired the next day's events.

Two years later, Sargant applied for study leave from 16 to 28 March 1959 'to attend and read a paper at a conference in Montreal (no expenses)'. St Thomas' General Purpose Committee minutes didn't give details, but a conference on 'depression and allied states' was hosted by McGill University on 19 to 21 March 1959. Cameron, on his home patch, spoke about the use of Tofranil (imipramine, a tricyclic antidepressant) in the elderly, which would have gone down well with its manufacturers, Geigy, sponsors of the conference. And Sargant led the discussion at the end of the conference's opening paper, on psychiatric concepts of depression.

Four months later, Cameron was back in Scotland to address the annual meeting of the Royal Medico-Psychological Association. He spoke at 11 a.m. on 15 July 1959, in the concert hall of the Glasgow Royal Mental Hospital. Sargant was in the audience, having just presented his annual registrar's report to the AGM at 10 a.m. After Cameron's talk, and lunch, Sargant then proposed, with three other people, that Cameron be elected an honorary member of the RMPA. (Sargant also proposed that his American friend Walter Freeman, champion of the transorbital lobotomy, be made a corresponding member.)

So there is no doubt that Sargant would have listened to Cameron's talk on 'Effects of Repetition of Verbal Signals upon the Behaviour of Chronic Psychoneurotic Patients', and heard all about the pillow speakers and electric shocks to the leg, and how patients were 'exposed to ten days of repetition of negative phase signals and ten days of positive phase signals and kept in a semi-sleep state by a combination of Sernyl and Largactil with occasional barbiturates'.

Ever mindful of sourcing funds, Sargant would also have made a note of Cameron's closing remarks, which were printed in the published version of his lecture. 'The work on this project was supported by a grant from the Society for the Investigation of Human Ecology, Incorporated.'

It's worth contemplating exactly what happened in Glasgow that day. Cameron gave a talk to the future Royal College of Psychiatrists on a brutal treatment called psychic driving – the research for which was funded by the CIA – and was made an honorary member thanks to Sargant's personal nomination. Despite Sargant's best efforts to airbrush Cameron from his life (denouncing his work as 'blacker than black' and 'wrong, wrong, wrong'), the two men were in reality as thick as thieves. It was not as if Cameron was acting in secrecy either. In a press release about his talk, he made bold claims about the new technique. 'We have shown that the reorganisation of the personality can be achieved not only by eliminating an older pattern, but by putting it out of circuit and putting in its functioning place an entirely new pattern.'

In June 1961, Cameron returned the favour. Sargant was made an honorary member of the Canadian Psychiatric Association at its AGM, held during the third World Congress of Psychiatry in Montreal, when Cameron was made president of the newly formed World Psychiatric Association. Sargant was also appointed one of the WPA's two 'associated secretaries'. The other was a Spanish psychiatrist, Juan José López-Ibor, who would become the second president of the WPA in 1966. During the Franco regime, he had used ECT and lobotomy to 'cure' patients of homosexuality. 'My last patient was a deviant,' López-Ibor said at a conference in Italy, but he now 'appears more slightly attracted to women', even if he had 'disorders in memory and vision'. Sargant described López-Ibor as 'a great personal friend'.

To seal his friendship with Cameron, Sargant returned to Montreal in May 1964 to address the staff of the Allan Memorial Institute on the subject of brainwashing. 'The atomic stalemate in which we live is primarily a battle for the mind of man,' he thundered. 'Anger and fear are disruptive influences on the emotional stability of the nervous system and these are used in brainwashing.' Cameron himself added: 'The intensity of the powers and passions which lie just below the surface are restrained by a thin layer of logical thinking.' And it was the thinness of that layer, and the danger of it being exploited, that was the cause of human anxiety, Sargant concluded.

It was as if the two men were finishing each other's sentences.

One aspect of Sargant's Sleep Room in London is often said to have differed from Cameron's in Montreal: the use of tape-recorded messages. Sargant didn't strap helmets with built-in speakers to his patients' heads; nor did he secrete speakers beneath pillows, or make people listen to a quarter of a million negative messages about their mother. But he did make much more use of tape recorders on Ward Five than is generally thought.

In the fourth edition of *An Introduction to Physical Methods of Treatment in Psychiatry*, when Sargant wrote about the use of LSD in drug abreaction, he said that it was best to wait until the day afterwards to talk to the patient about his experiences. He would still be in a 'heightened state of suggestibility' and suggestions could 'now be offered and will be accepted, which would have been rejected out of hand before treatment'. He then drops a bombshell: 'It is sometimes desirable to have the conversations and the abreactions which occurred under LSD recorded on tape, and play them back next day or later in order to reinforce therapeutic suggestions.'

The use of the word 'reinforce' in this context has disturbing echoes of what Ewen Cameron was doing to his patients. Val Orlikow was suffering from post-partum depression when she was admitted to the Allan Memorial Institute at the end of 1956. Cameron gave her LSD mixed with a stimulant or depressant, and then left her alone to listen to recorded extracts from a previous therapy session. This happened fourteen times. As she told John Marks: 'It was terrifying. You're afraid you've gone off somewhere and can't come back. You become very small.' So small she felt like Alice in her Wonderland, or a squirrel trapped in a cage, and that someone was going to kill her.

Val, who died in 1990, couldn't bear the treatment. Yet she idolised Cameron, no matter what he put her through. Every time she tried to leave the hospital, Cameron would put his arm around her and say, 'Lassie, don't you want to get well, so you can go home and see your husband?' Eventually, she did leave, but returned as a private patient. In 1963, Cameron subjected her to psychic driving, during which she listened to messages that included: 'Did you hate your mother? Did you hate your father?' 'I thought he was God,' she said. 'I don't know how I could have been so stupid.'

Val returned home with 'about 20 per cent of her capacity', according to her husband, David Orlikow, a member of the Canadian parliament. Later, he sued the CIA, and his wife was one of the nine patients who won compensation in 1988.*

Did Sargant, another idolised psychiatrist, subject any of his patients to something similar? In 1960, the Local Hospitals Committee approved the purchase of a £100 tape recorder, to be paid for by the Special Ward Five Account. 'It was noted that the tape recorder would be used primarily for diagnostic purposes.' The Endowment Fund had also signed off on a tape recorder, for £90, back in 1952, 'for the purpose of making abreaction recordings which would be of value for research in progress in his department'. A further tape recorder was purchased in 1963 for £78.

He also liked to use tape recorders during aversion therapy. It was a controversial treatment that tried to associate something unpleasant with a patient's bad habit: smoking, nail-chewing, drugs, drinking etc. In Anthony Burgess's 1962 novel *A Clockwork Orange*, Alex, the teenage protagonist, is subjected to the Ludovico Technique, a form of behaviour modification that

* The Agency settled out of court and did not accept any liability.

bears uncanny similarities to Sargant's take on aversion therapy. Injected with emetics while watching violent films, he is conditioned to be ill whenever he has an aggressive thought.

Sargant saw aversion therapy as a perfect way to disrupt patterns of behaviour (usually drinking to excess) by using a shock treatment: making the patient throw up every time they had a drink. But he took it a stage further. Repeated vomiting so weakened the patient that they eventually became amenable to suggestions such as going teetotal and joining Alcoholics Anonymous. 'As the treatment proceeds, reversal of previous attitudes and suggestibility may become much more pronounced,' he wrote in 'The Mechanism of "Conversion"', his controversial paper for the *BMJ* in 1951.

The paper caught the attention of Ewen Cameron, who referred to it two years later in one of his own papers, 'The Transition Neurosis'. Talking about how subconscious patterns of behaviour could be stimulated, he noted that Sargant had used 'depleting' emetics. 'We have explored this procedure in one case, using sleeplessness, disinhibiting agents, and hypnosis.'

Aversion therapy on Ward Five was conducted in one of the small private rooms at the end of a long corridor, beyond Sargant's own office. It was here that Julia Ross worked when she was a newly qualified nurse in 1967. 'The room was a very unpleasant place to be in,' she recalls. 'A tape-recording machine sat on the side and the floor and walls were completely covered in urine and vomit and smelt of stale whisky, cigarette smoke and unwashed body.'

She soon understood why. Her first patient, Mr Smith, was an alcoholic in his late forties with a heavy beer belly. He was divorced and had little contact with his two children. This was his final attempt to stop drinking. 'We had to wake him up and give him a tumbler of neat whisky, followed by an emetic to make him throw up, at which point we would play a tape recording. I'm pretty certain it was Sargant's voice – Sargant made sure he wasn't actually in the room during the treatment. The voice was rich and low.'

Afterwards, everything that Mr Smith had evacuated from his body was left in the room with him for twenty-four hours. 'As he was throwing up, he was told on the tape recording to look around, see what a disgusting, unpleasant human being he was.' Once he had finished vomiting, Julia turned off the recording and let him sleep. Six hours later, the whole routine started again.

Julia went on to work in health and social care for forty years and is the current chair of the British Association of Social Workers. She has also written a book, *Call the Social*, about her life and career. As she says, aversion therapy can be successful while the patient is under the direction of a therapist, but relapses are high. 'One of the major criticisms is that it lacks rigorous scientific evidence demonstrating its effectiveness,' she adds. 'Ethical issues over the use of punishments in therapy are also a major point of concern.'

Peter Tyrer also remembers the aversion therapy room, and how one side of it had been converted into a pub. 'It wasn't much bigger than a broom cupboard and there was definitely a tape recorder in there.' As soon as the patient started to vomit, the tape recorder was switched on. 'Everyone told him how terrible he was . . . We were competing with the awfulness of the recording to make it even worse for the patient.' It's not clear who paid for the bar or the booze, but Tyrer suspects it wasn't the NHS.

30

Anne White

When I arrived at Scutari, St Thomas' outpatient psychiatric ward, in March 1970, I was transferred immediately to Ward Five on the top floor of the Royal Waterloo. A mother of young children – at one point I had three children under three and a quarter – I was suffering from depression and had tried to take my own life. My husband was a doctor and we were living in Zambia, where he worked at a hospital in the Copperbelt. Dr William Sargant was considered the best person to get me well again and I had flown back to London to be treated by him.

I was initially seen by Sargant's deputy, Dr John Pollitt, who told me that my brain needed a rest and that I was going to be put into the Sleep Room. What he didn't tell me was that I'd also receive twenty-six electric shocks that would wipe my memory. I was twenty-eight years old but I don't remember signing any consent forms. I must have seen Sargant too, but I was in no condition to question him. Sargant was all-powerful on Ward Five.

The only thing I was told was that sleep would obliterate the negative feelings that I experienced when I was depressed and reinforce the positive feelings. That effectively amounted to 're-patterning' and I'm pretty sure it's the exact word they used. I was put into the Sleep Room, where I think there were six beds, but only three others were occupied. I don't remember ever talking to any of the other patients. We were all too drugged. I subsequently discovered that I was given Largactil, an antipsychotic, and Seconal, a barbiturate, to sedate me. I was also given two different types of antidepressant: Nardil and Tryptizol. It was Pollitt who later told me that I'd received twenty-six bilateral treatments of ECT during my time in the Sleep Room.

I don't remember being given any of the shocks, eating meals or being taken to the bathroom. Unfortunately, I was so drugged up that every time I tried to stand, I passed out, because my blood pressure was down in my boots. As a doctor, I now know that low blood pressure is a common side effect of psychotropic drugs. They also poured what seemed like a jug of water down me whenever they woke me up to keep me rehydrated.

As the weeks passed, I became increasingly resistant to the drugs they were giving me. I found myself strangely unable to sleep, no matter how much medication I was given. I just lay there, sedated but awake, in a sort of twilight state of consciousness, surrounded by these other sleeping women. For day after day, with no sensory input, really – and not sleeping. Everything became a blur. I was so tired and desperately wanted to sleep, but I couldn't. I couldn't do anything. I just lay there in the semi-darkness, watching the hours go by. This went on for day after day. It was almost like I was being abused, or tortured – I was, in effect, suffering a form of sensory deprivation.

Eventually, I'd had enough and begged to be taken out of the Sleep Room – the whole thing, my treatment, felt odd, not right – but I was told that I had to stay there. It was like being patted on the head. I must have got quite angry at that point, complained that I was no longer sleeping. Eventually, they put me in a single white room on my own. They also took me off the Seconal that had kept me sedated and I was left to my own devices as I went through barbiturate withdrawal for a week. Withdrawal effects can be very severe if you just suddenly stop taking a heavy sedative. It causes seizures and even death. I felt as if I was being punished because I had dared to challenge the system.

For the next week, I lay there in that tiny room with severe muscle aches, shaking so badly that the whole bed rocked. It was an absolute nightmare, but nobody seemed to care that much. Towards the end of the week, Pollitt gave me Artane to counter the shakes – but it's used to treat Parkinson's disease, not drug withdrawal. Finally, the symptoms passed and I was allowed out of my room. I really did sense the staff's displeasure while I was in there, as if I hadn't obeyed the rules.

I then recall spending a bit of time in the day room, looking out across at the Festival Hall as 'Cecilia' by Simon and Garfunkel was played over and over on the record player. It's funny what little things you remember. A lot of the other people who were in there were young women with troubled childhoods. I'm convinced that we'd been selected for a reason – we were more susceptible to being manipulated by dominant people like Sargant. In my case, I'd been abused by my father until I was twelve, leaving me vulnerable to male authority figures for the rest of my life. I certainly never questioned them. Whatever they told me to do, I would do. And in the early 1970s, doctors were the dominant males. They were treated like gods. So when I was admitted to Sargant's care, in 1970, I never stood a chance.

Just before I was discharged from the Royal Waterloo Hospital, my father came to see me. He was allowed to take me out to lunch on the South Bank. I'd been kept heavily sedated and given ECT for eight weeks, so I probably wasn't looking my best, but he was absolutely shattered when he saw me. He told me I looked like a 'walking zombie'. But what my father failed to acknowledge, then or later, was that I might never have ended up in the Sleep Room if he or my mother had hugged or kissed me as a child. Shown me some affection, a sign that they loved me.

My father still thought I looked like a zombie when I was finally discharged from the Royal Waterloo on 11 May 1970. The ECT had destroyed my memory prior to treatment and my recollections today of that period of my life are almost zero. The ECT wiped my brain clean of much that happened before I was admitted into the Sleep Room. Maybe that's a blessing. When I look back on my childhood, I realise I went through hell. Sadly, though, I can't recall much about my own children's childhoods either. I can't remember when they were babies at all. You know, those little moments that people normally rejoice in. First steps. First words. Nothing. It's all gone.

I was born on 31 December 1941 – a Wednesday child, full of woe – in Bicester, Oxfordshire, where my father, a photographer with the RAF, was stationed before going off to the war. In April 1945, he photographed the famous image of a dead Benito Mussolini and his mistress hanging from their feet in a square in Milan. I was an only child and didn't know my father until I was five years old, when he came back from the war.

After my father had returned from the war, we moved to Shirehampton, on the edge of Bristol. My father, demobilised from the RAF, worked as an aeronautical engineer at the Bristol Aeroplane Company. Later he moved to Shell and became very senior – he was so driven, at work and at home. He would ask me a question, and I'd answer it as best as I could, and then he'd always ask a follow up question. He'd carry on firing questions at me until I could no longer answer them. When I was only ten years old, he tried to teach me logarithms. Can you believe it? He made me feel an idiot because I couldn't make my own logarithm tables. As a result, I went through school thinking that I was stupid, that anything I did wouldn't be good enough. I lived in fear of getting something wrong.

I think my father was one of those people who made themselves feel good by putting other people down. If you step on a person, you're higher than them. He did the same to my mother, who had been an apprentice theatrical hairdresser. She'd married my father to get away from her abusive mother, but not all escapes lead to paradise, as she found out. I can remember when she lost the key to our front door and he just verbally ripped into her, telling her how stupid she was. When we finally got into the house, I stood in the hallway, looking into the living room. There he was, strangling her. He stopped when he saw me.

It was during this time that he abused me. It happened when my mother went out, for instance, to see a film by herself and I was in the house alone with him. My mother never knew. It would have devastated her if she had ever found out. She was already a very vulnerable person. I was never close to her. I don't think I was close to anyone. As an adult, I went back to visit both of them, but that was because I was their daughter, rather than because I wanted to see them.

I went to a grammar school in Bristol, before we moved to Swansea when I was thirteen. My memories of this part of my life are also vague, because of all the ECT I was later given. I can paint the bigger picture, but if you asked me who my friends were, or who my teachers were, I couldn't tell you. All those deep memories have gone. I've got superficial memories – like I know I went to school in Swansea – but I can't remember the actual details.

I do know that I went through high school doing very well in languages and the life sciences. It's then that I got accepted at three medical schools – St Mary's, the Royal Free and Cardiff – and turned them all down. Throughout my childhood, my father had repeatedly told me that I was stupid. Who was I to become a doctor? Instead, I went into physiotherapy. I did OK, but it was then that I had my first psychiatric problem. By now, I'd suppressed all memories of my abuse. I was admitted, aged twenty, to hospital with depression – something that I would wrestle with for the rest of my life. I was admitted for a week or two, but then I was let out and managed to become a chartered physiotherapist.

I met my husband-to-be, a med student, while I was a physio

student in Bristol. We knew each other for three years before we got married. Again, a lot of that time is kind of blurry. After we married, we moved to Gloucester, where he went into family practice as a GP, but we were only there for two years before my husband got fed up with the NHS and we moved to Mufulira, in the Copperbelt province of Zambia. He worked as a medical officer for one of the mines.

I worked part time as a physio, and I'd also had three children in quick succession. Unfortunately, I suffered from post-partum depression after each child was born. I felt tired all the time, even after getting sleep. Weepy, worthless as a mother, guilty that I wasn't doing a good job. Everything was an effort, including looking after the baby. I lost all pleasure in things I normally loved. I couldn't concentrate enough to read. I couldn't enjoy music. I was intermittently suicidal and thought that I was a drag on my family. As soon as I became pregnant again, however, my mood lifted and I felt good. I'd had my first two children thirteen months apart, then there was a gap of two years before the next one was born. The baby ended up in an incubator for a week. Again I became depressed, but this time there was no reprieve with a subsequent pregnancy and my mood spiralled.

My depression went untreated for two years, because no one diagnosed the problem, but then I was sent down to Johannesburg for some ECT. It wasn't excessive, just a regular normal dosage. I still believe, after all I've been through, that ECT, when it's given in the correct quantities, and at the right dose, can be beneficial for some people who are drug resistant, particularly the elderly. In my case, though, it didn't work, and the depression returned. It went on and on. You could have told me that I had won the lottery and there would be no feeling. Nothing. It was almost like a hibernation state. Eventually, I tried to take my own life by slitting my wrists, and my husband's medical insurers took over.

On New Year's Eve 1969, I flew back to from Lusaka to London on my own with my three young children and stayed with my parents in Rickmansworth for a while. Then, on 9 March, I had an appointment at St Thomas' Scutari outpatient ward. My husband had consulted with other doctors and it was decided that Sargant would get me better. I didn't know what to expect, but I was reassured that St Thomas' was at the cutting edge of modern medicine. I'm horrified that I did this, but I left my daughter with my parents and sent my two sons to stay with my in-laws in Somerset. Thinking back, I must have just blanked out everything, as I would never have put my daughter, who was just two at the time, with my father.

After twenty-six shocks and two months of narcosis on Ward Five, I went back to stay with my parents before returning to Zambia. They were appalled at the state I was in. I could barely function. It took me a good three months to get over my treatment at the Royal Waterloo, none of which had been helpful. I was, however, put on lithium, a treatment for bipolar depression. Much later, a psychiatrist diagnosed me as bipolar, so Sargant or Pollitt at least got that right, although lithium is quite a toxic medication.

We spent another four years in Zambia before we returned to the UK for six months and then emigrated to Thunder Bay in northern Ontario, Canada, where my husband worked at as a family doctor in private practice. Two of our children were now at school, so I did some part time physio and also taught nurses at Lakehead University. Because I was teaching there, I could study for free, so I decided to do an honours degree in biology and zoology and got the gold medal, the highest marks in the faculty of science. That was really important to me – at last, some external validation that maybe I wasn't so stupid after all.

We then moved to Hamilton, near Toronto, where my husband had a new job, and I decided to go to graduate school at McMaster University. It had a very good medical school so I thought I might as well apply. I'd always wanted to study medicine, ever since I'd been offered three places at medical school when I was eighteen. The first year I applied to McMaster, I was told I was too old. I applied again the next year and, aged thirty-five, I was accepted. I did pretty well and ended up becoming a fellow of the Royal College of Physicians and Surgeons of Canada.

I'd finally become the doctor I always wanted to be, and life was pretty good, but I was getting fed up with internal university politics. I kept on with the teaching but opened a private methadone practice, often dealing with recently discharged prisoners. By 2000 I'd had enough and went to work in the Middle East to pay off my mortgage. I'd left my husband and was mortgage free, but there was three feet of snow piled up outside my house when I returned to Canada. I thought, bugger this, and I took a job in the Caribbean, where I could indulge my lifelong love of scuba diving.

For two years, I worked at the school of medicine on Saba, a small island off Saint Martin. I also took the opportunity to complete a masters in hyperbaric medicine, to help divers who got into problems. I was then headhunted by Ross University on Dominica, where I worked for the next twelve years and became dean of students and a full professor of internal medicine.

The thing about scuba diving is that you're isolated from all your worries. It's always been an escape for me, a relief from my depression. Once you get to neutral buoyancy, you're just floating. When you look up, you can't see the sky – the surface of the sea is like a mirror. You are totally enclosed by the sea. And I only dive in tropical waters, where the colours are amazing. It's so tranquil, totally separated from the daily demands. Unfortunately, I've had to give it up recently. A couple of years ago, I had nine hours of surgery – I've got rods and plates and screws in my back now. I can't say one way or the other if a lifetime of back problems has been caused by my ECT and the accompanying fits.

For years, I'd put my experience in the Sleep Room to the back of my mind. It was a suppressed memory. And then, in 2000, I read *The Assets*, a thriller by Ted Allbeury, which was all about the CIA and MKULTRA, its drugs and mind control programme. It was a work of fiction, but he'd based it on well researched real events. At the end of the book, Allbeury said that if you thought his novel was far-fetched, look up MKULTRA. So I did, and I hate to say this, as I know I sound like a paranoid conspiracy theorist, but I thought, my God, that's exactly what happened to me under Sargant. I hadn't even thought about the Sleep Room until then. It was like a door had been shut on it for all those years.

I was particularly shocked by the similarities between what the CIA had done to innocent members of the American public and the medical treatment that we'd been subjected to in the Sleep Room. Reading about MKULTRA brought it all back to me: the drugs, the ECT, lying there on Ward Five for days on end in a distressing, semi-awake state, deprived of all senses. To me the whole thing suddenly slotted together. I'm absolutely sure that a government agency funded the Sleep Room and that we were part of some sort of psychiatric experiment – narcosis is an incredibly dangerous treatment. Sargant had enough connections with the British intelligence services. His friend Ewen Cameron had a similar Sleep Room in Montreal which was financed by the CIA as part of MKULTRA.

In 2004, I hired a solicitor and tried to sue St Thomas', but I was advised that there was a statute of limitations – too much time had passed. I wasn't interested in money, I just wanted to expose St Thomas'. I was really angered by the judge's decision. I'd only been aware of what had happened to me for a handful of years, as the memory had been buried up until then.

These days, I've retired from medicine and I'm back living in Hamilton, where the autumn colours are glorious. I have four grandchildren, all of whom are adults, and now a great-grandson and I have written an illustrated children's book, *The Cat Who Thought He Was a Mouse*. My eldest son, Chris, followed his parents into medicine and my daughter, Sara, is currently here looking after me. Tragically, I recently lost my younger son, Nick, which has plunged me into the worst depression I have ever experienced. Nick was an extremely gifted person. He ran the web architecture and security for the government of Ontario. He was an outstanding guitarist and loved scuba diving. He is missed so much by his family and friends.

I've met Mary Thornton, another one of Sargant's patients who was in the Sleep Room.* I travelled to Cumbria and stayed with her after a visit to London. It's been very therapeutic to talk about what happened to both of us. She's been a great comfort and friend. Now, as I look back on what happened to us all those years ago on the top floor of the Royal Waterloo, I can say, as a doctor and as a patient, that Sargant's treatments did nothing for me. Absolutely nothing. Maybe if my self-esteem had improved and my depression had never returned, I would think differently, but all he did was destroy much of my memory. I've been admitted to hospital with crippling depression off and on ever since – hardly an endorsement of Sargant and his treatments.

I have been left with nothing but anger that Sargant was never held responsible for the torture he put young vulnerable women through, and that St Thomas' covered it up. I wish our paths had never crossed, but then, as a Wednesday child, perhaps I had no choice. My life was lived under the shadow of two dominant men who nearly destroyed me. I am so lucky to have an intrinsic strength that has overcome the destruction those two men wrought – and been able to use the gifts I was given at birth.

---

* See Chapter 8.

31

'The thing to do is to give continuous sleep'

The absence of any letters to, or from, Ewen Cameron is by far the most troubling omission in Sargant's personal papers. The author Dominic Streatfeild interviewed Peter Roper in 2005 about his experiences working with Cameron in Montreal. Roper recalled visiting Sargant in the UK in the 1970s and being given the cold shoulder. 'Sargant had changed completely,' Roper told Streatfeild. 'At one time he was very friendly, advising me, but now he was distant. He didn't really have much to talk about.'

In a subsequent phone call, Sargant flatly denied that he had ever corresponded with Roper about Cameron. Roper, however, had a letter in front of him, signed by Sargant. 'Why did Sargant deny the connection, and to similar treatment to Cameron?' he asked Streatfeild. 'I wonder if Sargant's estate, or Sargant himself, might worry about being sued, even at this late date.'

The source of Cameron's funding came to light on 2 August

1977, when the *New York Times* revealed in a front-page story that the Society for the Investigation of Human Ecology was a front for the CIA. The article was based on thousands of classified CIA documents that John Marks had secured through numerous freedom of information requests. (They consisted mainly of financial records, which had been overlooked when the order was given in 1973 to destroy all MKULTRA records.) The expossure would have deeply troubled Sargant, regardless of whether the two men shared the same paymasters. Cameron's treatments, as we have seen, were similar to Sargant's in many key respects. They had now been publicly discredited in a major news story that soon went global.

There might not be any correspondence between them in Sargant's personal papers, but there are letters aplenty in the archives of the American Psychiatric Association: ten from 'Ewen' to 'Will' and thirteen from 'Will' to 'Ewen', written between December 1964 and March 1966 and mostly concerning World Psychiatric Association matters and minutes. Sargant organised its first European symposium at the Royal College of Physicians in London, on 28–30 September 1965, and there was much discussion about the billing. (They settled on 'The Psychiatric Disorders of the Aged and their Treatment'.) They also discussed the symposium's sponsor, Geigy, which had sponsored the 1959 conference in Montreal. Geigy was 'turning up trumps', according to Sargant, putting 'the whole of their publicity department' at the WPA's disposal. Sargant was delighted that 'all seats' were taken, 'overflow meetings' would be required and that people were 'coming from all over the world'. Cameron didn't attend in person, but he sent a congratulatory cable to Sargant. Cameron was also keen to push forward with other regional meetings, including in Sudan, India and Taiwan, discussing whether to approach Smith, Kline & French or stick with Geigy.

In among all the committee chat there are some more

revealing exchanges. Cameron concluded an administrative letter, dated 26 February 1965, by adding that he'd like to catch up with Sargant on his travels. Sargant had written ten days earlier to say that he would be lecturing in St Louis and Chicago, before going down to Trinidad and Haiti for 'abreactive research', followed by a lecture in Los Angeles. Cameron, who was now working at the Veterans Administration Hospital in Albany, New York, was keen to intercept him to 'talk a little bit about various matters'. Whatever it was that he wanted to discuss with Sargant, he felt unable to commit it to paper. Was it about funding? Or Sargant's work in Haiti, where the CIA was active? (According to Peggy, Sargant managed to get into Papa Doc's presidential palace.)

In another letter, dated 21 January 1966, Cameron tells Sargant that it was 'very sound' to get Juan José López-Ibor to talk at the European Symposium in London. But it's in a letter from Sargant to Cameron, dated 17 November 1965, that we see the first real evidence of the two men's complicity in extreme physical treatments.

They agreed to share patients.

'About that girl aged 21,' Sargant wrote in reply to a letter from Cameron that's not in the archive, 'one can never throw in one's hand in cases like this until all the treatments have been tried.' The patient in question was suicidal with depression – a suitable candidate for the Sleep Room. 'The thing to do is to give continuous sleep, and under sleep treatment give ECT and the antidepressant drugs,' Sargant said, adding that he had used this method effectively on patients who had been ill for a considerable time. They must, however, be of 'good previous personality'.

Sargant also suggested that she should consider being seen by him in Britain, where treatment 'was far more intense' than in America because 'they are so scared of combining anything with anything'. He asked Cameron to tell the parents 'either to bring her over here and let me see her, or it may be cheaper if I saw her on one of my trips to the USA'. Lobotomy was another option, followed by further ECT and narcosis – 'you may find that the treatments she did not respond to before the leucotomy will now do the trick'.

Cameron replied twelve days later, thanking Sargant for his suggestions. He gave the patient's name and location, and said that he had asked her mother to contact Sargant directly and decide whether the treatment would be done in London or America. It's a remarkable exchange. If Cameron had still been at the Allan Memorial Institute, both men knew that he could have treated the patient there, but he had resigned suddenly from his post in Montreal in the summer of 1964 and no longer had his own Sleep Room.

In 1967, their friendship was once again in evidence, in the pages of Sargant's autobiography, *The Unquiet Mind* – or at least in the US edition. Intriguingly, there is no reference to him in the British edition, but the first American copies carried a glowing preface written by Ewen Cameron himself. 'Sargant is an extraordinary man, living through extraordinary times,' he enthused. 'There is hardly a major discovery which has been made within the great upward surge of psychiatry in which Sargant did not take part and to which he did not add . . . The wellspring of his life is an intense compassion for his suffering fellowmen . . . Many of the things that appalled those of us who entered psychiatry in the early twenties have gone . . . The doors have been opened, the smells, the screams have gone.' Patients at the Allen Memorial might beg to differ about the screams.

A few months after he wrote these words, Cameron was dead. 'It is difficult to think of his not being with us any more,' the *British Medical Journal*'s obituary eulogised. 'Ewen Cameron, by his work and example, helped not only many psychiatrists to become much better doctors but directly and indirectly helped hundreds and hundreds of patients, both personally and through those he had inspired and taught . . . I have lost a much admired and inspiring friend, and so have many other people.'

The obituary was written by one 'W.S.'

32

'I don't suppose it's breaking the Official Secrets Act to say this . . .'

From the moment Sargant took up his post at St Thomas' in 1948, he had been adamant that his department would be dedicated to three things: treatment, clinical teaching and research. It's the last of these that has aroused most suspicion over the years, amid allegations that Sargant shared his research with Porton Down, MI5, MI6 and the CIA, or was even funded by them. Ewen Cameron's own researcher and technician, after all, were funded by the CIA between 1957 and 1960.

Ward Five was part of the Royal Waterloo, which had joined St Thomas' in 1948. Both hospitals were run by the NHS, which paid the doctors' and nurses' salaries. One exception was the researchers, some of whom were paid for out of St Thomas' Endowment fund. Sargant was adept at persuading various hospital committees to give him money. The minutes of St Thomas' Research Advisory Committee, for example, show how he fought hard to have a research registrar. He even convinced the Endowment Fund Sub-Committee to pay for a research secretary. In June 1958, the Finance Committee approved 'the grant of £1,200 for the salary of a full-time research registrar in the department of psychological medicine be renewed for a further year, subject to review at the end of that time'. And in a long letter to the chairman of the Medical Committee in 1959, Sargant applied for a grant to renew his psychiatric research registrar, which the endowment funds 'have been kind enough to recommend' in recent years.

His department, he wrote, had been 'extremely fortunate' to have the services of Dr Peter Dally and several research projects were 'coming to fruition'. Sargant went on to justify Dally's appointment, describing his work on anorexia nervosa* and the success of combining 'large doses of Largactil' with modified insulin. 'This research registrarship continues to be of the very greatest importance to the department,' Sargant added, 'for it enables us to investigate all these new drug treatments.'

Research was also good for Sargant's own reputation – and bank balance. The more papers that were published, the more private patients would come knocking. And there was no question that Sargant liked to make money. According to one former colleague, he was more than happy to be paid in cash by his overseas patients. If someone wanted to pay by cheque, 'Sargant with two a's' was a phrase never far from his lips. But there could be another explanation for his interest in hiring researchers. Two of them were certainly no run-of-the-mill medics. And one of them, Peter Dally, would go on to work for MI6.

Dally had been Sargant's house physician in 1955 before he

* On his retirement from the Westminster Hospital, the anorexia clinic was named after Dally; it was later renamed, after a scandal that had nothing to do with him.

became his research registrar. Asked about truth drugs by Dominic Streatfeild, he replied: 'Experimentation took place in a vague sort of way ... At the Royal Waterloo Hospital, part of St Thomas', we used to experiment in whether or not we could get confessions from people ... who were suspected of this or that. But it wasn't done in any sort of scientific way.' Dally left St Thomas' in 1961 to be consultant psychiatrist at the Westminster Hospital, but not before attending the Third World Congress of Psychiatry in Montreal in June of that year, where Cameron announced the formation of the World Psychiatric Association. Dally remained in close touch with Sargant, helping him with the fourth edition of *An Introduction to Physical Methods of Treatment in Psychiatry*. He also took care of Sargant's private patients when he was given free use of his consulting room at 23 Harley Street for six months in 1961.

It was during this time that he most likely began to work for the intelligence services. His ex-wife Ann told Streatfeild: '[Peter] saw an awful lot of spies. I mean, he used to vet them, you know. I know there was one – I don't suppose it's breaking the Official Secrets Act to say this – but there was one that they were very proud of. They had a splendid spy and they sent him to see Peter for vetting and Peter said he thought he'd changed sides. And they were rather cross about that because he was their special spy. Anyway, he did change sides.' According to Ben Spears, Sargant's former registrar, Dally also treated Kim Philby's third wife, Eleanor. She told him that the former MI6 officer, who defected to the Soviet Union in 1963, had taught her 'how to swallow messages on paper'.

Sargant, it seems, was already fulfilling a similar role for potential employees of the intelligence services. 'A candidate would be invited to spend a weekend at a country house, and I would cast an eye over him or her,' Sargant told Gordon Thomas. He would then write a report, 'noting whether the chap or girl drank a drop too much, was too talkative, or too familiar with others in the house party'. And Ann Dally herself saw a few MI6 employees in the 1970s who were depressed or 'otherwise disturbed'. 'It was only occasional. We didn't have whole clinics of spies or anything. But it was a sort of interesting aspect to the work. Made a change.'

The intelligence community had good reason to call upon the services of psychiatrists. Maintaining a cover story in the field could be stressful; so too an agent's day-to-day work in a clandestine office. 'Many senior officers in MI5 had counselling of one form or another during their careers to assist them in carrying the burdens of secrecy,' said the late Peter Wright.

Wright had first-hand experience. In 1964, he was asked to look into the background of Michael Hanley, who had been promoted to the level of 'Director C' in MI5 four years earlier and was widely tipped to be a future Director General. (He indeed became DG in 1972.) In 1964, however, there were fears that a Russian mole had penetrated the middle ranks of MI5. Hanley was a 'perfect fit'.

Wright looked into Hanley's background and discovered that he had been visiting a Harley Street psychiatrist since the early 1950s. His childhood had been 'most distressing', following the break-up of his parents' marriage. He was left with 'deep-seated feelings of inferiority', which, according to his record of service, required psychiatric treatment in the 1950s, when he was a young MI5 officer, a fact that Hanley had made known to his employers at the time.

The Director General, Martin Furnival Jones, duly wrote a letter to the unnamed psychiatrist, asking him to lift his oath of patient confidentiality. Wright was then dispatched to talk with the psychiatrist. He showed no hesitation in pronouncing Hanley 'a determined, robust character' who had learned to live with his 'early disabilities'. When Wright asked him if he could ever conceive of Hanley as a spy, the psychiatrist, with 'total conviction', replied 'Absolutely not!'

Sargant was nothing if not a man of total conviction. Could he have been the unnamed psychiatrist? If he was the private shrink of the future Director General, it would explain why he went on to work so closely with the intelligence services. Wright's book, *Spycatcher*, caused a huge stir when it was published in 1987.* But what people often forget is that the book was ghostwritten by Paul Greengrass, who went on to become one of Hollywood's most successful film directors (*Bloody Sunday*, three Jason Bourne films, *United 93*, *Green Zone*, *Captain Phillips*, *22 July*, etc). Did Greengrass, perhaps, know the identity of Hanley's psychiatrist?

'I never knew the name,' he told me. 'All I knew is that there was – according to Peter Wright – an in-house psychiatrist in Harley Street. He was very clear on that, and of course it makes total sense. I can't see that someone in Hanley's position would go outside the service. He was already a high-flyer at that time. As to whether it was Sargant – who knows? Though based on your research, it seems a heck of a coincidence.'

Hanley's son, Peter, now living in Spain, says that, understandably, he knows 'next to nothing' about his father's professional life. 'I do, however, remember him being highly disapproving of psychotherapy in general,' he says. '"They do more harm than good!"' Sceptical words that, once again, could have been spoken by Sargant. Peter Dally, another possibility, was less against it.

---

* The British government initially managed to prevent the publication of *Spycatcher* in Britain, on grounds of national security. Peter Wright had not only alleged that a former Director General of MI5 had been a Soviet mole, but that a cabal of disaffected MI5 agents had plotted against Harold Wilson when he was prime minster. It was explosive stuff. Margaret Thatcher, then prime minister, famously sent her Cabinet secretary, Robert Armstrong, to Sydney in late 1986 – in vain as it turned out – to prevent its publication in Australia. Armstrong was subsequently credited with coining the phrase 'economical with the truth' (although he always claimed it was first used by Edmund Burke). Documents recently released by the National Archives reveal that Thatcher was left 'utterly shattered' by the book's sensational claims.

'Every patient needs psychotherapy,' he once said. Dally was, however, central to another spy scandal in 1964, when he was asked by MI6 to sedate the British businessman Greville Wynne, who had been released in a prisoner swap with the Soviet spy Gordon Lonsdale. Back in London, Wynne was manic and talking too much, posing a threat to national security. Dally oversaw his care in a private room at the Gordon Hospital, an acute mental health facility in Westminster, where he was kept 'under heavy sedation'.

The historian Nigel West is certain that Sargant's patients included the occasional spook. 'Sargant was undoubtedly on the X list – an index of approved professionals and contractors who are cleared to work for the intelligence services,' he says. 'I know that he took over from Harold Dearden as MI5's go-to psychiatrist – someone whose services they could call on, twenty-four hours a day, to assess the mental health of employees or, occasionally, potential defectors.'

Sargant's other researcher in 1960 was Peter Rohde – one of three that Sargant had managed to persuade the committee to pay for. (John Pollitt, recently returned from a year in America, was another.) Rohde's research involved following up on ninety-five patients with schizophrenia who had been treated at St Thomas' between 1950 and 1959. The findings were published in the *British Medical Journal*, which stated that Rohde had been 'working on a grant from the Endowment Funds of St Thomas' Hospital, London'. Rohde left in September 1960, after two years as Sargant's researcher. His next job was an interesting choice: a military psychiatrist. For four years, he was based in Hong Kong, running a research project that studied sick soldiers and army prisoners.

Sargant's research jobs clearly opened doors, whether it was to the intelligence services or the military. In September 1963, Sargant once again raised the subject of a research grant for a senior registrar at a Research Advisory Committee meeting, this time explaining that an anonymous donor had stepped forward.

The committee's clerk reported that the donor had offered to contribute a sum of £3,000 towards the salary of a research registrar in the department of Psychological Medicine. The donor had also indicated that more money could be found to continue the appointment for a further two years. Perhaps to add a veneer of respectability, the anonymous donor had asked for the post to be advertised in the *Lancet* and the *British Medical Journal*. The successful applicant 'would be appointed by the governors in the usual way'.

£3,000 in 1963 is the equivalent of £80,000 today – a decent salary, in other words. Who was behind the donation? And why the secrecy? The Research Advisory Committee seems to have had its own concerns: 'As soon as the research registrar is appointed, the nature of the problem on which he is to work be made known to the committee and a detailed report be submitted to the committee at the end of the first year.' The Medical Committee also had to 'be informed of the nature of the work'.

Both committees had good reason to be cautious. Unbeknown to them, the CIA had paid the salary of a 'full time research psychiatrist' for Ewen Cameron, making payments through its front organisation between 1957 and 1960. The amount? $7,000, which equates to around $77,000 today.

Could the CIA have been behind the donation to pay for a researcher at St Thomas'? A declassified Agency report from 1963 had specifically said: 'A number of the grants have included funds for the construction and equipping of research facilities and for the employment of research assistants.' Unfortunately, the Agency refuses to confirm or deny the existence of records on foreign nationals. According to Gordon Thomas, Allen Dulles had talked of the need to crack the mystery of brainwashing, which is why he set up the Society for the Investigation of Human Ecology as a cover organisation to coordinate research.

Turning to Sargant at one of his cocktail parties, Dulles had asked if the British psychiatrist 'would continue to act as liaison between the foundation and similar research going on in Britain at Porton Down'. Sargant had apparently agreed.

The CIA-backed society/fund was certainly active in Britain in the sixties. Records are incomplete but there is evidence that it financed two academic projects in the UK. In 1961, Hans Eysenck, professor of psychology at the Institute of Psychiatry, then based at the Maudsley, wrote a rather dry paper on how to measure human motivation. Eysenck and his co-author wrote that they were 'indebted' to the Society for the Investigation of Human Ecology for a grant that made their study possible. Sidney Gottlieb approved a grant of $27,360 for 1 June 1960 to 31 May 1962, and MKULTRA Subproject 111 was up and running in the UK.

There is no evidence that either author knew of the CIA's involvement. In 1996, however, Channel 4's *Dispatches* programme revealed that Eysenck had received more than £800,000 from a secret tobacco industry fund known as Special Account Number Four. When confronted about the source of his funding, he said, 'As long as somebody pays for the research, I don't care who it is.'

In April 1961, James Monroe of the Society for the Investigation of Human Ecology had also approached a colourful counter-culture character called Steve Abrams, a graduate student at St Catherine's College, Oxford. Chicago born, he had arrived in Oxford in 1960 to write a doctoral thesis on extra-sensory perception and had soon set up a (short-lived) parapsychology laboratory at the university. Later in the 1960s, he became a controversial cannabis law reform campaigner in Britain.

Monroe had heard about Abrams' parapsychology research and encouraged him to apply for funding. MKULTRA Subproject 136 was given the go-ahead in August 1961 and Abrams received $8,579 to 'support the research in Oxford of an "Experimental Analysis of Extrasensory Perception"'.

In particular, he was to explore how ESP could be used 'as a method of communication'.

Abrams filed his report in March 1963, but he had already worked out – using ESP, presumably – who his real paymasters were.

There is another explanation. Despite Abrams' professed indignation (he claimed he was driven out of Oxford when it emerged that his work had been CIA funded), he might have been closer to the Agency than he let on in public. He had a 'near uncle' who worked in military intelligence and had taken part in experiments while he was a student at Duke University that 'had been performed in connexion with a private interest of Mr Dulles'. His personal papers at the Wellcome Collection also include what appears to be a certificate of graduation (with merit) from the CIA 'Training Academy', dated 15 July 1959 and signed by Arnold Delaney, Director, Office of Training and Education.*

The Human Ecology Fund, as the CIA cut-out was now called, was disbanded in 1965, so it could theoretically have covered the first two years of Sargant's research registrar's salary – and the first years of his Sleep Room, which opened in 1964, the same year as Cameron's had closed. The fund certainly knew about Sargant's work. In 1960, it had published a paper entitled 'Brainwashing: A Guide to the Literature', which included two references to Sargant. One of them, not surprisingly, mentioned his 1957 bestseller, *Battle for the Mind*. The other was a paper that

---

* In July 1961, just before Abrams received his Oxford funding, he passed through Washington Airport and called Allen Dulles' office. Dulles was in his last few months as Director of Central Intelligence. Abrams spoke to someone called Bricker, whom he had apparently talked to in the past. Bricker arranged for Abrams to meet Richard Lashbrook, deputy head of MKULTRA (and the man who had handed Frank Olson his LSD-spiked Cointreau). Abrams was told to go to a coffee shop at the north end of the airport terminal and wait, holding an umbrella in his right hand. When Lashbrook arrived, they talked for three hours. Abrams asked if the CIA would fund his forthcoming trip to meet fellow parapsychologists in Russia, but the Agency declined.

Sargant had written almost twenty years earlier, in 1942, for the British Medical Journal, entitled 'Physical Treatment of Acute War Neuroses'.

There are no more details in St Thomas' minutes about Sargant's anonymous donor. Guy's and St Thomas' NHS Foundation Trust was also unable to shed any further light on the source of Sargant's funding. It couldn't even confirm whether the Sleep Room was private or funded by the NHS. 'The Trust does not hold this information,' it replied to a freedom of information request. Nor could it confirm or deny whether Sargant had destroyed patients' records when he left the NHS in 1972, as some have alleged. 'The Trust does not hold this information,' it repeated.

Guy's and St Thomas' NHS Foundation Trust did, however, apologise, for the first time, for what happened in the Sleep Room: 'We are very sorry for any distress caused to patients treated by Dr Sargant at his sleep service at St Thomas' Hospital and the Royal Waterloo Hospital. Due to the historic nature of this service we unfortunately do not hold any records from this time, but we fully acknowledge the impact that these treatments may have had on patients and their families.'

Sargant was usually quite open about his research benefactors. Writing in 1965 about his outpatient work in Scutari, he acknowledged that 'Funds of St Thomas'' and a 'special grant from Robert Sainsbury, the Governor General of St Thomas'' had financed a research registrar. Another paper (on lobotomy), co-authored by Sargant in 1966, also acknowledged a 'generous donation' from Sainsbury.

In an article for the *BMJ* in 1966, Sargant looked back on his achievements since 1948 and was adamant that he had received 'no official outside research support whatsoever'. However, he added, 'valuable help was obtained from the endowment funds of St Thomas'' and from 'gifts of money from private lay persons', a carefully worded phrase he repeated in his autobiography.

Lord Owen suggests that 'Sargant may well have steered some of his richer patients to make a donation to St Thomas' hospital trust'. Nita Mitchell-Heggs also dismisses any suspicion about anonymous donations. After working as a house officer on Ward Five for six months in 1968, she was a research registrar on Scutari until 1972. (She later moved to St George's, where she retrained and had an illustrious thirty-year career in occupational medicine.)

'Sargant had so many grateful patients,' she says today. 'There would have been countless donations. The department was always full of huge boxes of top-notch chocolates and biscuits, which the nurses and junior docs loved.' She is not surprised to learn that there was an anonymous donor, given that psychiatric illness was, at the time, something that families may have wished to keep private. 'Many of the patients we treated were well-known, and wealthy, public figures,' she says. 'I can think of a time when the small ward was treating two aristocrats, an MP's nephew, a prima ballerina and a foreign royal. All but one did well (they had an underlying untreatable medical condition) and one went on to marry his nurse!* Funding a post would have been peanuts. I could easily imagine their wanting to make a donation but not wishing an episode of mental ill health to become public knowledge.'

But donating top-notch chocolates was one thing; offering to pay someone's salary for three years was quite another.

---

* In 1969, Patrick Pakenham, the second son of Lord Longford, married Mary Plummer, one of the nurses who cared for him on Ward Five. A witty and compassionate criminal barrister with an extraordinary memory (he could recite the Latin Credo backwards, for example), Pakenham suffered from manic depression, which would eventually cut short his distinguished legal career. (His mother, Elizabeth, was the sister of John Harman, Sargant's close friend.)

33

'I couldn't imagine why the CIA would be interested in my work'

In October 1959, Sargant was awarded a 'medical achievement' travel prize for his 'studies of the mechanics of indoctrination, brain-washing and thought control'. The award was given by Purdue Frederick, the drugs company that had been purchased by the Sackler brothers in 1952 and would later become Purdue Pharma – manufacturer of OxyContin, the addictive opioid that has caused so many deaths in America. The three Sackler brothers, Arthur, Mortimer and Raymond, had already expressed considerable interest in the 1950s in the new physical treatments in psychiatry, editing (with Félix Martí-Ibáñez) an extraordinary little book that celebrated them in grand style.

In *The Great Physiodynamic Therapies in Psychiatry: An Historical Reappraisal* (1956), Ugo Cerletti, Ladislas Meduna, Egas Moniz and Manfred Sakel – a hall of fame or a rogues' gallery, depending on your point of view – were given a platform to wax lyrical about ECT, Cardiazol, lobotomy and insulin coma treatments. Perhaps Sargant's medical achievement prize was consolation for not being included in the book.

Some suspect that it was Big Pharma, rather than the intelligence services, which funded Sargant's work on Ward Five. Sargant, like the Sacklers, strongly believed that drugs were the key to curing most mental illnesses, prescribing them with unprecedented zeal. There is certainly evidence that two pharmaceutical companies in particular might have funded his Sleep Room.

In June 1972, Sargant published a paper with Chris Walter and Nita Mitchell-Heggs, entitled 'Modified Narcosis, ECT and Antidepressant Drugs: A Review of Technique and Immediate Outcome'. It looked back on six years of his signature treatment: deep sleep therapy with electric shocks. Published in the *British Journal of Psychiatry*, two months after he had retired, it bore all the hallmarks of a legacy project. There was also an intriguing footnote: 'We should like to express our gratitude to Geigy (UK) Ltd, and to Roche Products Ltd, for financial support throughout the study.'

Does 'throughout the study' mean from 1962 to 1968? It was, and continues to be, common for medical research to be externally funded, sometimes by charities. Individual researchers too were often financed by what was known as 'soft money' from pharmaceutical firms. Mitchell-Heggs, whose sole contribution to Sargant's academic papers was to provide statistics and proof-read them, says that her research psychiatry posts were 'entirely funded' by money from pharmaceutical companies. The money, she says, went directly to the hospital finance department. 'Finance paid me in the normal NHS way,' she says. 'I was part of the team. The donation covered, I believe, all expenses relating to my NHS post.' She says there was nothing secret about her research positions and she applied for them in the normal way. For her job at St Thomas', she was interviewed by the full medical board – 'about thirty medical people in the boardroom, plus HR people'. The source of the funding was not discussed. 'I didn't realise, until later on, well into my role, that there was pharma funding to the finance department.' As for the acknowledgement of Geigy and Roche at the end of her paper, she says it was always the 'done thing' to express thanks to any benefactors.

Sargant had a particularly close relationship with Geigy. He gave one of its drugs, Tofranil, to patients during narcosis, controversially mixing it with Nardil. Sargant had also arranged for Geigy to sponsor the World Psychiatric Association symposium in London in September 1965. According to Cameron's papers at the American Psychiatric Association, Sargant's contact at Geigy was its UK marketing director, Stewart Kipling, who liaised with head office in Basle. Geigy deemed the symposium a big success and afterwards, Kipling wrote to Cameron, then president of the WPA, expressing his wish to continue the 'splendid relationship' that Geigy had with Sargant.

Geigy was due to sponsor a second WPA symposium, to be held in Khartoum in spring 1966 and once again arranged by Sargant. Entitled 'Treatment in Psychiatry', it would be his swan song – he was due to step down from the WPA committee in September 1966. 'Geigy have really gone to town and we are getting people from all over Africa and the Near East,' Sargant wrote to Cameron. On both occasions, Geigy produced a newspaper that Sargant said was 'circulated to doctors all over the world'.

But then, it seems, the conference was put back to the end of the year, after Sargant would have stood down. The rescheduling did not go down well with Geigy, who would only collaborate with Sargant. 'We do hope that the officials of the WPA do understand that our desire to work with you on this symposium is based very much on the respect that we have for you as a result of our past co-operation,' Mr Kipling wrote to Sargant. Sargant duly brought the conference back to March and Geigy sponsored it to the tune of £6,000 (£140,000 today).

Sargant stayed on in Sudan after the symposium to film Nilotic tribes in the south. Ever since his experience of snake handlers in the American Deep South, he had become increasingly interested in possession, mysticism, trance, sexual ecstasy and faith healing, all of which he would explore in *The Mind Possessed*. Robert Graves couldn't be persuaded to help him with the writing; instead Sargant turned to Richard Cavendish, a historian who wrote about occultism, religion and mythology. The first half of the book revisited his theories of heightened suggestibility; the second chronicled his extensive travels in Africa, India, South America and Haiti.

With one eye, perhaps, on his future book, Sargant had made sure the Khartoum symposium included traditional healing – 'which used to be called witch doctoring', as he explained in a letter to Cameron. He wasn't keen on what he called 'transcultural psychiatry'. In his opinion, all mental illnesses were the same the world over, and were not influenced by society or environment, as others were arguing. He then added a comment that suggested he was dispensing antidepressant drugs as he travelled through Africa. 'I also found that the depressions in these tribes respond to Nardil and Tofranil in the same way as ours do over here.' Sargant's missionary zeal for prescribing drugs had gone global.

There might have been another reason for Sargant's trips to Africa. At the same time as he was dispensing drugs in Sudan, a Canadian psychiatrist, Dr Raymond Prince of McGill University, was studying Yoruba witchcraft in Nigeria. Prince had been working in the country since 1957, including stints with the Nigerian government and with fellow psychiatrist Professor Thomas Lambo in Abeokuta. In 1963, he undertook a one-year study of the Yoruba people and how they treated mental illness. What he didn't realise was that the source of his funding – the Human Ecology Fund – was in fact a CIA cut-out. (The Agency's financial support for Prince ran from 1960 to 1963 as part of

MKULTRA, Subproject 121.) 'I couldn't imagine why the CIA would be interested in my work,' Prince said later. 'Looking at indigenous healers in West Africa – that seemed really strange.' He concluded that the CIA had funded his research in Nigeria to lend credibility to the Human Ecology Fund.

The CIA had other ideas. A witch doctor's power to heal, or to curse, fell well within MKULTRA's remit. Putting a hex on someone was seen as a form of mind control that warranted further investigation. John Gittinger, the CIA psychologist (and Sidney Gottlieb's protégé), believed that anyone who could explain why someone might 'run amok in Indonesia', or 'die of a sickness from a witch doctor in Africa' was worth knowing, adding to the Agency's understanding of 'behavioural science'.

Sargant, like Prince, had published a number of papers on traditional healers, including 'Witch Doctoring, Zar and Voodoo: Their Relation to Modern Psychiatric Treatments' (1967), the research for which ended up in *The Mind Possessed*. Sargant was also a global authority on mind control, following the success of *Battle for the Mind*. In a letter to Cameron about the proposed symposium in Africa, he had said that there was a lot of evidence that witch doctors, or traditional healers, were capable of indoctrinating people at puberty and taking 'complete control' of their communities' beliefs.

If the CIA didn't fund Sargant's trips to Africa, Haiti and beyond, it had missed a trick.

PART 4

34

'There was nothing about them that was human'

Catherine Mountain was in her second year as a student nurse when she was sent to work on Ward Five in 1965. The radio in the communal room was tuned to Radio Caroline, the pirate station that had been founded the year before. 'Michelle' by the Beatles was being played all the time. 'It was like twilight in the narcosis room, with thin curtains,' says Catherine.

Other patients on Ward Five were understandably upset by the sight of patients being led to the bathroom in their hospital gowns. The matter was soon addressed by St Thomas' General Purposes Committee. According to the minutes, patients undergoing narcosis treatment had to be taken along the ward corridor and down steps to the lavatories. 'This was dangerous for them in case they fell and the other patients became reluctant to have this treatment themselves after seeing the effects during treatment.' A lavatory and small hand basin was subsequently fitted in an adjoining room.

By 1964, Sargant had twenty-two beds on Ward Five, including six in the Sleep Room. Later he would have up to twenty-six beds, with more squeezed into the Sleep Room when required. At one point there were eight; sometimes as few as four. Ward Five itself comprised a mix of one- and two-bed rooms, including two that were private, one amenity room, a dining room and treatment rooms. The private rooms were also occasionally used for narcosis and a two-bed bay was reserved for men. (Most patients and nurses can only recall a few men who had narcosis – the vast majority were women.)

The Sleep Room itself, immediately to the left as you entered the ward, operated from 1964 to 1973. Sargant made a point of recruiting general rather than psychiatric staff and many were young student nurses. 'We dreaded being put down for Ward Five because of the reputation of the narcosis room,' says Sue, who was sent there in 1972, during her third year of training. 'You knew it would be pretty grim, with loads of ECT and spending a lot of time in the dark.' Sargant, by contrast, felt that general nurses in training provided 'a tremendous psychotherapeutic boost'.

She remembers that the Sleep Room could hold up to eight patients. 'We had to wake them every six hours, day and night, and help them, confused and stumbling, to the bathroom, to eat and drink, and to take another huge cocktail of drugs to sedate them again.' Ann Rowland, who was a nurse on Ward Five in 1967, during her Nightingale year, says working in the Sleep Room was 'awful' and that there was something 'really odd' about it. The women were 'drugged up to the eyeballs' and unable to hold a conversation. 'We had to clean their teeth for them.'

Three shifts of young nurses covered the Sleep Room, with some overlaps for meetings and reports to be written up. 'It was a half life we all became accustomed to,' recalls Shelley, who was in her Nightingale year when she worked there in 1968. Visiting hours on the ward were from 2 to 6 p.m. and 7 to 8 p.m., except for narcosis patients. 'They went for weeks and weeks, not being seen by their nearest and dearest,' says Tish, who was assigned to the Sleep Room during her second year of nurse training in 1971. 'They were depersonalised – there was nothing about them that was human.' Medication was given at six-hourly intervals (7 a.m., 1 p.m., 7 p.m., 1 a.m.). Largactil was the main drug, given four times a day in doses of between 100mg to 400mg (up to 600mg in a one-off dose for 'very disturbed' patients). In 1972, Sargant suggested that he'd sometimes given even larger doses. 'Doses of up to 3,000mg a day have been reported,' he said, 'but we have rarely had to give more than 1,200mg a day.'*

He also sedated patients with between 100mg and 400mg of sodium amytal, the barbiturate he'd first used at Belmont twenty years earlier, given in six-hourly intervals. Ewen Cameron's own Sleep Room treatments are often perceived as having been more extreme than Sargant's. But in 1964 Cameron had administered similar drugs to his patients in markedly smaller doses: 50mg of Largactil three times a day combined with a mixture of barbiturates; Seconal (100mg), Nembutal (100mg) and sodium amytal (150mg). In other words, Sargant was giving patients more than *ten times* more Largactil a day than Cameron (1,600 mg vs 150mg) and at least 50 per cent more barbiturates (1,600mg vs 1,050mg).

Sargant also gave antidepressants to his patients while they slept. Initially, he administered tricyclics and MAOIs, a combination that many thought was dangerous; later he dropped the tricyclics when they were thought to cause potentially fatal constipation. By 1966, Sargant had conceded the dangers of sodium amytal too. 'Although anxiety was greatly reduced, this drug also led to confusion and a feeling of intense apprehension in the withdrawal period, and occasionally to withdrawal fits, and

---

* Sue has kept her drug book, in which nurses wrote down recommended doses for patients. As well as giving narcosis patients up to 600mg of Largactil, four times a day, anorexic patients on Ward Five were also being prescribed 400mg of Largactil, three times a day ('400mg tds', as she wrote).

we now rarely use it in narcosis,' he wrote. From 1966, Sargant used Mandrax as his preferred sedative. It proved an equally controversial choice, because of its addictive properties, which some experts said were on a par with heroin.

The one constant in the Sleep Room – Sargant's and Cameron's – was the use of ECT, which was initially given to patients at their bedside, and then later in a small room nearby. By the 1960s, the use of muscle relaxants was standard and bone fractures were rare. The treatment, though, remained an ordeal for patients as well as for the nurses. 'They still fitted horribly,' says Tish, who would accompany them from the Sleep Room. 'You were jerking their brain with electricity,' Sue says. 'Some of them might be sick.' Afterwards, she would watch over them in the Sleep Room, where they lay moaning, half asleep in the recovery position. 'It was awful actually, yet you were so persuaded by Sargant that this was the right way forward.'

One house officer who worked on Ward Five and wishes to remain nameless stresses the need to see these experiences of student nurses in a wider medical context. 'Coming *de novo* from general nursing, they would have found many things about being on a psychiatric ward very challenging,' they say. 'Some of the patients were disturbed. The Sleep Room was a bit spooky! Dim light with six sleeping bodies. It certainly might have struck very young student nurses as weird and almost dystopian.'

Sargant didn't seem too concerned if young nurses were spooked by the Sleep Room. Experienced psychiatric nurses might have questioned what went on in there and he didn't want anyone meddling. Now that longer periods of sleep could be induced more safely with Largactil, he believed that ECT combined with continuous narcosis was a winning formula – a dark alchemy of drugs and electricity.

The Sleep Room was the ultimate expression of Sargant's long held belief in shock therapy and 'heroic' doses of drugs, the twin pillars of his controversial approach to psychiatry. The treatment, he said, was best suited to patients suffering from schizophrenia. He also believed that it was good for treating mid-life or menopausal patients with depression, providing, of course, they were of 'good previous personality'.

It also existed at a time when patient consent had yet to become an issue. It would take the likes of R. D. Laing, the campaigning work of MIND (the National Association for Mental Health) and the engagement of the civil rights movement in America with detained patients (prompted, ironically, by Henry Beecher's 1966 paper on ethics) for consent to become enshrined in the Mental Health Act 1983, by which time Sargant had retired. Remarkably, the 1959 Act, under which the Sleep Room operated, made no reference at all to consent. And the power to detain and treat psychiatric patients no longer lay with magistrates but largely with the responsible medical officer (RMO) – a consultant psychiatrist such as Sargant. (Doctors were also protected from legal action.) Not surprisingly, he hailed the Act as enabling him and his colleagues to 'lead the world in implementing sane and practical psychiatric treatments'.

One of the ironies of the legislation is that it had tried to reduce the stigma of admission to a psychiatric hospital by making it easier for people to be admitted voluntarily. But these 'informal' patients often ended up with fewer rights than those who had been sectioned. As Phil Fennell, a Mental Health Act commissioner from 1983 to 1989, says, this is 'one of the central paradoxes' of the psychiatric system in England and Wales: the treatment of sectioned patients has long been subject to closer scrutiny than those who might nominally 'agree' to be admitted (or whose families agree).

It remains unclear exactly how many ECT treatments Sargant subjected his patients to while they slept or whether they were aware of their treatment before being admitted to the Sleep Room. (One of the inherent difficulties of seeking the consent of psychiatric patients and explaining their treatment is that the very illness that they are being treated for – and the drugs they have initially been given – often clouds their judgement and cognitive faculties.) In 1965, Sargant said that ECT was still being 'intensively used'. Sue remembers it was given three times a week in the Sleep Room in 1971. Writing a year later about narcosis and ECT, Sargant said that 'for some resistant patients who may have been ill for years, up to 20 to 30 ECT during the treatment many finally be needed. Many failures of the past seem to have been due to breaking off ECT too soon.'

Twenty years on from when he had first administered ECT with a primitive shock box, Sargant had refined his technique and equipment, although he still preferred a small portable unit with a 'well cleaned head and good electric contact'. Insufficient voltage produced sub-shocks – a 'momentary loss of consciousness, but no convulsion', which caused 'cardiac irregularities' that could subsequently deepen the patient's depression.

The biggest change from the 1940s was the development of new short-acting muscle relaxants that paralysed the body and prevented fractures. They were given once the patient had been anaesthetised with a rapid-onset barbiturate such as sodium pentothal. The effects of curare would last for up to forty-five minutes, whereas Scoline (suxamethonium chloride, known by medics simply as 'sux') would wear off after five minutes. Unfortunately, it wasn't just the limbs that were paralysed; the respiratory muscles stopped working too, which meant that the lungs had to be artificially ventilated. It was also essential that no food was taken for at least four hours prior to treatment, in case the patient regurgitated his gastric contents. Sargant warned that paralysis of the throat muscles could permit 'inhalation of the vomitus'. And it was important that the patient was unconscious before the muscle relaxant was administered. Otherwise, Sargant said, the feeling of 'progressive paralysis' would be 'terrifying'.

An oxygen mask was routine, especially if the patient was elderly or suffering from arthritis and full paralysis was required. In such circumstances, it was sometimes difficult to establish if a fit had taken place. 'Normally, however, the toes may be seen to be twitching slightly, and there may be slight movement of the facial muscles,' he wrote in 1972.

It was a benign, reassuring image of ECT and one that Sargant was keen to promote. And yet, in the same year, he also admitted that, 'for some special reason', ECT might still have to be given 'in the raw', without a muscle relaxant or sedation – just as it would be so disturbingly depicted three years later by Jack Nicholson in *One Flew Over the Cuckoo's Nest* (1975). Unmodified ECT had been used in Broadmoor in the 1950s as a form of deterrent or corrective, and continued to be 'open to abuse, in the guise of an emergency treatment', according to Fennell. If it had to be done, Sargant said, the patient needed to be restrained but instead of a straitjacket he had swapped in a 'special canvas restraining sheet', personally developed by him, to prevent 'the wilder and more dangerous bodily movements'. Once a sufficient shock had been administered to 'fire off a fit', it was essential to restrain the 'initial jerk on the back' and prevent it from flexing to avoid fractures. The restraining sheet was taken off after the fit had died down so as not to restrict breathing. 'If breathing does not rapidly recommence after the fit a few rhythmic compressions of the chest will cause it to begin.'

Sargant liked to play up the potential drama of ECT, in the raw or modified, but he also argued that the risk of death was usually negligible. 'Actual figures are hard to obtain, but the rate is probably well below 1 in 1,000 and is comparable with that of giving a general anaesthetic without other operative procedure.' He was more accepting of the damage that ECT could do to a patient's memory, particularly in elderly patients. He also urged caution when treating a patient 'who uses a highly trained memory in the exercise of his profession', comparing the effects of ECT to 'mild concussion'. There was no need to fear 'permanent impairment', however, because in most cases the damage was temporary. Besides, he argued, some slight degree of impairment 'may be a price worth paying for recovery from a severe depression'.

Given the raft of perceived dangers, perhaps it's no wonder that Sargant gave ECT to his patients while they were in the Sleep Room.*

---

* Even though narcosis patients were not given their morning sedatives on days when they were due ECT, it seems unlikely that they would have been sufficiently compos mentis before being anaesthetised to refuse the treatment. Largactil in particular has a long half-life.

35

'Actually, Dr Sargant, I feel suicidal this morning'

Christine will never forget her first day on Ward Five. She had been assigned to the Sleep Room in her final year as a student nurse in 1968. 'I went to wake the patients up, about eight of them, I think, and I was horrified to discover that I knew one of them.' Christine, then twenty, had just been on holiday with the girl as part of a group. She had been unaware that she had a psychiatric problem. Heavily sedated, the girl didn't recognise Christine. 'Here was reality – she was a real person,' Christine says.

Like other nurses, Christine remembers the 'quite distinctive' smell of Largactil in the Sleep Room. Shelley also says that the odour, sweet and musty, came back to her when she thought of the narcosis treatment. 'You'd just smell it and know what it was straight away.' There was something else in the airless room too. 'If they'd had anaesthetics for ECT, you'd get this anaesthetic smell when they were breathing,' remembers Jane, who was assigned to the Sleep Room for three months in 1970.

Nurses assigned to the Sleep Room did their best to improve the atmosphere. They used air fresheners and opened the windows when the patients were in the bathroom or being fed. (For the rest of the time all the windows on Ward Five were kept shut for safety reasons.) 'I do remember great care being taken to keep it fresh and nice,' says Catherine Mountain.

Julia Ross worked as a night matron on Ward Five at the 'ridiculous age of twenty-two' after she'd qualified as a nurse in December 1966. She only did one shift in the Sleep Room, but her memories are vivid. 'It felt uncomfortable,' she says. 'All you could hear was people just breathing. It was as though they were half dead, half living. It was a separate world ... The curtains were always drawn. I remember the portholes and swing doors.'

She also remembers being instructed not to get too friendly with the patients. 'We were not to call them by their first name or give them our first name.' Sargant, however, was apparently quite happy for patients to know his home address. Julia's late friend and colleague, Jenny, received a phone call one evening from Sargant about a 'highly disturbed' patient with multiple personalities. She had been admitted the previous day but was now standing outside Sargant's house on Hamilton Terrace, having turned up in a taxi.

Jenny had to go and fetch her.

Some of the nurses who worked on Ward Five are sadly no longer with us. In 2005, Dominic Streatfeild spoke to Jane, who told him that the three months she spent working in the Sleep Room, aged nineteen, was 'horrendous' and 'absolutely terrifying' – 'The sort of thing you'd expect in Hitler's time'. She felt that 'they were almost trying to take over these people ... Infiltrate them, change them, change their personalities, change who they were. Almost acting like a god ... Any of us who tried to defend them or question what was happening were just shouted down by the senior staff.'

Student nurses had little or no contact with Sargant himself, who would only speak with the ward sister or charge nurse. Julia Ross remembers his presence. 'He was a figure of authority,' she says today. 'You sort of admired him.' According to Ann Rowland, Sargant was treated 'like an emperor'. Shelley says that there was little kindness in his bombastic manner and recalls Sargant's 'overwhelming self-belief' that Ward Five was the way forward for mental health. There was, she thinks, a bit of Sir Lancelot Spratt (from the film *Doctor in the House*) about him. 'Sargant was a huge figure of a man with a very loud voice,' she says. 'Plenty of consultants were quite like him in those days – God's gift to St Thomas'. They didn't brook much disagreement from anyone. "You're on the mend," Sargant would say to a patient. "I can see you're on the mend." It was very difficult for a patient to say, "Actually, Dr Sargant, I feel suicidal this morning."'

R. D. Laing was similarly critical of Sargant's bedside manner, revealing that a senior nurse, Joan Cunnold, had once contacted him. 'She was the nurse in charge of all that electric shock stuff that Sargant would do,' Laing said, adding that patients were so terrified of ECT that they pretended to feel better on Sargant's ward round: 'He would say, "How are you today, are you all right?" And if you didn't click to attention and say, "Yes sir, fine, I'm OK", you would get another set of electric shocks. So he got a 95 per cent immediate remission rate.'

Laing and Sargant did, however, have one thing in common: a desire to make psychiatric units feel as far removed as possible from the overcrowded back wards of the old asylums – places like Hanwell Mental Hospital, which still haunted Sargant. For a bit of normality, Sargant arranged for a film night on Tuesdays, run by Nita Mitchell-Heggs with the help of her husband, who operated the projector. 'Patients did not sit quietly in rows,' she remembers. Some were in the throes of psychosis. Others were too depressed or anxious to stay for the whole performance. 'I let them do whatever was best for them, wandering about, speaking to their hallucinations, leaving and returning frequently.' Sometimes the only person left watching the film was her husband.

In early summer 1964, Sargant had a terrible row with his ward sister, after she had installed grilles over the electric fires in patients' small rooms to stop nurses from burning their stiff uniforms as they turned around. Sargant was incensed, arguing that the protective bars were 'institutional', but the sister got her way. The row had one unexpected consequence. It persuaded David Owen, then a senior neurology and psychiatric registrar at St Thomas', to switch from medicine to politics. Owen had enjoyed working with Sargant but felt that on this occasion he was acting 'like a spoilt child'. Suddenly he had a vision of himself in Sargant's position in thirty years' time, behaving in exactly the same irrational way. 'That night I wrote to the constituency Labour party accepting nomination,' he says.

Despite the vigilance of the medical and nursing teams in the Sleep Room, continuous narcosis remained an extremely high-risk treatment. Dangers included deep vein thrombosis, bladder, bowel and abdominal distension, chest and throat infections, and withdrawal fits. Pressure sores and muscle loss were also a problem. 'With hindsight it was a desperately dangerous thing to do,' says Maria Rollin, who was a junior anaesthetist on Ward Five in 1972. 'Being sent to work in the Sleep Room felt like a kind of punishment.' The biggest threat to life was severe constipation leading to paralytic ileus, a condition caused when the muscles that usually move food through the gut are temporarily paralysed.

Sargant admitted that five patients in total died during narcosis. His 1972 legacy paper reviewed the cases of 484 patients who had been treated with narcosis (sometimes more than once) between 1962 and 1968 at St Thomas' and Belmont. He reported four deaths, two of which were attributed to paralytic ileus. One patient 'died as a result of inhalation of vomit; she had become severely constipated and developed paralytic ileus during the fifth week of narcosis'. The second, a man, 'died during his second course of modified narcosis, at the end of the third week . . . the cause of death was again inhalation of vomit following paralytic ileus'. A third patient died after six weeks of modified narcosis 'as a result of acute haemorrhagic enterocolitis' – a bacterial infection that leads to severe cramping and bloody diarrhoea. The fourth patient died after three days of peritonitis – inflammation of the stomach lining – after a two-week course of narcosis. 'There has been one further death from bowel complications,' he revealed elsewhere, taking the total to five.

What these figures didn't include was patients who might have initially improved and then died of related complications after being discharged from Ward Five. Sargant was often criticised for overlooking relapses, preferring instead to focus on patients' immediate improvement. Anticipating such criticism, he promised, at the end of his 1972 report, a 'further paper' that would describe 'detailed long-term follow-up' of a group of narcosis patients. 'Treatment with Modified Narcosis: A Retrospective Controlled Study of 106 Patients' was credited to Sargant but never published. It was written by his senior registrar, Chris Walter, who had felt obliged to highlight that there was no meaningful equivalence, for ethical reasons, between the duration and severity of the two groups' illnesses. Furthermore, only 24 per cent of the patients were interviewed personally about their treatments, which had taken place many years earlier, between 1962 and 1964, at St Thomas' and Belmont. Sargant did his best to put a gloss on the findings – patients with agitated depression seemed to improve with narcosis – but sixteen of the 106 who had narcosis went on to have a lobotomy (compared to seven in the control group).

'Reading the paper now, I feel that it may not have been accepted by the *British Journal of Psychiatry*,' says Nita

Mitchell-Heggs. 'The results were statistically significant in favour of narcosis, but the two groups were not similar, the numbers were very small and the results could have been affected by "confounders", such as the number of ECTs. Chris Walter was hugely principled and conscientious – in highlighting the paper's flaws, he rather shot himself in the foot with regard to getting it published.'

Anecdotal evidence suggests that many people might have suffered in the months and years after passing through the Sleep Room. Tish says that her uncle's wife had two three-month periods in the Sleep Room in the 1960s. She was then given a lobotomy and sent back to a secure unit in Rugby, where she died. 'It was absolutely dreadful,' she says.

Nita Mitchell-Heggs has never forgotten what happened one night in early 1969. As a psychiatric house officer, she had her own room on the ground floor. She says that patients in the Sleep Room were never alone. 'They were very chronically ill, many with crippling symptoms.' Life for them and their relatives had become intolerable. Some had been referred for consideration for lobotomy. When they were woken every six hours, they were walked up and down the corridor. 'It was hugely important to avoid the effects of prolonged immobility, such as deep vein thrombosis and muscle wasting.'

To avoid the risk of paralytic ileus, the house officer would use a stethoscope to listen to the abdomen to ensure that bowel sounds (created by the gut's motility) were present. 'I did this, as instructed, a few times every day and just before I went to bed for the night.'

On the particular night in question, Mitchell-Heggs had a flu-like illness with a high temperature. When her husband, also a doctor, agreed with her that she was no longer fit to work for the rest of the day, she approached one of the other resident house officers and asked him to cover her role. 'I reminded him that he had to check all the Sleep Room patients before he himself went to bed,' she says. He told her that he would.

'As far as I recall, he said that all patients had audible bowel sounds when he had examined them.' A middle-aged woman (probably in her mid-forties) had, however, developed ileus with pain during the night. The nurse on night duty summoned the house officer who was covering for Mitchell-Heggs. Because the patient was vomiting, he called at once for surgical help.

'I believe the patient may have been near death, or dead, by the time the surgeon arrived. I don't think there had been an especially major delay. I was utterly shocked and hugely upset when I heard the news.' She couldn't help wondering whether, had she been present, she would have noticed something was awry.

The next day, she saw the patient's widower on the ward. There was no visible anger, she says. He just looked sad. 'I suspect that he might have been accepting of the fact that his wife had been very unwell for many years and that she had been given a treatment that might have helped her.' Looking back on the tragic events today, Mitchell-Heggs says she doesn't know if the patients or their families were apprised of potential risks. 'In those days most patients and their relatives were very trusting, did not question and very rarely sued medical professionals.'

Sargant insisted that she was not in any way to blame for the death and told her that she would not have to attend the coroner's inquest. (Sargant attended.) Later she was informed that no further action would be taken. 'I have never forgotten the case, but I have not worked in any roles in specialities that are associated with high death rates. So I recall all patients who died, especially the ones in paediatrics. These I found utterly heartbreaking.' She says she was unaware of any other deaths on Ward Five related to narcosis.

Did anyone really benefit from the Sleep Room? A senior sister on Ward Five, who remained friends with Sargant in retirement, told Dominic Streatfeild in 2005 about a psychotic girl who was 'so tormented by her voices that she was a terrible, terrible head banger'. To rid her of the voices, Sargant gave her narcosis that resulted, said the nurse, in 'quite a marked improvement'. Annabel Thompson also spent time in the Sleep Room during her three years being treated on Ward Five. 'I had my nineteenth, twentieth and twenty-first birthdays as an inpatient,' she says. She had been admitted in January 1969 with depression and anorexia and went on to have 'countless' ECT treatments.

Her memory of that time is 'not good', but she does remember Sargant. 'I was always admitted under his care. I remember being terrified of him – he had huge brown hands with lots of white hairs and loomed over the bed.' Her sisters have confirmed that Annabel was initially in the Sleep Room for twelve weeks, followed by one week on Ward Five, and then another twelve-week session back in the Sleep Room. 'I do not know if the experience helped or hindered my recovery but recover I did,' she says today. Fifty-one years later, she travelled to Canada for a happy reunion with Ben Spears, one of the psychiatrists who had looked after her during her recuperation.

In his 1972 paper, Sargant claimed that more than 70 per cent of patients suffering from 'chronic tension states', depression or phobic anxiety states were rated as 'symptom free' or 'much improved' following one course of combined narcosis, ECT and antidepressants. 'Encouraging results' were also obtained in patients with severe obsessional neuroses (43 per cent rated as 'symptom free' or 'much improved') and those with 'longstanding schizophrenia or schizo affective states' (41 per cent).

'What we're doing is breaking up long, set patterns of behaviour, which don't respond to so-to-speak quick treatments,' Sargant claimed. Others argued that he put dogma before clinical proof. 'It was a series of one-off individual case reports,' according to the late Professor Malcolm Lader. 'And that is not scientific evidence. The problem is his reputation was such that people were blindly following these dangerous practices.'*

Narcosis wasn't the only dangerous practice on Ward Five; nor was it the only place where patients died. Sargant also ran a controversial programme for patients with anorexia (some of whom spent time in the Sleep Room). After six weeks on the ward as a student nurse, Christine asked to be moved elsewhere. 'A&E was much more enjoyable.' Shortly before she left, however, Christine went into the bathroom and discovered an anorexic patient lying dead in the bath. 'She had a stocking around her neck and had drowned. She was a similar age to me.'

The resident medical doctor turned up in the middle of the night in his pyjamas and dressing gown. 'It was all very tragic and bizarre,' Christine says. Afterwards, new senior staff were brought on to the ward to improve patient safety. Sargant might have favoured the open, unlocked environment of a general hospital staffed largely by student nurses, but the tragic incident had highlighted a fatal flaw in his laissez-faire approach.

Anne was admitted to Ward Five for three months in January 1969, shortly after the anorexic patient's death in the bath. For the past eighteen months, she had stopped eating at Queenswood, her girls' boarding school in Hertfordshire, and started to hide her food. By the time a female psychiatrist in Harley Street had referred her to Sargant, she was barely five stone. 'I was in my own room and not really allowed to leave it,' she recalls. 'They told me it was because the more I moved, the more I wouldn't put on weight.'

Anne says she was put on Largactil to sedate her, as well as

---

* Sargant once took Professor Malcolm Lader on a guided tour of the Sleep Room. 'To be quite frank, I was horrified by what I saw,' Lader told BBC Radio 4. 'Here were people who were being kept deeply asleep for weeks on end. Firstly, you physically smelt all these people . . . I'm sure they did what they could for the hygiene but it's not an easy thing to do. There was no actual therapy being given.'

Nardil. She also remembers the screams of other patients. 'When I asked a nurse what was happening, she told me it was electric shock treatment.' Anne didn't have ECT herself, but at 4 a.m. each morning, she was given insulin as part of Sargant's modified insulin treatment, which sedated patients even more, sending them into a sopor – just short of a coma.

They told Anne it was to make her hungry. Later, she remembers ten pieces of buttered white toast lined up in front of her. 'I could choose what I wanted to have on it – my mum brought me in a tin of Golden Syrup. And they just sat with me and kept threatening that, if I didn't eat it, they were going to stick a tube down my throat.'

Her mother came in most days and sat beside her while she ate or slept – 'she was amazing'. After three months, Anne weighed eight and a half stone. Sargant would come into her room and talk to the nurses. 'I don't think he had much interaction with me, as far as I can remember,' she says. 'It's all so hazy because I was so drugged up. You're like a zombie. I just remember either sleeping or eating.'

At one point, Sargant asked Anne if she would go over to St Thomas' and talk to medical students. It was early on in her treatment and she was still quite thin. She had no idea that she was about to be subjected to the same experience that Celia Imrie had suffered a few years earlier, as a fourteen-year-old. Anne was just two years older.

'I was wearing a gown and they took it off and I was just wearing my bra and knickers in front of all these medical students,' she says. 'It was so humiliating. I felt under their control all the time. They wouldn't let me go unless I did what they said.'

Anne was eventually let out at Easter. She remembers one nurse, called Sue, who had been particularly caring. 'She was so kind to me, amazing, which is why I can remember her name.' Reflecting now, she doesn't feel particularly angry about her experience on Ward Five. 'I probably would have died otherwise.

I also realise I could have died from the treatment too. It was a horrible time in my life.'

Mitchell-Heggs believes that Sargant's physical approach to mental health was not suited to treating anorexia. Most patients, she says, want to recover from their psychiatric illnesses. The reverse is true for many anorexic patients. 'They want to stay thin and are often very reluctant patients, being treated at the behest of worried parents – against their own wishes.' She says that they don't see doctors and nurses as saviours but as cruel torturers, force-feeding them against their will. Sargant's physical methods were insufficient for their deep psychological needs. 'I am not surprised that teenagers found it a very difficult experience.'

It was narcosis, however, that proved most challenging for patients and nurses at the Royal Waterloo and at Belmont – where staff were beginning stand up to him.

36

'She told me that Sargant killed . . . a patient'

Belmont Hospital in Sutton, with its imposing watchtowers and Victorian gables, was Sargant's old stamping ground. He had forged his reputation here during the war, learning how to circumnavigate the London County Council's rules and regulations. And it was where he had lived with his new wife, Peggy, in a terraced house across the road from the hospital. The former workhouse was almost like a second home. It had joined the NHS in 1948 as a neurosis centre – the first civilian facility in the country. Initially it had more than four hundred beds for 'informal' (rather than detained or sectioned) psychiatric patients, treating them in a general hospital environment. Forty of them were under Sargant's supervision. And from 1939 to 1957, it was run by his old ally Louis Minski. Sargant had resumed part-time work as a consultant at Belmont on his return from America in 1948, working one day (two sessions) a week. Another familiar face, his former senior registrar Eric West, was appointed consultant in psychiatry and EEG in 1959.

Sargant would drive down from Hamilton Terrace every Thursday to Belmont. It was on these visits that he would employ one of his former patients to clean his car. He paid him properly and said that the car was cleaner than if he'd taken it to a garage. The man had been languishing in hospital for sixteen years before being transferred to Belmont. Sargant had given him a course of ECT and antidepressants, a lobotomy and a further course of ECT, after which he felt able to work again.

Belmont, like the Royal Waterloo, was out of the way. 'It felt like the "gloves were off",' says 'Freya', who spent nine months at Belmont in 1969 (see Chapter 37). 'It was far away from the scrutiny of a London teaching hospital ... I think Sargant thought he could do what he liked with me.'

It was undoubtedly a place where he could experiment with treatments that might not have been so readily tolerated at St Thomas'. 'Rosa', from Spain, spent her second year of nurse training at Belmont in the late 1960s. One summer, she was having her lunch on the hospital lawn when she heard a strange drumming sound coming from Sargant's office. 'We all jumped up, thinking that it was one of the patients, an African man,' she remembers. When they reached Sargant's office, they discovered it was Sargant who was playing the drums: an artefact from his global travels. 'There was this black patient – he was completely stiff and didn't react to anything. He was really schizophrenic, catatonic, and Sargant was running around, drumming.' Uncharacteristically, Sargant had decided not to give the patient any medication, opting instead to 'take him back' to his own country. 'How did he know that people played drums in his own country? It was just ludicrous, and we asked him, "Please, can you stop." We said, "Look, he's more frightened than anything."'

Belmont had its own Sleep Room, with six beds, and many believe it was where Sargant sent his most disturbed patients. According to Rosa, it was reserved for women and not a pleasant place to work. 'It was horrific, you know,' she says today. 'They were absolute zombies – complete zombies.'

Like her colleagues on Ward Five, Rosa's duties included regularly checking patients' vital signs and taking them for meals and to the bathroom every six hours. There was, however, one striking difference at Belmont: a groundswell of rebellion against Sargant and his methods.

On one occasion, a registrar became so concerned about a patient's reaction to modified insulin therapy that he told the ward sister he was going to take the patient off treatment. 'Under no circumstances were we allowed to tell Sargant that he'd done that,' Rosa says. 'When it was time for Sargant's ward round, we prepared the patient, told him to keep his eyes closed – "don't move". We were all pretending and Sargant would say, "You see how wonderful the therapy is."'

No one at Belmont personified this growing spirit of defiance more than Sister Brown. From her glass office, she would point a stick and call out what was wrong. 'She was fabulous,' Rosa says. 'She observed everything. She also stood up to everybody and wasn't afraid of anything or of any doctor.' Sister Brown had a particular problem with Sargant and his Sleep Room. On one occasion, a famous actress was being treated with narcosis and was taken for an enema to help her constipation. It had little effect. Sister Brown felt sorry for the 'poor woman' and was appalled by the treatment. 'She was going bananas,' Rosa remembers. 'She was swearing at Sargant.'

Sister Brown also refused to allow ECT to be given to narcosis patients on her watch, arguing that it destroyed 'billions' of brain cells. Rosa had similar reservations about the treatment. 'I mean, I'm Spanish – Franco would have loved to do these things.' On one occasion, she pressed Sister Brown on why she was so opposed to the treatment. 'She told me that Sargant killed ... her words were, "he killed a patient". She was a very big, powerful woman and she told Sargant, "You can go to hell and back again – you do not do that to my patients."'

And so patients didn't have ECT when Sister Brown was around. It was sacrilege even to mention Sargant's name in front of her. 'I'll never forget Sister Brown. She gave me the courage later on in life to stand up to bullies in medicine – told me that the patient was always the first thing you should protect.'

Sargant didn't help himself by being rude to his colleagues, particularly new doctors. 'He talked about himself most of the time and what he had achieved,' Rosa says. 'And he was so condescending to everybody else, with such narrow opinions.' At Belmont staff meetings, Sargant would try to battle with Jungian and Freudian psychiatrists, telling them they were stupid. 'Most of them just took it or ignored it . . . Amongst the nurses we regarded him as a joke.'

Rosa was particularly irked that Sargant never consulted nurses, even though they usually had more contact with patients than doctors. When he later invited her and other nurses to a Christmas party in London, none of them went because they had no respect for him. 'There was just something about him, we didn't trust him somehow, as a person – not as a doctor, just a person. We knew he had a reputation – he flirted a lot with the nurses.'

Rosa remembers one particular Christmas party where Sargant spent the entire time pursuing a nurse who had recently arrived from the West Indies. 'He just chased her all around the hospital, saying, "You are wonderful" and "Come and let me catch you", "You're so beautiful, come here." We were sitting in the dining room, filling ourselves with laughter. And she would scream, running away from him. She wanted to get away from him, you know.'

The story chimes with a more general perception of Sargant's attitude to nurses. Several people have spoken of a notorious group photograph of St Thomas' nurses and doctors at another Christmas party. A mirror had been placed in the middle of the group. Look carefully and a reflection of Sargant can be seen enveloping a young Nightingale nurse at the back of the room. 'William ... would not have survived long in the #MeToo movement of today,' says Peter Tyrer. 'He had more than wandering hands.'

Emma Dally recalls her mother Ann's experiences at St Thomas' parties and dances. 'I remember my mother complaining because she said that Sargant always wanted to dance with her. And I thought that was a bit funny, a slightly lecherous sort of thing.'

Patients were more vulnerable to Sargant's advances and Rosa remembers that he would see them unaccompanied at Belmont, after he had carried out a fast ward round in the presence of other doctors and nurses. 'We would wonder why and he would say, "I want to read the notes of so and so" and go to the patient and talk to the patient without anybody there. Sister Brown wouldn't let him do that.' Another registrar who worked with Sargant recalls the time when a medic walked in on Sargant as he was kissing a patient in her single-bed room. 'He stands up and walks out, saying, "That's the way to cure a patient."'

Sargant seems to have been at his most predatory in his private room on Harley Street. 'Liz' is an acclaimed artist in her eighties with a pin-sharp memory of her past – 'I just can't tell you what I went into the next room to get.' She'd married another artist and they ran a business together in southern England. Six years into the marriage, she realised something was very wrong. 'I was feeling strange, and nearly drove into the back of a car.'

When she went to see her GP, she didn't tell him that she was in a coercive relationship. She didn't even admit it to herself. 'I was a loyal wife and we were working together and it didn't actually occur to me that my husband was the cause of all my stress.'

Her GP diagnosed endogenous depression and put her on a low dose of Tofranil, but her mood failed to lift. Two years later, he proposed another solution: a trip up to Sargant in Harley Street. In his referral letter in 1970, Liz's GP gave Sargant detailed case notes. 'Her husband is a very pleasant, rather hairy individual, and appears articulate and artistic, altogether rather "way out". Mrs —— follows the same trend and style.'

In December 1970, Liz found herself taking a tiny lift to the fourth floor of 23 Harley Street, concerned to see Sargant's secretary pressing herself into the corner of the lift in case Liz attacked her. 'It was a very odd feeling,' Liz says. She was meant to have been there a month earlier but hadn't known about the appointment. 'By the time I turned up, I had this black mark against my name.'

She remembers entering the 'not particularly luxurious' attic room, full of old furniture and Persian rugs, and meeting Sargant. 'He was a big man, dark and very good looking,' she says. After reading the letter from the GP, Sargant explained his approach. He would stop the Tofranil and put her on a combination of Surmontil (another tricyclic antidepressant) and Parstelin (an MAOI). If that treatment didn't work, she would be given ECT.

Then something very strange happened. Sargant said that he had to examine Liz to ensure the drugs he would be prescribing were suitable – if her heart would cope. 'So he made me take off my top and then my bra and stood me around for quite a long time.' He then asked her to sit down opposite his desk in a small armchair. 'I tried to squeeze myself in – I'm not used to sitting around with my tits hanging out.' Sargant talked to her for about half an hour, without suggesting she should get dressed. 'I don't suppose he got many tits to look at in his line of business,' she says. 'I was remarkably close to him and he was just talking to me. All he did was sort of gaze at me while I was answering his questions.'

Was it punishment for Liz's earlier no-show? Or simply him taking advantage for his own gratification?

Sargant prescribed the antidepressants and saw her for two more, fully clothed sessions, after which Liz felt no improvement. The prospect of ECT made her nervous so she herself suggested lithium. That seemed to do the trick. Ten years later, she divorced her husband and embarked on a very successful solo career as an artist. Reflecting on what happened, she says that attitudes towards sex were different in those days. 'It was the sixties. He didn't touch me or do anything, but I wouldn't have been surprised if he had, because that's what people did. I really do believe he liked looking at tits.'

Sargant's attic room at 23 Harley Street was also implicated in a second case of sexual impropriety. In 1987, a year before Sargant died, a woman filed a complaint with the General Medical Council. A few years later, she contacted another psychiatrist, explaining that she was dependent on benzodiazepines, originally prescribed by Sargant, and was desperate to come off them. 'In the course of our assessment,' the psychiatrist remembers, 'she said, "Of course Sargant seduced me, he seduced me in Harley Street. It went on for years. He told me I was the only person who could cure his impotence with his wife."' The woman told the psychiatrist that she had felt she had to report Sargant to the GMC. Eventually they had written back with thanks but explained that as Sargant was retired they had decided not to pursue the matter further.

There is no way of verifying this account as the psychiatrist has long since lost contact with the patient. But corroborating evidence indicates that one of Sargant's former female patients did contact the GMC to discuss the details of her grievance, before lodging an official complaint. Responding to a freedom of information request, the GMC confirmed that it had a record of one complaint about Sargant that was received in 1987. It concerned Sargant's treatment and behaviour dating back to 1971, which was when he first began to see the patient in question. The allegations in the complaint were that 'Dr Sargant initiated and engaged in an inappropriate sexual relationship with a patient and there were also concerns from the patient about the effects and dosage of medication prescribed'.

The GMC went on to confirm that the complaint had been considered by a fitness to practice preliminary proceedings committee. It added, however, that, 'due to the passage of time', it unfortunately no longer held a copy of the PPC findings and the complaint outcome. 'Therefore, it is important to note that we can't confirm whether the allegations were found proved.' It's unusual for a case report to go missing. Following further FOI requests, a spokesperson subsequently confirmed that Sargant had remained registered with the GMC until his death in 1988. The case also wasn't referred on to the Professional Conduct Committee, the next stage in any fitness to practice proceedings action. Sargant's lawyers were involved – they wrote to the GMC – but there is currently no way of establishing if a warning letter was ever issued to the eighty-year-old Sargant, who by that time was seriously unwell.

37

'Freya'*

Dr Sargant was very kind towards me when I first arrived as an outpatient at St Thomas' Hospital in 1969. I was twenty-two and had just suffered a total psychotic breakdown. My initial response when I met Sargant – I hated all psychiatrists at this point – was to fly at him and attack him. But as I hammered my fists against his chest, he wrapped his arms around me. It was a memorable act of kindness. He thought there was no need to hear me speak: he believed all mental illness was physical in origin.

Unfortunately, I failed to respond to the ECT and medication that he subsequently gave me on Scutari, the outpatients' ward. The ECT left me with blinding headaches and I was so despairing that I would try to throw myself over the edge of my high-railed bed onto my head in order to kill myself. It was then that I was sent to Belmont, where I was admitted with psychosis and schizophrenia – I was very deluded and hallucinating. Things changed dramatically after I arrived. It felt like the 'gloves were off' at

---

* Some details and names, including Freya's, have been changed to protect privacy.

Belmont, a place where Sargant could do what he liked. Trauma was piled on trauma, and it soon became evident that I was trapped. I was held there for nine months, including three months in isolation in my own Sleep Room.

Sargant began by giving me drug-induced narcosis, combined with ECT and insulin coma therapy. My family wasn't allowed to visit me for the first couple of months. When my mum finally managed to come, she said afterwards that she'd looked at the chart at the bottom of my bed and saw that I'd received well over a hundred ECT treatments in two months – almost two a day. For many years afterwards, I had chronic pain in the back of my neck due to whiplash from all the convulsions.

My mother also said that Sargant used to send the staff away to have their lunch and then come into the room on his own to talk to me. (She said that I told her this after I had left Belmont.) I have no recollection of any conversations with Sargant while I was in bed, but I do remember asking the nurses a number of times during narcosis why my genital/pelvic area was very sore and painful. It was only later, when I was made to go and see Sargant in Harley Street and he repeatedly attempted to take advantage of me, that I began to wonder whether those symptoms were due to abuse that he had perpetrated – and ensured I couldn't remember.

I was kept in a stupefied state a lot of the time, my narcosis interspersed with ECT and insulin treatment, which put me into a more extreme coma. It felt like I was dying. All the strength would gradually leave my body, which felt increasingly heavy until I could no longer move at all, and my consciousness would very slowly shut down. It was a horrible process, invoking a profound, primitive terror. Eventually I lost consciousness completely. And then, at a certain point, they'd wake me up, making me eat great bowls of cornflakes smothered in glucose and drink sickly sweet tea. Getting me to remember my name was always a big deal. I didn't have a clue who I was when I came round, which was a terrifying feeling, especially as I had so little general recall of my life by then.

I'd had a traumatic upbringing in north London, complicated by a physical disability – I was born with very severe deformities of the lower limbs. The painful treatment, which started three days after I was born, involved splints day and night, operations and long stays in hospital until I was nine to enable me to walk (and later run and jump). Home life was very chaotic. I loved my parents, but they both had many problems. There was constant physical, psychological and emotional abuse from both of them, but it was all hidden.

My father had been doing sensitive scientific work for the government during the war, which prevented him from leaving the UK. As a result, he was unable to help his immediate family, who all died under very distressing circumstances in Europe. The tragedy greatly affected his mental health. At school I became very isolated and withdrawn. PE teachers would comment on how many bruises I had all over my body and a form teacher eventually realised that something was wrong.

Occasionally I spoke to the teacher, but my parents didn't listen to her when she said that I needed help. When I was nineteen, I referred myself for help through my GP, having twice left home for rented accommodation. I was very depressed and anxious and afraid that I was going mad. But the doctors thought I was lying, perhaps because of the extreme nature of some of my experiences. There was also a chronic lack of understanding of child abuse in the mid sixties. They refused to speak to my teachers, who could have confirmed what I told them.

Many years later, I realised that the doctors had been projecting a stream of negative female stereotypes onto me. I think psychiatry was very naive in those days, lacking in self-insight. It was misogynistic in an unconscious way, underpinned by a lot of harmful Freudian theories about hysteria and the female psyche. I became more and more desperate – none of my issues were being dealt with. Being repeatedly accused of lying was the most devastating experience in itself. I found it very confusing and deeply humiliating to be branded as a person devoid of moral and ethical values. As the weeks passed, and the validity of my own memories and perceptions continued to be aggressively undermined, it was increasingly difficult to tell what was real. I became very angry, then violent. I began to self-harm and couldn't stop crying; I had a total breakdown.

The nursing care I received during narcosis at Belmont was mainly one on one. If I was taken to the toilet or for a bath, someone was always there watching me. It was a complicated relationship and depended on me being frequently made to forget – thanks to the ECT – a great deal of what happened. All I can remember is constantly agreeing to things, because I didn't want anything done to me because I'd been overpowered. It left me with a deep sense that all resistance was futile. So I would walk into the ECT room, but then, when they tried to give me the general anaesthetic, something would kick in and they would have to hold me down. All the resistance that I had been trying to suppress would hurtle up just as the anaesthetic started to take effect. I would struggle like crazy as I was going under, desperately trying to get away. Subsequently, there was always this group ritual of one person pinning down each limb and another holding my head whenever I went for ECT. The staff would try to make light of it.

The nurses were nice and kind, particularly a Filipino nurse called Chantale. And the general medical atmosphere was a brisk and bright indifference, but with a dark undertow. For me, there was always this sense of mystery about why I was there: all these strange procedures that I was not aware I had agreed to. Sargant and the staff just thought I should be grateful they were 'making me better', but the treatments struck me as so violent and dark. It didn't help that I once had to be rushed to a heart unit in Reading because they had overdosed me with narcosis drugs to 'get me under'. I also got severe double pneumonia while in Belmont.

I think my room may have been down a corridor on the first

floor. There was one window set high up in the wall, too high and too small to climb out of – as I often noted. All the window showed was sky – no trees, houses or fields, no sun or moon. Nothing. So the colour of the sky itself became incredibly important. It told me day from night, but it was also the only feature that changed – whether it was blue or cloudy, pale or bright, calm or stormy. I was meant to be asleep all the time so I wasn't allowed out of bed. When I couldn't sleep, I was terribly bored and the changing colour of this patch of sky often became my sole focus: for me, it represented the entire outside world, the whole of normal life.

After my time in this Sleep Room, I could never find my way round the hospital – I always seemed to get lost. The directional bit of my brain had been very damaged by ECT. As you entered the hospital on the ground floor, I think there was an imposing kind of polished wood reception cubicle with a uniformed porter. I felt I had to get past him in order to escape. And I did manage to escape a few times, somehow making my way back to my parents' home in north London. I told my parents they were destroying my memory at Belmont, but they couldn't believe me, such was Sargant's standing at the time. Much later, they told me that each time I escaped, Sargant would send a special ambulance from Belmont to collect me from north London and take me back. There must have been some ghastly scenes.

I did do some occupational therapy while in Belmont, in a modern annexe attached to the main building. I would often get lost trying to find it. Both my memory of the hospital and the annexe have conflated over time with memories of other asylums and the years of nightmares I have subsequently had. In these I am wandering around this vast, endlessly confusing hospital building, either looking for a way to escape or urgently trying to find the annexe. The Belmont that has survived in my mind's eye doesn't look much like the photographs, though its distinctive watchtowers were always a very sinister feature, common to both.

I have some other, isolated memories from Belmont, devoid

of sequence or context and from when I assume I was no longer under narcosis. The most important one is of an Irish cleaner called Sally, who mopped the floors. She was middle aged with a beautiful, tired face and straight dark brown hair to her shoulders. She had a strong Irish accent, and often used to talk to me – a great beacon of homely warmth and sanity in that place. I think she sometimes hugged me.

For a while, there was also a girl of about thirty with long pale brown hair. An aspiring folk singer, she would sit in some kind of dining area when it was empty, singing and playing her guitar. She had a beautiful voice. I was her sole audience. Once a large bunch of flowers arrived for her from her 'agent'. I was very impressed.

The other important memory for me is of a young boy of about six or seven, who appeared one day accompanied by his mother. He never spoke, but sometimes he screamed a lot. I understood he was autistic. He had blond hair and blue eyes and looked like an angelic child from *The Midwich Cuckoos*. Sometimes, when I regained consciousness after a procedure, I would find him standing by my bed just staring into my eyes, in complete silence. I would lie there looking back at him, neither of us speaking. Speech didn't feel necessary.

I also have a couple of memories of trying to explore the hospital, but they have a bizarre feel to them, as if I was very drunk at the time. In both memories I am wandering down a featureless corridor and come to a door in the wall made of thick, glossy wood with a glass porthole window near the top at eye level. I look through it and see a large clean and tidy ward, with two rows of beds all occupied by middle-aged women, knitting. They are happily chatting to each other.

In the other memory, as I walk down another corridor I am hit by the most awful smell. It gets worse and worse as I come up to a different door. This time, when I look through the glass porthole, I see a very large ward with many beds in a chaotic state: it is full of terribly neglected, filthy and incontinent old people, who are obviously demented, wandering around in a most pathetic and shocking condition. This made a great impression on me at the time, and I became permanently afraid of ending up in there if I was sent to a locked ward.

And I remember a strange new event that began at some point after I emerged from the Sleep Room. It was meant to be a monthly dance, to enable some of the women in Belmont to have a chance to enjoy the company of the opposite sex. Our dance partners were from Henderson Court, a centre for psychopaths next to Belmont. The dances took place in a large room with a few small bare tables by one wall. Each one had a white saucer with a single white candle on it, and plain tall glasses of orange squash. Burly male nurses, arms crossed, stood around the edge of the room, keeping an eagle eye on the psychopaths. This was obviously someone's bright idea of how to give a girl a good time. The blokes behaved fine, as far as I remember, but the whole scene was just so grim and contrived – not even Terry Pratchett could have dreamt it up. I called it the Psychopaths' Ball and I don't remember whether I managed to enjoy the dances, but I was very aware that I must have been regarded in the same vein as the psychopaths.

I know I also had (so-called) intelligence tests because Sargant said later that they showed I was a lot more intelligent than he thought I was – gosh, thanks. Using EEGs, he had been surprised to find my brain waves were highly anomalous. I remember having ink-blot tests too, because I was very afraid they would reveal something horrible about my mind or personality that I wasn't aware of.

I got to know Sargant well during my stay as he oversaw my treatment. I used to have conversations with him when I was a bit better. Nervously, I started to question him about what the ECT was doing to my memory. Sometimes he'd claim that nothing he did affected the memory and that I must have hysterical memory loss, which really angered me. He was quite self-deluding about what he could and couldn't do. One day, he'd deny that he was affecting memory at all; the next, he'd forget to deny it, and say that he could selectively destroy bad memories and leave only the good ones.

I was only partially recovered (much fewer delusions or hallucinations) when Sargant finally sent me home for a trial weekend. But life at home was still very difficult. In all this time no one had addressed the basic issues at all or advised me how to handle them. I came back at the end of the weekend and smashed some windows in the hospital: they symbolised this invisible barrier between me and the doctors' ability to understand, so a lot of windows got smashed. The staff then said I had to go into a locked ward, at which point Sargant decided he'd dope me up so much that I wouldn't be a problem to anyone. 'We'll send her home.'

So that's how I finally got out after nine months, but I was continually threatened with being sent back to a locked ward at Belmont if I didn't take all the drugs that Sargant had prescribed. I was being injected once a fortnight with antipsychotic medication and taking fifteen pills a day. I'd put on loads of weight by then. As for my hair, it had been kind of Pre-Raphaelite when I went in, but I came out with so much hair loss, so bleached and thin at the temples from ECT, that I had to have it completely cut off. My health was ruined. I couldn't walk for more than five or ten minutes without being exhausted and, ironically, I had to sleep a great deal of the time.

I was so brain damaged that I'd lose my way when I went out, even in places I had been completely familiar with before. It was as if, at the age of twenty-two, I had severe Alzheimer's – I'd lost all sense of direction. Several times I was picked up by the police as I was wandering disorientated in the street. I'd also forgotten a great deal of knowledge. At school, I'd done A-level maths, but I now had difficulty doing the simplest arithmetic. I still have difficulty with certain forms of abstract thinking.

I couldn't remember or recognise friends I'd known all my life.

The inner history of shared emotions and experiences was all gone – and has never come back. I had to get to know people again from scratch, which was deeply troubling. I lost good friends who couldn't cope with me treating them like strangers. If people told me things, I'd forget them the next day. I was constantly being told that I had said or done things that I had no recollection of. There was no context to anything, no sequential connection between events.

My mum was totally shocked when she discovered I had so much memory loss. She had been in awe of Sargant. Feeling very guilty, she spent a lot of time trying to feed memories of my childhood back to me, as well as repeatedly explaining what had happened to me while I was in hospital. These second-hand memories were like empty eggshells – devoid of any inner, subjective substance, with no sense of personal relevance: like dry historical facts from a textbook. The degree of memory loss was so vast that it caused me a great deal of inner panic and anxiety. Apart from some vague generalised memories, I was just living with this huge, very largely blank space where all the myriad memories of my past life should have been. I had very little sense of identity left.

I was determined, however, to go to university after I left Belmont. I had been accused by the medical profession of, among other things, inventing all my troubles as an excuse not to go to university and I wanted to prove them wrong. After working with an educational psychologist on my memory, I re-took my A levels and was accepted on a degree course at Oxford. The effects of the medication made studying extremely difficult. Most of the time I had to set an alarm clock at fifteen-minute intervals to keep me awake – I repeatedly fell asleep soon after I sat down. It was a pretty hopeless ambition, but I managed to get a distinction in the only final exam I took – before my university education fell apart. I am still in touch with my old college tutor and her husband, who have been very good to me.

While I was at Oxford, I had to see Sargant at Harley Street every so often. He would regularly 'try it on' with me on these occasions. It made me very angry that I was forced to see him under pain of being sent back to a locked ward at Belmont when he behaved in that sort of way. On a couple of occasions, I went to the appointment and a dozen or so middle-aged men in suits were sitting there. I felt I was on display, and Sargant would be asking me staged questions as if he was showing me off: here was the patient who had recovered enough to go to university. I still wonder what that was all about.

The only message I got from Sargant and my parents was that I would become psychotic again if I didn't take the drugs, which I must take indefinitely. But I had begun to remember that the dysfunctional nature of my family life lay at the root of all my problems. I managed to switch to a different psychiatrist, this time in Oxford: if I became his patient, I reasoned, Sargant would not be able to lock me up for refusing to take all those drugs. It transpired that three of them were physically addictive. I was given the choice of coming off them one at a time (which could take years) or off all three at once and doing cold turkey as an inpatient in an Oxford clinic. I chose the latter. I became very ill, and the damage to my eyesight that ensued from weeks of withdrawal led me to lose my university place. I had hoped that, drug-free, I could re-take my finals, but it wasn't to be.

Eventually, having left the clinic and Oxford, I went home, where I met my future husband. Although he had been living in my parents' house as a lodger for six years, I had no memory of him. He was familiar with my family dynamics, however, and understood where I was coming from. He had also inherited profound problems in his family, so we understood one another. Shortly before, I had been introduced to the work of R. D. Laing. Reading the Glaswegian psychiatrist was the first time I managed to get any kind of handle on the complexities of home life and my own reactions to it. We soon moved away. My trust in the mental health services was shattered, so I was effectively on my own as far as any kind of therapy went, with just my partner and a couple of much-valued friends for back-up. I also began to read Jung, Freud, Szasz and Foucault, and explored other forms of consciousness.

The legacy from my time in the Sleep Room proved long lasting. The antipsychotics left me with a permanent Parkinsonian tremor. I also suffered from a form of acute chronic fatigue when I left Belmont, which lasted until my late forties. As a child, once all the operations on my feet were finished, I had set myself the goal of winning my primary school sports medal and cup. I trained hard, despite the inevitable pain, and managed to win both. I loved sport. Later, in my forties, I wondered if I could kick-start my metabolism by taking up karate. It did help a bit. I also suffered from very severe migraines during and after my stay at Belmont. Sometimes they required medical intervention and didn't go away until my late fifties (when I was helped by a fine Chinese herbal practitioner), and they greatly affected my work prospects and income.

It was my memory, however, that was most affected by Sargant's treatments. I lost virtually all individual memories of my childhood, retaining only a generalised photographic recall of what things had been like. Short-term memory, which was initially catastrophic, has improved over time, but long-term is very damaged. The only plus side is that – to my knowledge – I am the only person to have ever had the pleasure of reading *The Lord of the Rings* for the very first time, twice.

Virtually all 'Proust Effect' types of memory went too: those linked by association to the senses, like taste, smell or atmosphere, also memories dependent on emotional association were much diminished, although intellectual association is now much more intact. I also have a great sense of having lost a large portion of my emotional range and the subtler range of emotional responses after Belmont: it's a bit like a musician only having access to one octave of a piano.

In the months and years after I'd left Belmont, I don't think I would have survived without the great love, sympathy and support of my partner. I remained incredibly confused and traumatised by everything that had happened. I could never understand why I had not been believed in the first place, nor why I had emerged from Belmont in such an awful state. All these questions – and a terrific sense of injustice – troubled me for many years, however much I tried to 'put it behind me' and 'move on'. I felt very sure something strange had being going on at Belmont.

It was only when I saw a TV programme around the year 2000, about MKULTRA, the CIA's mind control programme and its connection with Dr Ewen Cameron in Canada, that I got an inkling of what Sargant was doing. The condition of brain-damaged patients in the TV programme, their accounts of the treatment they had had, was so similar to mine. In 2003, I went to the Wellcome Collection, where Sargant's personal papers are kept, and made forty-five A4 pages of notes, documenting parallels between his work and British and American areas of mind control research. Then I edited the glowing Wikipedia entry on Sargant to incorporate some of what I had found.

In 2020, I nearly died from an excruciating non-aneurysmal subarachnoid brain haemorrhage, of unknown cause. It was during lockdown, and I found myself back in a room on my own, hallucinating from additional encephalitis. The evocation of my earlier experiences in the Sleep Room was very strong. After Belmont I had suffered from a lot of pain in the back of my neck and head, often associated with migraine. The haemorrhage occurred at the back of the base of my skull.

My partner, who very sadly died in 2014, had a successful career in the arts. After living for fifteen years in London, we managed to fulfil our dream of moving to the country. We bought a house in the West Country visited by all kinds of wildlife – a wonderful place where I became an artist, poet, environmentalist and gardener. The impact of Sargant and the events of my early life were all-pervasive, and the aftermath has been enduring and catastrophic, despite therapy in later life. It is very isolating. Most people have never heard of Sargant.

Birds, animals and the natural world, art, family and friends: these are the things that sustain me. I have to feel it was worthwhile to survive, so I build meaning into my life in whatever way I can. I feel very grateful to those who have helped me over the years and I'm a great believer in simple kindness.

38

'There was a Russian man . . . it was the talk of the hospital'

Ward Five was much more public than 23 Harley Street, but Sargant was known to drop his guard after he'd finished his afternoon ward round and hint at his work for the intelligence services. 'He would sit down and be quite expansive about what he'd been doing,' Mo Harvey, Sargant's ward sister between 1968 and 1972, confided to Dominic Streatfeild. He never gave any details, preferring instead to report how 'funny' they all were in 'MI5 or MI6 – whichever one had a house somewhere for debriefing people. He thought that the people there were – to quote him – "in need of treatment"!'

Rosa, the nurse at Belmont, also remembers Sargant being involved with MI5. In particular, she recalls a strange case in September 1967 involving a potential Russian defector. 'It was the talk of the hospital.' The Tkachenko affair was a major diplomatic incident involving Soviet and British intelligence services. Sargant was called in to assess the mental health of Vladimir

Tkachenko, a twenty-five-year-old postgraduate researcher, after he appeared ready to defect.

The drama began to unfold at 11.30 a.m. on Saturday 16 September, on the Bayswater Road in London, where three members of the public saw Tkachenko being bundled into a car and shouting for help, before being driven away at high speed. The police traced the diplomatic number plate to the nearby Soviet embassy.

Tkachenko was in the UK to research low-temperature physics using helium gas at the University of Birmingham, as part of a Royal Society exchange programme with the Academy of Sciences of the USSR.* He had travelled to Cambridge the previous day to spend two weeks at the university's Cavendish Laboratory. His wife, Galina, who had recently arrived to visit her husband, later claimed that he had started to behave strangely: he objected to staying in a room at Churchill College hostel with the number 13. Instead, the couple went to London that evening and booked into the Embassy Hotel on Bayswater Road, where Tkachenko had a disturbed night's sleep.

Here the Russian version of events diverges from the British one. The Russians maintained that Tkachenko tried from 4 a.m. onwards to raise staff at the Russian embassy, also on the Bayswater Road, before wandering off. Galina had got into an embassy car and set off with concerned staff to find him. After picking him up on the Bayswater Road, they took him back to the embassy, where a doctor decided he was unwell and gave him a 150mg shot of Largactil to calm him down. He

---

* In one of the more bizarre details of the Tkachenko case, it was reported that he had made several phone calls a week to Russia from his lodgings in Edgbaston, a suburb of Birmingham. Enid Banks, his landlady, told one newspaper that he adopted 'a strange high-pitched voice unlike his own' during these conversations. As part of his work with low physics, he used helium gas. Did he inhale on the gas before ringing home, perhaps to confuse – or amuse – anyone listening in on his call?

was then taken at high speed to Heathrow, cleared through immigration as a sick passenger and driven straight onto the runway, where an Aeroflot plane was waiting to fly him back to Moscow.

Meanwhile, Special Branch officers had been alerted and rushed to Heathrow too. Suspecting that Tkachenko had been kidnapped, they boarded the plane and prevented it from taking off. Tkachenko, by this time 'semi-conscious with his head lolling from side to side', asked to speak to British officials in private, saying that he didn't want to return to Moscow and had been drugged against his will in the embassy. An argument ensued between Heathrow's chief immigration officer and the Soviet consul.

After a scuffle with Soviet officials, the police eventually escorted Tkachenko off the plane. MI5 whisked him away to an undisclosed location, described in the media as a 'secret nursing home', possibly the Priory in Roehampton, where he was assessed by British doctors, including an 'eminent psychiatrist'. Enter Sargant, his identity later confirmed by a subsequent Royal Society report. He was also named in the press, including an article in the *Daily Sketch* that referred to the 'beetle-browed 59-year-old physician' and 'one of the world's greatest authorities on mental illness'. (It was the only cutting on the Tkachenko affair that Sargant kept.) According to other press reports, Sargant attended to Tkachenko twice on Sunday, concluding that the Russian had been drugged and was also suffering from psychotic episodes. In short, he was a political innocent in need of medical attention. Sargant, however, appears to have been uncharacteristically reluctant to prescribe further drugs. The British were also wary of being accused by the Soviets of using drugs to extract information from him.

In a strange conclusion to the whole affair, Tkachenko was delivered back to the Soviet embassy at 10.30 a.m. on Monday, less than forty-eight hours after he had apparently been kidnapped.

A few hours later, he was on a plane bound for Moscow with his wife.* Was Sargant wrong in his assessment? If he was, it wouldn't be the first time that the Soviets had covered up a potential defection with the cloak of mental ill health and a syringeful of drugs.

Sargant no doubt enjoyed his central role in what had become a global story. The affair was amplified by the arrival in Britain of Andrei Gromyko. The Soviet Union's Minister of Foreign Affairs was on his way to meet his British counterpart at a United Nations meeting in America, prompting a possible turf war between the Foreign Office and the Home Office. The Foreign Office/MI6 was keen not to rock the international boat, and arranged for the prime minister, Harold Wilson, to write personally to Tkachenko's wife. Meanwhile, the Home Office/MI5 suspected a genuine defection attempt and Russian poisoning, and was upset by the prompt return of Tkachenko to the Soviet embassy. 'MI5 Indignant Over Tkachenko Affair Haste' said one newspaper headline.

On this occasion, Sargant chose to do MI6's bidding rather than MI5's. Either way, the episode demonstrated his close links to the intelligence services at a time when the Sleep Room was in full swing.

* It later emerged that the deal to return Tkachenko back to Moscow was brokered by Ivan A. Schischkin, a senior KGB official who had been involved in the high-profile release of U-2 pilot Gary Powers in exchange for Colonel Rudolf Abel in 1962.

39

'Reduced him to a zombie, poor dog'

He might have been a keen rugby player in his youth, but the only time anyone saw Sargant move at speed at St Thomas' was when the BBC was on the phone. 'He'd run down the corridor to take the call, pill bottles rattling in his pocket,' remembers Ben Spears. 'He loved publicity.' Sargant had also worked out that it was important to suck up to the cameraman – the one who removed his wrinkles. As the 1960s drew to a close, however, the phone rang less often. Sargant's star was on the wane, his Sleep Room falling out of fashion. In the early 1960s, he had been asked to lecture all over the world, publicising his Pavlovian theories of brainwashing in America and Australia, but those invitations had also dried up.

Since his appearance on the first, ill-fated episode of *Panorama*, he'd participated in a number of high-profile BBC programmes, including the popular *Your Life in Their Hands* in March 1962. Other programmes had included an episode of the BBC's *Sunday Break*, entitled 'Battle for the Mind', in May 1962, as well as his appearance with R. D. Laing on *Late Night Line-Up*. He'd also appeared on the Third Programme in December 1965 with the singer P. J. Proby. According to Sargant, Proby's wild and gyrating antics on stage induced increased suggestibility among his hysterical teenage fans, culminating with an infamous concert at the ABC Croydon, where his velvet trousers had split.

Sargant had drawn similar conclusions about Beatlemania. 'From the Stone Age to Hitler, the Beatles and the modern "pop culture", the brain of man has been constantly swayed by the same physiological techniques,' he wrote in his last book, *The Mind Possessed*. 'Reason is dethroned, the normal brain computer is temporarily put out of action, and new ideas and beliefs are uncritically accepted.'

His last prominent appearance was in a 1968 episode of the documentary strand *Towards Tomorrow*, entitled 'People Like Us'. It was filmed on Ward Five and included a short sequence in the Sleep Room. The nurse sat at her small table, the patients lay still in their beds as if frozen in time, their skin clammy from the Largactil. It was a haunting piece of footage. Only forty-five seconds long, the sequence didn't go into detail about the treatment, but it might well have hastened the end of the Sleep Room.

Life wasn't a bed of roses either in the picturesque Dorset hamlet of Pentridge, where he and Peggy were renting the Old School House as a weekend retreat. They had spent money on improving the property but someone in the village, a former colonial police officer, objected to the rental arrangement between Sargant and the village hall. Sargant eventually handed the house back, wrote off the costs and moved across the A354 to the nearby hamlet of East Woodyates, where in 1969 he bought his own house for £21,000 (c. £300,000 today).

The large property, complete with stone-mullion windows, was set in three acres of land. It was big for a couple with no children, but the kitchen was tiny and antiquated. The back of the house had originally been an eighteenth-century deer lodge.

In 1929, one of the previous owners had extended the building at the front and created 'a cod gentleman's residence, a slightly peculiar Arts and Crafts house where none of the fireplaces were opposite the windows', according to the current owner, who has since converted it into an elegant country residence.

Sargant decided to close off the back third of the house (it had once been the servants' quarters) and just live in the new front portion. Neighbours remember it was packed with furniture, paintings and artefacts collected on his travels. Much like his father had done in Highgate, the Sargants filled the house with guests at the weekend – his old Cambridge friend John Harman and his wife were regulars – and threw large drinks parties as they did at Hamilton Terrace. 'Will enjoyed his success,' a neighbour says. 'He was always very conscious of his father's and grandfather's fluctuating fortunes.' Another describes Sargant's presence in the rural community as 'lordly'.

Sargant didn't endear himself when he first arrived. He soon found himself at loggerheads with a neighbouring landowner over two beech trees, beyond his boundary, arguing that they obscured his view of the rolling Dorset countryside. Others felt the trees made the view. 'There was an element of entitlement about Sargant's controversial position,' another neighbour says. But the landowner knew his trees, recognised that they had been planted too close together and compromised by cutting down one of them. It wasn't the outcome that Sargant was looking for but the remaining tree stands to this day.

The only other evidence of Sargant's twenty years at the house is a garden fountain and semi-naked Italianate statue on an outside wall. The pornography has long since gone too. When Peggy was showing the property to a prospective buyer, a Conservative peer, he was surprised when he tried to take out a book from the library. 'Will's collection of pornography cascaded around Peggy's feet,' a neighbour says. 'It was no surprise to Peggy.'

Locals were more surprised by Sargant's lack of general

medical skills. 'When old Mrs Groves fainted in church, Will was no help at all,' the same neighbour recalls. 'Others had to revive her. This was not Will's type of medicine. He did treat an elderly cousin of mine for severe depression, but he failed, explaining the condition was too longstanding.' The entire family agreed with him.

The neighbour also remembers Sargant's dogs. Sargant loved animals – he was anti-bloodsports, disapproving of the local shoot – and dogs in particular. The first one, Perkins, was a miniature poodle and a Londoner who never took to country life. Perkins soon died. His second dog was a terrier, Perkins 2, who was frightened of the sound of gunshots and bird scarers. Sargant put him on Valium. 'Reduced him to a zombie, poor dog,' he told neighbours.

And then there were Sargant's cars. The first to grace Dorset's narrow country lanes were Bentleys, including a Mark VI, which Peggy crashed at a local crossroads. Sargant was a much worse driver. He was prone to frequent crashes – as demonstrated by his misreading of the traffic lights in Trafalgar Square. He also assumed that others were prone to accidents too.

'I remember Will calling at my parents' house on one occasion,' the same neighbour says. 'Will was distraught and tearful in the kitchen with my mother.' He and Peggy had driven down in separate cars. When Sargant had arrived and discovered that Peggy hadn't appeared, he went to pieces, 'imagining every horror'. Peggy appeared some time later. She'd had a puncture, pulled into Popham Services, and Sargant had driven past without realising. 'Peggy gathered up the great and famous man and took him home.'

The Bentleys were soon replaced by a series of beaten-up Renaults, perhaps because of too many collisions. And then, in the mid 1970s, the black Rolls-Royce Silver Shadow appeared. 'Peggy declared she would not drive it,' a neighbour recalls, but within two weeks she was driving the car down from London and collecting Sargant from Salisbury train station. 'An elegant blonde driving a Rolls – people frequently asked who she was.'

She is remembered with genuine affection. 'Peggy was an absolute darling, a really sweet, lovely woman,' says the current owner of their old house. 'And a keen, if old-fashioned, gardener.' He bought the property from her in 1989, and she moved to Bowerchalke, where she lived until her own death in 2009.

Sargant drove the Rolls too but not for long. After a while, the local garage advised him that the front wing would need to be replaced if he crashed it again. There was one other striking feature about the car: its distinctive number plate. Some remember it as ECT1, which would have been a tasteless reminder of the medical treatments that had paid for the life of luxury he and Peggy now lived.* But that might just be gossip. The source of the Rolls-Royce itself, however, was another story altogether.

---

* Others remember the number plate as ECT2 or possibly ECG1. The DVLA is unable to confirm, because of data protection, whether any of these was ever attached to Sargant's Rolls-Royce.

40

'The Narcosis room appeared to be particularly overcrowded'

Sargant had expected a landslide victory when he stood to become the first president of the Royal College of Psychiatrists in 1971. He was initially against a separate college for psychiatrists, believing they should sit within mainstream medicine, but once he'd put his name forward, he was desperate to win. To his great disappointment, however, he was passed over in favour of Martin Roth.

'Perhaps he was too individualistic for the College to vote him their first President,' Peter Dally mused later. Ben Spears has another theory. 'I explained that Roth would get the Jewish vote, correctly I think, and I felt obliged to tell Sargant – it was not realistic to think that someone as divisive as him could be voted in.'* Roth was knighted in the following year's New Year

* Sargant sat next to Dr Maria Rollin at a dinner after his defeat and told her that 'all the Jews in the College had ganged up on him', preventing him from being elected. 'It was said with great bitterness, in the most virulent, antisemitic terms,' according to Rollin. When she pointed out that she herself was Jewish, 'it went completely over his head – I'm not sure if he was sober'.

Honours list. Despite being the most famous psychiatrist of his day, Sargant never received any honour from the Queen, nor was he ever made an emeritus professor. He told himself that awards didn't matter. 'In medicine, establishment honours mean so little compared to the happiness you earn by helping others rather than yourself.' He was, however, elected a Foundation Fellow of the RCP in 1971 and an Honorary Fellow in 1973. 'He wanted to be an honoured person, but he also, I would have thought, wanted the money,' Lord Owen says. 'He enjoyed private practice.'

Colleagues such as Professor Malcolm Lader and Dr Henry Rollin felt that Sargant distanced himself from the college after his defeat, publicly accusing the 'talkers' (psychotherapists) of having too much say. He couldn't let the college go, however. In 1984, he arranged for *The Unquiet Mind* to be privately reprinted and complimentary copies to be sent to all 1,500 members and associates of the RCP. It was 'one of the most extraordinary and egomaniacal things I've ever known,' recalled John Hughes, former chairman and CEO of the Priory Group.

Meanwhile, there was a sense that the Sleep Room itself was beginning to feel tired, even if Sargant himself was more keen on narcosis than ever. Extra mattresses had been wedged into the cramped space and the whole of Ward Five had a dilapidated feel. Its time had passed. Lady Seebohm, one of St Thomas' trustees, visited in September 1971 and reported back to the General Maintenance Committee that 'the Narcosis room appeared to be particularly overcrowded'. All the furniture on the ward looked old and worn, she observed, and was in urgent need of replacement.

Two months later, a fire survey of the Royal Waterloo Hospital revealed further shortcomings. Ward Five was an accident waiting to happen. Sargant agreed to an expenditure of £770 from 'his Ward V fund' for additional refurbishing, but some people were still deeply troubled by what was happening on the top floor. A young medical student tried to raise a complaint about Sargant but was quickly shut down. Dr Vincent Argent, who trained at St Thomas' between 1971 and 1974 and went on to become a senior consultant in A&E, described Ward Five as 'like a living mortuary'. But when he reported it to the hospital authorities and the General Medical Council, he said he was 'taken aside' and told that Dr Sargant had friends in high places. 'I would lose my place at medical school if I took it any further and that far worse could happen to me.'

In April 1972, thirty-seven years after he had entered medicine, Sargant retired from his role as Physician in Charge of Psychological Medicine at St Thomas', a title he had fought so hard for in 1948. But Sargant still had much to do, not least shoring up his reputation as Britain's most influential post-war psychiatrist. It's no coincidence that the final edition of *An Introduction to Physical Treatments in Psychiatry* came out in 1972. So too his legacy paper on narcosis, ECT and antidepressants.

John Pollitt, Sargant's loyal right-hand man, took over Ward Five. He had first joined St Thomas' in 1953 and had worked at the hospital full time since 1958, apart from a year at Harvard on a Rockefeller travelling scholarship in 1959 (the same as Sargant's in 1938). Shortly after his return from America, he was appointed to the consultant staff at St Thomas'.

There's a common perception that Pollitt was the quieter, more reasonable foil to Sargant's forthright, reckless character – a pale shadow. 'Pollitt was a mild, courteous chap who came across as distinctly colourless,' remembers Ben Spears. 'He was also highly obsessional.' His hobby on retirement was said to be repairing clocks. Mild and courteous he may have been, but in 1973, with Sargant no longer around, Pollitt remained fully committed to ECT, modified insulin treatment, ether abreaction, MAOIs and tricyclic antidepressants in combination, aversion therapy (including 'treatment of homosexuality and perversion') and lobotomy, all of which were recommended in his 1973 book, *Psychological Medicine for Students*. The only treatment that he didn't endorse in print was narcosis, but it didn't stop him continuing with the Sleep Room for a year before it was finally closed down. 'Pollitt was not a natural ally but the ambience around Sargant made sceptics into believers,' says Peter Tyrer.

Susannah was admitted to the Sleep Room in January 1973, nine months after Sargant had left. The twenty-two-year-old was from a working-class family in King's Cross and had a difficult relationship with her mother, who had come over from the west of Ireland on a one-way ticket when she was fourteen. She already had a child from another relationship, before having Susannah with someone whom she felt obliged to marry. She always blamed Susannah, and it was a complicated, unhappy childhood.

'There wasn't a day when my mother wouldn't bully and humiliate me,' Susannah says. So far as her mother was concerned, everything was wrong with her daughter, particularly the way she looked. Susannah was born with a spinal deformity and her mother called her 'the hunchback'. 'She used to call me that every flipping day. She laughed at me.'

In her late teens, Susannah went to visit her GP, who concluded she had 'lost contact with reality'. At the time she was working in market research. She had met Peter, who was at art school, when she was eighteen and they would later marry. Susannah was doing well in her job, but then she was headhunted for a new role and felt unable to cope. After eighteen months as a psychiatric outpatient at St Bartholomew's Hospital, and an attempt to jump under a train, she was admitted to Halliwick House, part of Friern Barnet mental hospital. Two months later, she was referred to Ward Five by Dr John Bradley, who specifically recommended the Sleep Room. He diagnosed her as schizophrenic – wrongly, in Susannah's opinion – and decided that a lobotomy might be the only answer.

Susannah was on Ward Five for two weeks before she was moved to the Sleep Room. Her memories are hazy, but she recalls that there were six beds with chairs wedged between them. People were at different depths of sleep and nurses would fetch bedpans for the patients at all times of the day and night – not just every six hours. The bedpan was placed on the chair, where patients were obliged to use it, within three feet of the next patient's head. The process was the same for enemas. 'The nurses would get you out of bed, sit you on the chair and raise the end of the bed with blocks,' Susannah says. 'Then they'd put you back into the bed that they'd covered with a rubber sheet and administer the enema. If I'm remembering this properly, it breaks every rule of hygiene, dignity and infection control.'

The nurses, she says, were understandably fed up with the patients, who protested about being woken up and put back to sleep. They weren't always kind either. 'We weren't washed carefully and tenderly and tucked up – it wasn't like that,' Susannah says. 'I don't really blame them. We weren't great patients.'

Susannah was supposed to spend three months in the Sleep Room, but she was removed after eight weeks, because she had 'euphoria and incongruity', a possible indication of brain damage. For many years afterwards, she felt lucky to have been treated on Ward Five. 'Narcosis was a terrible experience and I can remember begging the staff to let me go home,' she says. But once she was out, she began to think she had been fortunate, as a working-class woman, to have had so much care lavished on her. In her mind, the drastic nature of the treatment meant that it was specialised and rarely available – 'a measure of the severity of my illness'.

It wasn't until many years later, in 2010, when she heard about the Sleep Room on a Radio 4 programme (*Revealing the Mind Bender General*, presented by James Maw), that she began to think her narcosis treatment had been abusive. 'It seems ridiculous to say that some patients might not realise that they were abused on Ward Five, but I really believe that that's true.' She had never heard of William Sargant or his treatments until the BBC programme. 'I was absolutely disgusted. As I listened, I just couldn't believe it – I was so shocked. And I thought, Actually, no, I didn't consent, I didn't want the treatment and it didn't make me any better.' She says they had no right to impose narcosis on her because she had never been sectioned – for good reason. 'The moment you're sectioned, the law gives you some protection.'

Susannah was determined to find out exactly what treatments she had been given. Two years later, she managed to extract some information from St Thomas' Medical Records Department about her stay on Ward Five and subsequent referral as an outpatient to Scutari. A copy of her outpatient record had been kept on microfiche, which included the referral letter that got her admitted to the Royal Waterloo and the letter that was sent to her GP when she was discharged.

Susannah had received thirty-four ECT treatments – far more than Sargant had publicly recommended. 'You could hear them bringing oxygen cylinders, clanking down the long corridor, coming nearer and nearer,' she remembers. As well as Largactil and antidepressants (Nardil, Melleril, Surmontil), she was given ether abreaction – an outdated treatment that Sargant had pioneered in the Second World War. It didn't work. She also believes she was given modified insulin treatment because of her extreme weight gain, despite eating so little in the Sleep Room.

To anyone who thinks that they might have been patients on Ward Five, either under Sargant or Pollitt, Susannah's advice is to contact their GP and ask to see their discharge letter. When patients were discharged from the Royal Waterloo a letter detailing their treatment, including any time spent in the Sleep Room, would have been sent to their GP, which they have a legal right to see.

Susannah has campaigned tirelessly for greater transparency over the past fifteen years. She has contacted other patients, setting up the Ward Five Association, and has also tried to encourage a class action against St Thomas' – but it has proved difficult. Her biggest problem with what happened to her is that Sargant and his acolytes always claimed that only patients of 'good previous personality' could be cured. And she wasn't like that. She'd been struggling since she was a little girl.

41

'Can I buy you a Rolls-Royce?'

Sargant was devastated when the Sleep Room finally shut its doors in 1973. 'The minute I left, the Royal College of Nursing closed the wards,' he said in his last ever interview in 1987. 'Now, for twenty whole years, I had used general hospital nurses in training, and St Thomas' nurses, they really are the salt of the earth, but they had to be replaced by nurses from a mental hospital. My sleep treatment ward, which I had specially designed for that treatment, was converted to a television room, and it was all very distressing.'

He wasn't to be defeated, however. 'The trouble is that since my retirement from St Thomas', my private practice has increased enormously,' he wrote to a journalist. As well as doing four half days a week at 23 Harley Street, he set up another Sleep Room – this time exclusively for private patients – and wasn't afraid to talk about it in the medical press, even if he never revealed publicly where it was.

In a letter to the *BMJ*, he said that, following his retirement from St Thomas', he had been able to re-establish a 'narcosis ward' in an unnamed psychiatric nursing home. '25 often considered "chronic" schizophrenics have had the full combined narcosis and ECT treatment with additional insulin sopor when needed,' he wrote. It had sometimes needed 'over two months' of narcosis and 'more than 20' ECTs, to bring twenty-two out of the twenty-five patients into remission.

In another letter to the *BMJ*, he boasted that he had used various forms of continuous sleep treatment since 1940 on 'several thousands of patients'. More recently, he had kept patients under narcosis for two or more months, during which time 'intensive electric convulsion' therapy could also be given. The longest course of narcosis had been 'over four months', he said, adding that 'at present I have 10 patients on this regimen at a nursing home'.

The anonymous nursing home was in fact the Priory Hospital in Roehampton, south-west London. It was an obvious fit for Sargant. It had long been popular with celebrities, including Eric Clapton and George Best (and later, Kate Moss and Amy Winehouse). Dr Saeed Islam worked closely with Sargant for five years when he ran the acute service at the hospital, and later served as its medical director from 2005 to 2015. He confirmed that Sargant had been a visiting consultant since the 1950s, and that he had admitted his private patients to a narcosis unit from 1972 to 1982. (The unit was renamed the North Wing after the hospital was bought by an American healthcare provider in 1980.) 'Modified narcosis as a term was dropped in the mid 1980s,' according to Dr Islam, who says that acutely disturbed patients are still semi-sedated for two to three days, using a combination of atypical antipsychotics and benzodiazapenes. 'In very severe cases, they may be sedated for up to a week, with close monitoring of their mental state, vital signs, nutrition and hydration.'

Dee Bixley worked as the PA to one of the Priory's medical directors, Desmond Kelly, in the 1970s and 80s. (Kelly had been Sargant's senior registrar at St Thomas'.) She interviewed a number of Sargant's former colleagues for her book, *Inside the Priory*, including Sister Eileen MacAuley, who was asked by Sargant to run the narcosis unit when she joined in 1972. It had between six to eight patients at that time and the average stay was six weeks. The daily routine was similar to the Ward Five Sleep Room, except patients, who were on 'massive' doses of medication, were woken for three two-hour breaks each day for a big cooked breakfast, lunch and dinner.

'We might give them a wee walk up and down,' MacAuley told Bixley. 'We had to escort them physically and it was very hard work.' Drugs included two types of antidepressant, heavy tranquilisers and sleeping tablets. (The use of Mandrax was later stopped, because drug addicts were abusing it.) ECT was also given as well as enemas. Murphy remembered patients selling their jewellery to pay for their treatment because they'd been through many other hospitals and nothing had worked. Many were suicidal and suffering from severe psychotic breakdowns.

She was initially wary of the 'weird' treatment, but became convinced that it worked, even though it seemed to go completely against her training. 'There were patients that I thought would never ever get better, could not get better. And they did get better.'

Sargant visited the narcosis unit on Friday afternoons, when everything had to be ready. His patients had not been sedated that afternoon to ensure they were awake for Sargant's round. 'He would instruct: "continue treatment", "stop treatment", "reduce treatment",' MacAuley recalled. In those days, ECT was usually carried out 'two to three times a week and not on consecutive days', confirms Dr Islam, who was also lead consultant for the ECT service at the Priory until 2015.

Sargant was clearly adored by some of his patients. According to MacAuley, one company heiress arranged for nighties to be delivered from Harrods especially for his visits. Middle Eastern royalty took a particular shine to him. 'He would sit on the bed beside them and hold their hand,' MacAuley said. 'He always had a smile and a twinkle in his eye. It was all done very professionally.' Another patient, a 'gorgeous Arabian princess', arrived with two veiled assistants who fed her by hand. 'I remember the princess saying to Dr Sargant: "Can I buy you a Rolls-Royce today?"'

She wasn't joking.

According to gardener Brian Suter, who was interviewed by Bixley, five different coloured Rolls-Royces later drove up to the Priory entrance and parked outside. The driver of the first car got out and asked for Sargant. When he appeared at reception, the driver asked him what colour he would like. Sargant replied that he'd always liked the classic black. 'So the driver handed over the keys, with Sheikh do-da do-da's compliments!' Suter said.

At one point Sister MacAuley herself was suspected of having fallen for Sargant's charms. 'I admired this man,' she explained to Bixley. 'I didn't have an affair! I must get this point in.' She conceded, however, that there was a certain aura about him. 'He was a great big Daddy, a gentle giant.'

Dr Morven Thomson was a registrar and visiting consultant at the Priory between 1976 and 1997, who looked after Sargant's narcosis unit in between his weekly Friday visits. 'It was tricky putting people to sleep like that,' she told Bixley. 'It was difficult – both the nursing and the medical supervision.' Thomson, however, had total confidence in Sargant – 'he was an outstanding man' – and his mixing of MAOIs and tricyclic antidepressants. 'All the textbooks said never mix these two, but he had no disasters.' Nor did she have any hesitation about Sargant's frequent use of ECT on his 'very ill' patients, who in many cases were manic and suidical. She said that three times a week was standard, but Sargant would administer it on consecutive days if a patient was failing to respond.

Dr John Cobb was a consultant psychiatrist at the Priory from 1985 to 2004 and had also worked there as a locum in previous years. He told Bixley that he was amazed by Sargant's bedside manner. 'He almost bullied the patients into getting better:

“You will get better! You have had the best treatment in the world!”’

Desmond Kelly became medical director of the Priory Group in 1979. He confessed to Bixley, his PA, that when Sargant introduced junior doctors to the narcosis treatment, they were ‘frightened silly’ by the potential risks. ‘But when they saw the results, they changed their minds.’

Despite the pay and the gifts, Sargant missed his Sleep Room on Ward Five. In a letter to Dr Eric Cunningham Dax, a friend in Australia, he wrote that he had ‘plenty of beds at the Priory’ and made ‘much more money’. But the work ‘wasn’t so interesting’.

When Sargant wasn’t attending to his private patients he was busy writing – firing off letters to *The Times* (referring to himself as ‘Honorary Consulting Physician’ at St Thomas’) and penning provocative articles about his favourite subjects: Pavlov, brainwashing, exorcism, M’Naghten rules of madness (a defendant is presumed to be sane and accountable for his actions unless it can be proved otherwise) and religious conversions. He knew how to catch the eye of a commissioning editor. In one article, he warned that ‘drug traffickers in central London watch for ecstatic dancers to find their prey’. In another, he speculated what would have happened if his approach to psychiatry had been available earlier. ‘Jesus Christ might simply have returned to his carpentry following the use of modern treatments,’ he wrote. The philosophical implications of lobotomy – the ability to remove memories – also raised troubling issues, potentially enabling pilots to drop atomic bombs without any lingering guilt. ‘Conscience can now be eliminated surgically without any impairment of day to day working efficiency.’

It was double-blind trials, however, that had long upset him the most – particularly the *BMJ*’s support for them. Back in 1965, he had written to the journal, fuming that ‘we are never going to learn how to treat depressions properly from double-blind sampling in an MRC statistician's office'. He saw them as a direct challenge to all that he had achieved in the Sleep Room, a place built on clinical intuition rather than statistical analysis. In 1973, the Medical Research Council had carried out a double-blind trial on Moditen, a long-term 'depot' antipsychotic, to see if it could prevent recurrent schizophrenia. The '"statistical" experiment' had involved giving a placebo to half the patients. Sargant was appalled, writing an article for *The Times* asking 'Should patients be tortured in the name of progress?' The project was 'Belsen-like', driven by 'armchair writers' and 'laboratory technicians' who had done so much to hold back new treatments by physicians such as himself. Those patients who had been given an inert substance 'immediately went mad again, and were violently precipitated back into asylums'.

One of the MRC's investigators was Peter Rohde, Sargant's former researcher. Rohde clarified in a subsequent letter that anyone who had relapsed on placebos had been withdrawn from the trial, but Sargant never let the matter drop. 'Whenever [Sargant] met me after this,' Rohde remembered, 'he would shake his head and say, "You wouldn't do it to your wife, Rohde, you wouldn't do it to your wife."' (Sargant always claimed that he never administered any method of treatment to patients that he wouldn't use on himself or his family – including a lobotomy. 'I wouldn't let myself stay for twenty years in a mental hospital without having a modified leucotomy,' he told the BBC in 1968.)

The biggest riposte to Sargant, however, was from Anthony Clare. In many ways, Clare would go on to replace Sargant as Britain's most well-known psychiatrist, largely thanks to his long-running BBC Radio 4 series, *In the Psychiatrist's Chair*. In 1975, he wrote a stinging article in *World Medicine*, in which he accused Sargant, with his 'flashing mop of grey white hair' and 'brooding presence', of displaying 'petty tactlessness' in his *Times* article on double-blind trials. Sargant had made the basic error of believing that 'improvement *after* treatment is *due* to treatment' (an example, he said, of the *post hoc ergo propter hoc* fallacy that wrongly assumes a causal relationship based on the order in which two events happen); the only way to establish why someone felt better was through a control trial. He finished by comparing Sargant to Franz Mesmer, the eighteenth-century German physician (and philanderer) whose theory of invisible animal magnetism was widely adopted before being proved useless by a royal commission. The changing of the guard had begun.

Sargant saw an opportunity to salvage his reputation in November 1975, when Randolph Hearst, the fourth son of William Randolph Hearst, media magnate and founder of the Hearst Corporation, invited him to America to help his daughter. The previous February, Patty, a nineteen-year-old student at the University of California, Berkeley, had been kidnapped at gunpoint by the Symbionese Liberation Army.

The SLA was a left-wing revolutionary group, largely made up of white middle-class Americans, whose communiqués ended with their signature slogan: 'Death to the fascist insect that preys upon the people.' Hearst was kept in a closet for almost two months while the SLA made various ransom demands, including the distribution of food to California's poor. Eventually, Patty was given a choice: she could leave or stay with the group. One of the leaders told her: 'You're kinda like the pet chicken people have on a farm – when it comes time to kill it for Sunday dinner, no one really wants to do it.'

Patty stayed. Two weeks later, in April 1974, she was caught on camera, wielding an M1 carbine semi-automatic rifle as the gang robbed a bank in San Francisco. America was gripped. In May, she was firing shots in the air to free gang members who had been caught shoplifting in Los Angeles. When she was finally arrested on 18 September 1975, she gave her occupation as 'urban guerrilla', pumping the air with a fist salute.

At the heart of her trial, set for November 1975, was the question of whether she had been brainwashed or had willingly taken up arms with the SLA. Enter Sargant for the defence. He had already made clear his Pavlovian views on Patty, arguing in *The Times* that that it was entirely possible for someone to change their whole viewpoint on life 'suddenly and dramatically'. The article was enough to convince Patty's legal team to get the author of *Battle for the Mind* on board.

The defence counsel set about assembling an intriguing team of psychiatrists to act as expert witnesses, two of whom had been involved in the MKULTRA programme. Louis Jolyon 'Jolly' West, chair of psychiatry at UCLA, had been a beneficiary of Sydney Gottlieb's largesse in the past while at the University of Oklahoma (MKULTRA Subproject 43). He was also the one who killed Tusko the bull elephant with a massive dose of LSD (see Chapter 24). Martin Orne, professor of psychiatry at the University of Pennsylvania, had hypnotised scores of students while at Harvard for John Gittinger, the CIA psychologist (MKULTRA Subproject 84). Robert Jay Lifton, meanwhile, had been a psychiatrist for the US Air Force in Korea, working with brainwashed returning POWs. Given his own intelligence connections, both in the UK and in America, Sargant must have felt quite at home in such company.

Having burnished his credentials two days before with another article for *The Times* about suggestibility, Sargant touched down in California on Friday evening, 14 November 1975. 'As you know, I know quite a lot about brainwashing,' he said on his arrival. The media lapped it up and he loved the attention. Sargant visited Patty the following afternoon at the San Mateo County Jail, south of San Francisco, and was horrified. Her IQ had dropped dramatically, and she reminded Sargant of the patients he'd seen at Belmont. 'She's pathetic now,' he said later. 'She resembles a person during a war who has just come back from battle.'

Sargant saw Patty for a second time on Sunday. He couldn't resist talking to the admiring American press again. The 'tall, craggy faced physician' said that Patty had been 'extremely co-operative'. Sargant had been told not to speak but it was clearly proving a challenge. 'She is not being difficult in any way but beyond that I cannot say anything for the time being, at the request of her defence lawyers.' After five visits, he returned to the UK, where he gave more comments to the press, following the postponement of the trial until January. 'I found her a very charming person – extremely helpful and cooperative,' he told the *Guardian*, claiming that he had personally helped to get the trial postponed because of her depression. 'I am forbidden to give information as to whether or not I think she was brainwashed, because I may be called as a witness.'

In the end, he was never called. Publicly, the defence team said that a British expert might not play well with an American jury, but Sargant had become a liability with his leaks to the media. Desperate to be part of what had become the trial of the decade, Sargant continued to argue Patty's case back in Britain. He had prepared a detailed witness statement, some of which he used in an article for *The Times* in January 1976, on the third day of the trial: 'There will never be any doubt in my mind that Patty Hearst was "brain-washed", "forcibly converted", "coerced in thought and deed" or whatever other expression one chooses to use for the same thing,' he wrote. Under the prolonged stress of her incarceration, he argued, 'One's behaviour and ideas become the opposite of those normally held, just as the exhausted rabbit finally turns and runs into the mouth of the stoat.'

Patty's family had clung to the brainwashing defence, unable to accept that their daughter's decision to reject her bourgeois upbringing and join the SLA had been an act of free will. The jury disagreed. Patty Hearst was convicted of armed robbery in March 1976 – a 'moral outrage', according to Sargant – and was later sentenced to the maximum thirty-five years, which was subsequently reduced to seven. But the Hearsts were well connected. President Jimmy Carter reduced her sentence to twenty-two months and she was released at the beginning of February 1979. On his last day in office, President Bill Clinton pardoned her. Today, she is only in the news when her French bulldogs win prizes at the Westminster Kennel Club dog show in New York.

42

'Wanted: information on William Sargant'

Sargant stopped his work at the Priory and Harley Street in the early 1980s, when he suffered a stroke. Already concerned by the damaging revelations in America about MKULTRA, and in particular the work of his old friend Ewen Cameron, who had died in 1967, he now had another threat to deal with. In 1981, the Scientologists had the Sleep Room in their crosshairs, alleging that Sargant's private patients were still paying £500 a week for narcosis treatment at the Priory.

On Saturday 19 September, an advert appeared in *The Times*. 'WANTED,' it announced. 'Information on the psychiatrist William Sargant in the fields of ECT AND DRUG TREATMENTS, LEUCOTOMY AND PSYCHOSURGERY, MODIFIED NARCOSIS.' Readers were invited to call the Citizens Commission on Human Rights on Tottenham Court Road in London. The commission, set up in 1969, was a well-known front for the Church of Scientology, with a mission to expose 'atrocities' and eradicate 'brutality' in the field of mental health.

The advert appeared in *The Times* on four consecutive days the following week. It also ran in a wide range of other national and provincial newspapers. The appeal proved fruitful. The Scientologists published a series of articles on Sargant's work in its magazine, *Freedom*, including allegations that he had been subject to complaints to the General Medical Council. In the December issue, an article, 'State Secrets on the Couch' alleged that Sargant had become a national security risk, thanks to a photo of him cavorting with naked young people at a party. On the next page, another piece, 'The Russian Connection', attempted to link the World Psychiatric Association to the Soviet Union.

The lurid photo was displayed on the cover, with the banner caption: 'Blackmail photo of top psychiatrist? – See inside'. It was printed again on page 2, alongside another from the same sex party. It certainly looked like Sargant. Stripped to the waist, he struck a distinctly Jimmy Savile-esque pose, with his shock of swept-back white hair. His hands were around a topless young woman, who had her hands on his arms as she gazed up at him. The caption read: 'Close associates had no hesitation in identifying the central figure in these photographs as Dr William Sargant, founder member of the World Psychiatric Association.' It also said that 'discreditable photographs such as these' could be used for blackmail by foreign intelligence agencies and that copies had been sent to the Home Office.

It was a textbook example of tabloid trickery – denouncing a photo while publishing it – but it remains a deeply disturbing image, not because of its blackmail potential, which was minimal, given all the stories about Sargant's drinks parties, but in the more serious context of sexual allegations made by patients.

The magazine also mentioned a six-page article on sexual ritual that Sargant had written for *Man, Myth & Magic*, a publication edited by Richard Cavendish, who had helped Sargant to write *The Mind Possessed*. And it quoted Alex Sanders, 'an authority in the field of witchcraft as practiced in Britain', who had met Sargant in a TV studio green room ten years earlier. When the conversation had turned to Wiccan sex rites, in particular the 'Great Rite', which involves sexual intercourse between a priest and priestess, Sargant had apparently invited Sanders and his wife, Maxine, back to dinner – for research purposes. 'He explained that he wanted to watch us perform the intercourse, and for us to have simultaneous orgasms, at which point he would photograph our eyes ... Needless to say, my wife and I refused his proposition.' According to the *News of the World*, an unnamed 'eminent psychiatrist' had made a similar suggestion to Maxine, who had slapped him in the face. Today, Maxine confirms that the psychiatrist in question was indeed Sargant. 'All true, I'm afraid,' she says. 'The few contacts I had with the man were most unpleasant, leaving me with the opinion that he was a deviant and a dirty old man.'

Sargant had a convenient cover story for his interest in other people's sexual habits. For *The Mind Possessed*, he had travelled the world to study trance states and sexual ecstasy, observing that 'lovers in orgasm behave as if they were possessed, trembling, writhing, groaning, crying out, as blind and deaf to everything around them as if they were no longer on any earthly plane'. He'd also compared orgasm to Pavlov's 'collapse phase', which was similar to what happened in 'abreaction, ecstatic dancing and convulsion therapy'.

Time Out picked up on the 'wanted' adverts and contacted the Citizens Commission on Human Rights, which said it was compiling a dossier on Sargant's own sex life and alleged interest in black magic. *Time Out* chose not to publish the photo, but it later emerged in the *Express* and continues to circulate online today.

It must have all been deeply humiliating for Peggy, who personally dropped off a copy of *Freedom* magazine at the offices of the Medical Defence Union. Its secretary 'took a very serious view on this latest attack' and promised to look into the matter – once he'd read *The Mind Possessed* and Sargant's article on sex rites. 'The scientologists are torturing me,' Sargant told *Time Out*. 'I have had a stroke and what good they think they can do, I cannot imagine.' Seeming to distance himself from his own career-long approach to psychiatry, he explained that he had recommended only two cases for lobotomy during his last five years of private practice. 'Now we know that we can get people better by other methods, I am the first person to applaud the advance of treatment and research,' he said. 'All my life I have had only one aim – to help people.'

It was all too late and an ignominious end to Sargant's career. But there was one more person from his past who was about to come back to haunt him.

Some time in 1955, a young Australian psychiatrist called Dr Harry Bailey had passed through Britain on a World Health Organization fellowship that enabled him to study sedation. While in London, the hard-drinking, charismatic doctor met Sargant and was apparently impressed by his narcosis treatment. Fast-forward to 1963 and Bailey was back in Australia, working as a psychiatrist at Chelmsford Private Hospital, a mental health institution in a suburb of Sydney. For the next sixteen years, he subjected patients to his own version of deep sleep therapy and ECT – with catastrophic results. A royal commission, set up in the late 1980s to investigate Bailey, concluded that twenty-four patients had died under his care, a further twenty-four committed suicide, and twenty-two died unexpectedly within a year.

Bailey had always seen himself as a disciple of Sargant. According to the author Brian Bromberger, the two men remained in constant contact for almost thirty years. 'A nurse at Chelmsford during the 1970s, Rosa Nicholson, recalled that Bailey often spoke of the competition between them to see who could keep their patients in the deepest coma without killing them.'

Nicholson passed her information to the Citizens Commission on Human Rights, which launched a campaign against Bailey.

A powerful episode of *60 Minutes* that aired on ABC in 1980 investigated the death of one of Bailey's female patients. Three years later, he was charged with her manslaughter. The charge was subsequently dropped but the media scrutiny had become intense and other cases were coming to light. His defence team soon realised that his deep sleep treatment appeared to have much in common with Sargant's modified narcosis and called him to testify in Bailey's favour. There were, however, some key differences. Although both men were giving ECT and narcosis, Bailey was not waking his patients every six hours. They were kept in a much deeper sleep, given a more toxic cocktail of drugs and fed via stomach tube.

Sargant, one eye on his own reputation, refused to support his disciple. In a letter to Bailey's lawyer, he explained that if he'd travelled to Australia to give evidence under oath, he would have found himself 'supporting the prosecution and not the defence'. He added that stomach feeding and not waking patients regularly for food and fluid had resulted in the deaths of two of his own 'earlier patients'. Presumably he was referring to wartime fatalities, when he was tube-feeding narcosis patients at Belmont; he abandoned the practice in the 1940s.

Bailey was devastated. His mental health had been poor in recent years – at one point he was himself given deep sleep treatment by a colleague, apparently without his knowledge – but Sargant's letter tipped him over the edge. Bailey drove out of Sydney and took his own life in a deserted lay-by. In his suicide note, he wrote: 'I've had enough. I've learnt today that they've sent police today to interview Sargant. Always remember that the forces of evil are greater than the forces of good.'

Sargant's own health continued to deteriorate. On 3 October 1985, Desmond Kelly arranged an event to celebrate Sargant's life and work. In the afternoon, a series of lectures were given at the Priory, followed by dinner. Every psychiatrist who had ever worked with Sargant, dating back to the 1930s, had been invited. 'We had a turnout that filled the room,' recalled John Hughes, who admitted that everyone who encountered Sargant either loved or loathed him. 'These people came from all over the world – Cairo, Canada, Australia. It was an amazing thing.'

Lord Owen was there too, and wrote to Peggy after his death. Sargant, he said, was 'the most important figure in post-war psychiatry', adding that he had been a 'major influence' in his life and looked back on their time working together with immense pleasure. 'All of us, if the need arose, would have put those nearest and dearest to us in his care. He was a rebel *with* a cause.' (In the past, Lord Owen has been criticised for his comments about Sargant, whom he once described as a 'dominating personality with the therapeutic courage of a lion'. Today he says he is 'not an apologist' for Sargant. He believes that he was 'a very considerable pioneer' who wasn't perfect, but 'a driving force is often a necessary element in progress'.)

In 1986, two years before he died, Sargant moved to live full-time with Peggy at East Woodyates. According to a former nurse who knew him well, he was very ill, couldn't speak or swallow properly and was 'embarrassed being seen'. Sargant had been hounded out of London by the Scientologists, destined to be a polarising figure until the very end. (Blue plaques abound on Hamilton Terrace today, but there isn't one for Sargant.)

Sargant maintained throughout his career that he was motivated by a desire to do something for patients who would otherwise have been left to languish in overcrowded asylums. His patients in the Sleep Room – women like Celia, Mary, Linda, 'Sara', Anne and 'Freya' – would beg to differ. They wonder how anyone would willingly submit themselves, or a loved one, to what they were forced to endure. They would also like to know if Sargant's work for the intelligence services had affected their treatment. Were they ever subjected to experiments conducted at their request? And why was he allowed to work, unchecked, for so long in the NHS, which has only now apologised for his behaviour, more than fifty years later?

Sargant continues to polarise opinion today. The Royal College of Psychiatrists still has an annual William Sargant Lecture and carries a glowing tribute by Desmond Kelly on the 'inspiring physicians' section of its website. (The RCP has now qualified its historical obituaries as 'products of their time'.) St Bernard's Hospital, an acute mental health facility built in the grounds of the old Hanwell asylum in Southall (where Sargant was admitted as a patient and possibly worked as a locum), had a William Sargant ward until 2014. However, his name remains in gilded letters on the wooden panel at St Thomas' that honours past physicians and surgeons. And in 2019, his 1957 bestseller, *Battle for the Mind*, was re-released by an Indian publisher as a self-help book. 'He had a very lucky streak about him,' said Ann Dally. 'He did a lot of very dangerous things with his patients but they never seemed to die on him.'

There's no question that some of his changes were for the good. He helped to end the era of overcrowded Victorian asylums, bringing psychiatry into the medical mainstream. Many patients were discharged from Ward Five feeling better – at least in the short term – and ECT continues to be administered today, if in a very modified way, to almost two thousand people a year in the UK and Ireland. For some the treatment is undoubtedly a lifesaver.* Sargant also introduced an innovative training rotation for his senior registrars, equally divided between neurology and psychiatry. And he did much to advance the cause of antidepressants, for better or worse. He also wasn't the only doctor to embrace extreme physical treatments such as lobotomy, insulin coma and narcosis – all were briefly front and centre of post-war

---

* In 2023, Dr Tania Gergel, Director of Research at Bipolar UK, revealed in a BBC Radio 4 programme, *Shocking*, that she had willingly had 'close to two hundred' ECT treatments for her depression, psychosis and mania. ECT, she said, had saved her life on numerous occasions.

psychiatry in Britain. But only briefly. That was the difference. They were soon widely discredited by his contemporaries. Sargant persisted with them, like the lone man at the bar, still drinking heavily long after closing time.

Sargant died on 27 August 1988, leaving behind £750,000 – more than £2 million today. Psychiatry had served his bank balance well. His body was buried at St Rumbold's Church in Pentridge, a tranquil spot bordered by green fields in a fold of Dorset chalk downland. Peggy would leave £5,000 in her will for the church and graveyard's upkeep. The grave is on the right of the path that leads up through the grassy graveyard to the Victorian church. Worshippers would struggle to miss it. One of the church windows also has a small *in memoriam* etched in a leaded pane.

It's the gravestone's simple inscription, however, that catches the eye. 'Loving memory, William Walters Sargant FRCP FRC PSYCH, 1907–1988. Writer and Physician.' The reference to 'Physician' is understandable. Sargant's job title was 'Physician in Charge' when he joined St Thomas' in 1948, a reflection of his lifelong desire to bring psychiatry into the medical mainstream. Ditto the letters after his name. He had become a Fellow of the Royal College of Physicians, a rare honour, as well as a Fellow of the Royal College of Psychiatrists. 'Writer' is more intriguing, particularly as it comes first. *Battle for the Mind* was a global bestseller, but Robert Graves didn't consider him much of a writer.

Peggy knew what sort of husband she wanted to remember. It wasn't the pills or the shocks, the insulin or the narcosis. It was his pen. Even more telling is the gravestone itself. The dedication to Peggy, 'his beloved wife', is hard to read, hidden by grass. Sargant's headstone is sinking, soon to disappear into the English soil. His Sleep Room has long since gone too. The Royal Waterloo hospital is now owned by the University of Notre Dame. Known as Conway Hall, it provides accommodation for international students. On the top floor, formerly Ward Five, the Sleep Room has been converted into a dormitory.

Acknowledgements

I couldn't have written this book without the help, cooperation and extraordinary courage of the patients who shared their experiences of being treated by Dr William Sargant. Some were happy to be named; others have chosen to remain anonymous, a reminder of the social stigma that still, regrettably, surrounds mental illness.

Celia Imrie, Mary Thornton, Linda Keith, 'Sara', Anne White, 'Freya', 'Liz', 'Ruth Chadwick', 'Susannah', Annabel Thompson, 'Anne' – I am incredibly grateful to you all for your patience, honesty and bravery. It has been a privilege to tell your stories, for so long unheard, and I know they will be a source of great comfort and hope to the many others, mostly women, who suffered at Sargant's hands. I am also hugely indebted to Christina Berry, who generously shared her many years of research. Her tireless efforts to expose Sargant have been inspirational.

Many former Ward Five nurses also agreed to speak, and I am thankful to Shelley, Pippa Ecclestone, Catherine Mountain, Ann Rowland, Tish, Sue, Christine, Julia Ross, as well as 'Rosa' (Belmont) and Monica (Atkinson Morley). Ditto Sargant's other St Thomas' colleagues who kindly agreed to talk to me. Specifically, I'd like to thank Peter Tyrer, Emeritus Professor of Community Psychiatry at Imperial College London, for his recollections of being Sargant's house physician in 1966; and Dr

Ben Spears, who spent fifty years in private practice in Prince Edward Island in Canada, after being Senior Registrar and Chief Assistant in the Department of Psychiatry at St Thomas' between 1969 and 1972. Ben has been incredibly generous with his time, insights into Sargant's character and considerable knowledge of psychiatry. Nita Mitchell-Heggs, who worked on Ward Five in 1968 as a post-registration house officer, has also been a formidable sounding board. We have occasionally agreed to differ, but she has offered invaluable wisdom and perspective, as well as sharing her own memories of her brief experience working with Sargant. Nita (and her husband Peter) have answered numerous medical queries of mine in confidence and with great diligence and humour. Lord David Owen, Sargant's registrar in 1965, has also been generous with his time. None of the above are apologists for Sargant, and they only briefly crossed paths with him in their long and distinguished careers, but they reminded me of the need to judge Sargant's work in the context of the era in which he worked.

Sadly, I can't name all the people who have helped, as some have asked to remain anonymous, but I'm grateful to you all. Those I can mention include Dr John West, consultant cardiologist, whose father, Dr Eric West, was Sargant's senior registrar at St Thomas' before he was appointed consultant in psychiatry and EEG at Belmont in 1959. John has written *The Psychiatrist*, a fascinating novel inspired by his father's experiences in the Second World War. I am very grateful for his advice and support. He was also an eagle-eyed 'beta reader' – any mistakes are, of course, mine. I must also thank Justin Robbins (and Mary Thornton for the introduction). He kindly introduced me to St Thomas' redoubtable 'Class of 66', many of whom were good enough to share their memories of Sargant as medical students and as newly qualified doctors and nurses in the 1960s; Dr Maria Rollin, MBE, a retired consultant anaesthetist who worked on Ward Five in 1972, allowed me to quote her late husband, Dr

Henry Rollin, one of Sargant's fiercest critics; Emma Dally, daughter of Peter and Ann Dally, gave me permission to use her mother's nascent biography of Sargant; Professor Andrew Lees, consultant neurosurgeon at the National Hospital for Neurology and Neurosurgery, Queen Square, London; Joanna Moncrieff, Professor of Critical and Social Psychiatry at UCL; and Diana DeFalco, for her help and trust.

Writing non-fiction after many years in fiction has been an enjoyable gear change, but not as dramatic as it might sound. My spy thrillers, published under my own name (and written when I was a journalist), and my psychological thrillers, written under the pen name J. S. Monroe, already feature a lot of real-world research. The only noticeable difference has been greater interaction with other authors (novelists tend to be solitary creatures). Dominic Streatfeild was the first person to subject Sargant's career – and intelligence connections – to serious scrutiny. The research he did for a section on Sargant in his acclaimed book, *Brainwash* (2006), has been invaluable. I carried a well-thumbed copy around with me in the early days of my own research. I am also indebted to him for subsequently sharing his interviews with Sargant's colleagues (published and unpublished), many of whom have since died.

James Maw picked up the baton a few years later and presented a compelling thirty-minute documentary about Sargant for BBC Radio 4 (*Revealing the Mind Bender General*, 2009). I am grateful to him and to his producer, Neil George, for their help. Mike Jay has been unfailingly helpful, full of encouragement and kind advice. 'Over the Edge' (2013), his dazzling essay on Sargant, was a source of great inspiration, and set a very high bar. Barbara Davis, who wrote about Sargant for the *Daily Mail* in 2013, was also generous with her contacts. William Graves, son of Robert Graves, took time out to show me and my wife around his father's house, Ca n'Alluny in Deià, and share memories of Sargant, a regular visitor to Majorca. He and his son Philip are in the process of digitising all of Robert Graves' correspondence, which will be available for free to everyone at robertgravesletters.org.

Other academics, writers and broadcasters who have helped include John Marks, whose seminal book, *In Search of the 'Manchurian Candidate'*, is the *ur*-text for anyone wanting to know about MKULTRA; Harvey M. Weinstein, whose father was a victim of Ewen Cameron (his book, *Father, Son, CIA* is a must read), was very supportive and, crucially, introduced me to one of Sargant's most eloquent patients; Egmont R. Koch helped with Frank Olson's passport as well as Sargant's connection with Henry K. Beecher; Rob Evans of the *Guardian* shared his forensic digging into Porton Down and LSD; Lisa Ellenwood, producer of the fascinating *Brainwashed* podcast about Ewen Cameron, gave me time and leads; Professor William Douglas Woody at the School of Psychological Studies, University of Northern Colorado, sent me his impeccable research into the psychology of Cold War interrogation techniques; and Duncan Cameron, son of Ewen Cameron, steered me towards his father's papers at the American Psychiatric Association, offering to help me get access to them in the APA's archives. I'd also like to thank David H. Price, Professor of Anthropology at St Martin's University in Lacey, Washington; Elizabeth Roberts-Pedersen, Senior Lecturer in History at University of Newcastle, New South Wales; Andy Beale; Damien Lewis; John Lancaster; Dee Bixley; Kitty Hauser; Robert Miller; Gerry Luckett; Saeed Islam at the Priory Group; Khaleelah Jones; the anonymous author behind ECT Statistics; Jonathan Gaisman and Tim Palmer in the West Country; Kevin Barnes and K. Ram at Conway Hall, University of Notre Dame, London; Neil Berrett; Jay Joseph; Peter Hanley; Laurena Grant; Professor Christopher Griffiths; fellow committee members of Marlborough LitFest; and Eric Gow, who has done so much for the victims of human experiments at Porton Down in the 1950s.

Thanks too to Louise Harrison at the London Metropolitan Archives; Nicola Cook, Collections Information librarian, and

Ross MacFarlane at the Wellcome Collection; Deena Gorland, archivist/librarian at the American Psychiatric Association; Ann Trevor, researcher, at the National Archives in Washington DC; Rebecca Williams, archives librarian at Duke University Medical Center; Rupert Baker, Library manager, the Royal Society; Polly Clint and Frances Paine at the Royal Society of Medicine Library; and Claire Hilton, honorary archivist at the Royal College of Psychiatrists.

I edited this book in various warm and welcoming libraries: Marlborough town library (where I often wrote to the sound of 'The Wheels on the Bus' – a soothing antidote to the darkness of Sargant's Sleep Room), Hungerford Library, Newbury Library and the Morrab Library in Penzance, where I was given endless support – and my own writing room – by the wonderful Lisa di Tommaso and her team.

Special thanks to my top agents at Janklow & Nesbit, Will Francis (UK) and Kirby Kim (US), and Corissa Hollenbeck; the great team at Little, Brown: my peerless editor, Sameer Rahim and forensic copy editor Zoe Gullen; publicity manager Katya Ellis; proof-reader David Bamford; and indexer David Atkinson; big thanks too to Sarah Robbins at Abrams in New York; Sharon Hughff at Scott Free; Oskar Söderlund; Chris Kennedy; Emily Hayward Whitlock and Rhiannon Davies at the Artists Partnership; the Royal Literary Fund; and Jeremy Parr for his impeccable legal advice.

Most of all I'd like to thank my family: Dinah, my mother-in-law, let me stay in the Nook in Cornwall, where I wrote some of this book; Maya typed up many of my interview transcripts; Felix and Jago were full of encouragement, as were my brothers and brothers-in-law; and my wife Hilary put up with me disappearing down so many rabbit holes that I grew whiskers. I'm eternally grateful for her love, patience, wisdom and humour.

Bibliography

Albarelli, H. P., Jr, *A Terrible Mistake: The Murder of Frank Olson and the CIA's Secret Cold War Experiments* (Walterville: Trine Day, 2009)

Baxter, James Phinney, III, *Scientists Against Time* (Boston: Little, Brown, 1946)

Bixley, Dee, *Inside the Priory: Roehampton Priory Stories Told by Doctors, Staff and Patients* (Sandy: Bright Pen, 2012)

Bromberger, Brian and Fife-Yeomans, Janet, *Deep Sleep: Harry Bailey and the Scandal of Chelmsford* (London: Simon & Schuster, 1991)

Burgess, Anthony, *A Clockwork Orange* (London: William Heinemann, 1962)

Burrough, Bryan, *Days of Rage: America's Radical Underground, the FBI and the Forgotten Age of Revolutionary Violence* (London: Penguin, 2015)

Calahan, Susannah, *Brain on Fire: My Month of Madness* (New York: Particular Books, 2012)

Clare, Anthony, *Psychiatry in Dissent: Controversial Issues in Thought and Practice* (London: Tavistock, 1976)

Collins, Anne, *In the Sleep Room: The Story of CIA Brainwashing Experiments in Canada* (Toronto: Lester & Orpen Dennys, 1988)

Conant, Jennet, *Tuxedo Park: A Wall Street Tycoon and the Secret*

Palace of Science that Changed the Course of World War II (New York: Simon & Schuster, 2002)

Corera, Gordon, *The Art of Betrayal: Life and Death in the British Secret Service* (London: Weidenfeld & Nicolson, 2011)

Dally, Ann, *A Doctor's Story* (London: Macmillan, 1990)

Deighton, Len, *The Ipcress File* (London: Hodder & Stoughton, 1962)

de Young, Mary, *Encyclopedia of Asylum Therapeutics, 1750–1950s* (Jefferson, NC: McFarland & Co., 2015)

Dimsdale, Joel, *Dark Persuasion: A History of Brainwashing from Pavlov to Social Media* (New Haven: Yale University Press, 2021)

Dorril, Stephen, *MI6: Fifty Years of Special Operations* (London: 4th Estate, 2000)

Ellingwood, Finley and Lloyd, John Uri, *American Materia Medica, Therapeutics and Pharmcognosy* (Chicago: Ellingwood's Therapeutist, 11th edn 1919)

Fennell, Phil, *Treatment Without Consent: Law, Psychiatry and the Treatment of Mentally Disordered People Since 1845* (Abingdon: Routledge, 1996)

Filer, Nathan, *The Heartland: Finding and Losing Schizophrenia* (London: Faber & Faber, 2019)

Freeman, Hugh (ed.), *A Century of Psychiatry* (London: Mosby, 1999)

Fry, Helen, *The London Cage: The Secret History of Britain's World War II Interrogation Centre* (New Haven: Yale University Press, 2017)

Graves, William, *Wild Olives: Life in Majorca with Robert Graves* (London: Hutchinson, 1995)

Harris, Robert and Paxman, Jeremy, *A Higher Form of Killing: The Secret Story of Gas and Germ Warfare* (London: Chatto & Windus, 1982)

Hearst, Patricia Campbell (with Alvin Moscow), *Every Secret Thing* (New York: Doubleday, 1982)

Hilton, Clare and Stephenson, Tom (convenors and eds), *Psychiatric Hospitals in the UK in the 1960s. Witness Seminar 11 October 2019* (London: Royal College of Psychiatrists, 2020)

Holden, Wendy, *Shell Shock: The Psychological Impact of War* (London: Channel 4 Books, 1998)

Hopkins, Linda, *False Self: The Life of Masud Khan* (New York: Other Press, 2006)

Imrie, Celia, *The Happy Hoofer* (London: Hodder & Stoughton, 2011)

Jay, Mike, *This Way Madness Lies: The Asylum and Beyond* (London: Thames & Hudson, 2016)

——————, *Psychonauts: Drugs and the Making of the Modern Mind* (New Haven: Yale University Press, 2023)

Jacobsen, Annie, *Operation Paperclip: The Secret Intelligence Program that Brought Nazi Scientists to America* (New York: Little, Brown, 2014)

Jones, W. L., *Ministering to Minds Diseased: A History of Psychiatric Treatment* (London: Heinemann, 1983)

Keefe, Patrick Radden, *Empire of Pain: The Secret History of the Sackler Dynasty* (London: Picador, 2021)

Kesey, Ken, *One Flew Over the Cuckoo's Nest* (New York: Viking, 1962)

Kinzer, Stephen, *Poisoner in Chief: Sidney Gottlieb and the CIA Search for Mind Control* (New York: Henry Holt, 2019)

Klein, Naomi, *The Shock Doctrine: The Rise of Disaster Capitalism* (London: Allen Lane, 2007)

Knight, Sam, *The Premonitions Bureau* (London: Faber & Faber, 2022)

Koch, Egmont and Wech, Michael, *Deckname Artischocke: Die geheimen Menschenversuche der CIA* (Munich: Bertelsmann, 2002)

Lewis, Michael L., *Inventing Global Ecology: Tracking the Biodiversity Ideal in India, 1947–1997* (Athens, OH: Ohio University Press, 2004)

Lindley, Richard, *Panorama: Fifty Years of Pride and Paranoia* (London: Politico's, 2003)

Llewellyn, Sheila, *Walking Wounded* (London: Sceptre, 2018)

Macintyre, Ben, *A Spy Among Friends: Kim Philby and the Great Betrayal* (London: Bloomsbury, 2014)

McCoy, Alfred, *A Question of Torture: CIA Interrogation, from the Cold War to the War on Terror* (New York: Henry Holt, 2006)

——————, *Torture and Impunity: The US Doctrine of Coercive Interrogation* (Madison: University of Wisconsin Press, 2012)

Marks, John, *The Search for the 'Manchurian Candidate': The CIA and Mind Control* (New York: Times Books, 1979)

Mitchell, S. Weir, *Fat and Blood: An Essay on the Treatment of Certain Forms of Neurasthenia and Hysteria* (Philadelphia: J. B. Lippincott, 1898)

Moncrieff, Joanna, *The Bitterest Pills: The Troubling Story of Antipsychotic Drugs* (Basingstoke: Palgrave Macmillan, 2013)

Mullan, Bob, *Mad to be Normal: Conversations with R. D. Laing* (London: Free Association Books, 1995)

O'Prey, Paul (ed.), *Between Moon and Moon: Selected Letters of Robert Graves 1946–1972* (London: Hutchinson, 1984)

Otterman, Michael, *American Torture: From the Cold War to Abu Ghraib and Beyond* (Melbourne: Melbourne University Press, 2007)

Owen, David, *Time to Declare* (London: Michael Joseph, 1991)

Pincher, Chapman, *Their Trade is Treachery* (London: Sidgwick & Jackson, 1981)

Pollitt, John, *Psychological Medicine for Students* (Edinburgh: Churchill Livingstone, 1973)

Porter, Roy (ed.), *The Faber Book of Madness* (London: Faber & Faber, 1991)

Pressman, Jack D., *Last Resort: Psychosurgery and the Limits of Medicine* (Cambridge: Cambridge University Press, 1998)

Price, David H., *Cold War Anthropology: The CIA, the Pentagon, and the Growth of Dual Use Anthropology* (Durham, NC: Duke University Press, 2016)

Rodman, F. Robert, *Winnicott: His Life and Work* (Cambridge, MA: Da Capo, 2003)

Ronson, Jon, *The Men Who Stare at Goats* (London: Picador, 2004)

Ross, Colin A., *The CIA Doctors: Human Rights Violations by American Psychiatrists* (Richardson, TX: Manitou Communications, 2019)

Ross, Julia, *Call the Social* (London: Best Books and Films, 2022)

Sackler, Arthur M., Sackler, Mortimer D., Sackler, Raymond R. and Martí-Ibáñez, Félix (eds), *The Great Physiodynamic Therapies in Psychiatry: An Historical Reappraisal* (New York: Hoeber-Harper, 1956)

Sargant, William and Slater, Eliot, *An Introduction to Physical Methods of Treatment in Psychiatry* (Edinburgh: Churchill Livingstone, 5 edns 1944, 1948, 1954, 1963, 1972)

——————, *An Introduction to Somatic Methods of Treatment in Psychiatry* (Baltimore: Williams and Wilkins, 1944)

Sargant, William, *Battle for the Mind: A Physiology of Conversion and Brain-Washing* (London: Heinemann, 1957)

——————, *The Unquiet Mind: The Autobiography of a Physician in Psychological Medicine* (London: Heinemann, 1967; Boston: Atlantic/Little, Brown, 1967)

——————, *The Mind Possessed: A Physiology of Possession, Mysticism and Faith Healing* (London: Heinemann, 1973)

Schmidt, Ulf, *Secret Science: A Century of Poison Warfare and Human Experiments* (Oxford: Oxford University Press, 2006)

Scull, Andrew, *Desperate Remedies: Psychiatry and the Mysteries of Mental Illness* (London: Allen Lane, 2022)

Shephard, Ben, *A War of Nerves: Soldiers and Psychiatrists 1914–1994* (London: Jonathan Cape, 2000)

Shields, James and Gottesman, Irving I. (eds), *Man, Mind, and*

Heredity: Selected Papers of Eliot Slater on Psychiatry and Genetics (London: Johns Hopkins University Press, 1971)

Shorter, Edward and Healy, David, *Shock Therapy: A History of Electroconvulsive Treatment in Mental Illness* (Toronto: University of Toronto Press, 2007)

Streatfeild, Dominic, *Brainwash: The Secret History of Mind Control* (London: Hodder & Stoughton, 2006)

Summerscale, Kate, *The Book of Phobias and Manias: A History of the World in 99 Obsessions* (London: Wellcome Collection, 2022)

Talbot, David, *The Devil's Chessboard: Allen Dulles, the CIA, and the Rise of America's Secret Government* (London: William Collins, 2015)

Tallis, Frank, *The Sleep Room* (London: Pan, 2013)

———, *The Act of Living: What the Great Psychologists Can Teach Us About Suriviving Discontent in an Age of Anxiety* (London: Little, Brown, 2021)

Thomas, Gordon, *Journey into Madness: Medical Torture and the Mind Controllers* (London: Bantam, 1988)

———, *Secrets & Lies: A History of Mind Control & Germ Warfare* (London: JR Books, 2008)

———, *Inside British Intelligence: 100 years of MI5 and MI6* (London: JR Books, 2009)

Thomas, R. W. and Wilson, I. G. H., *Report on Cardiazol Treatment and the Present Application of Hypoglycaemic Shock Treatment in Schizophrenia* (London: Board of Control for England and Wales, 1938)

Tooth, G. C. and Newton, Mary P., *Leucotomy in England and Wales, 1942–1954* (London: HMSO, 1961)

Urban, Mark, *UK Eyes Alpha: The Inside Story of British Intelligence* (London: Faber & Faber, 1996)

Valenstein, Elliot S., *Great and Desperate Cures: The Rise and Decline of Psychosurgery and Other Radical Treatments for Mental Illness* (New York: Basic Books, 1986)

Watson, Peter, *War on the Mind: The Military Uses and Abuses of Psychology* (London: Hutchinson, 1978)

West, John, *The Psychiatrist: Conscript, Prisoner, Interpreter, Healer* (London: Fortis, 2021)

West, Nigel, *The Circus: MI5 Operations 1945–1972* (New York: Stein and Day, 1983)

——————, *Molehunt: The Full Story of the Soviet Spy in MI5* (London: Weidenfeld & Nicolson, 1987)

——————, *The Friends: Britain's Post-War Secret Intelligence Operations* (London: Weidenfeld & Nicolson, 1988)

—————— (ed.), *The Faber Book of Espionage* (London: Faber & Faber, 1993)

——————, *At Her Majesty's Secret Service: The Chiefs of Britain's Intelligence Agency, MI6* (London: Greenhill, 2006)

Wynne, Greville, *The Man from Moscow: The Story of Wynne and Penkovsky* (London: Hutchinson, 1967)

Wright, Peter (with Paul Greengrass), *Spycatcher: The Candid Autobiography of a Senior Intelligence Officer* (London: Viking, 1987)

Notes

Chapter 1

6 *'sofa merchants':* Streatfeild, *Brainwash*, p. 243.

7 *'cut the cackle':* William Sargant, 'Psychiatric Treatment in General Teaching Hospitals: A Plea for a Mechanistic Approach', *BMJ*, 2:5508 (30 July 1966), pp. 257–62.

7 *'What is also so valuable':* Sargant and Slater, *An Introduction to Physical Methods of Treatment in Psychiatry* (5th edn 1972), p. 89.

7 *a BBC documentary: Towards Tomorrow: People Like Us*, BBC One, first broadcast 22 February 1968.

8 *'Some people think':* 'The Work of the Devil', *Sunday Times*, 23 February 1976.

8 *'Of all the twentieth century':* Ann Dally, 'William Walters Sargant', *Dictionary of National Biography* (Oxford: Oxford University Press, 2004), p. 963.

8 *'There was a whiff of sulphur':* Streatfeild, *Brainwash*, p. 245.

9 *Over six feet tall:* According to his US immigration card in 1947, he was 6ft 2in.

9 *'If he'd been a gorilla':* Streatfeild, *Brainwash*, p. 243.

9 *'of whom legends are made':* Ibid.

9 *A man who claimed:* Owen, *Time to Declare*, p. 77.

10 *'not without its dangers':* Sargant and Slater, *An Introduction to Physical Methods of Treatment in Psychiatry* (4th edn 1964), p. 27.

10 *instead of being lobotomised:* 'Report on the Department of Psychological Medicine, St Thomas's Hospital, 1948–1965', Sargant Personal Papers, 'Institutions', Wellcome Collection, PP/WWS/B/2/5. The registrar who made the discovery was Chris Walter. Jim Birley, another registrar, had noticed that chronically tense patients who had been given leucotomies at St Thomas' became depressed after the operation, suggesting that an underlying depression might have been missed. All patients were subsequently given ECT, drugs and narcosis before any decision was taken to lobotomise them.

10 *one of Sargant's fiercest critics:* D. W. Winnicott, 'Ethics of Prefrontal Leucotomy', letter, *BMJ*, 2:496 (25 August 1951), pp. 496–7.

11 *'severely depressed, anxious':* Sargant and Slater, *An Introduction to Physical Methods of Treatment in Psychiatry* (5th edn 1972), p. 89.

13 *Some of the medical records:* Non-selective statistics are hard to find, but we know that 484 patients were given narcosis treatment at St Thomas' and Belmont Hospital in Sutton, where Sargant worked one day a week, between 1962 and 1968. C. J. S. Walter, Nita Mitchell-Heggs and William Sargant, 'Modified Narcosis, ECT and Antidepressant Drugs: A Review of Technique and Immediate Outcome', *British Journal of Psychiatry*, 120:559 (June 1972), pp. 651–62.

Chapter 3

25 *first announced in the* Lancet*:* Will Sargant, 'Treatment of Subacute Combined Degeneration of the Cord by Massive Iron Dosage', *Lancet*, 219:5657 (30 January 1932), pp. 230–1.

25 *invited to talk at Cambridge:* Letter from Samuel Squire Sprigge, 16 November 1927, Sargant Personal Papers, 'Autographed Letters from Eminent Medical Men', Wellcome Collection, PP/WWS/A/3.

25 *'The intention of this paper':* William Sargant, 'On the Treatment of the Nervous Disorders Accompanying Anemia by Intensive Iron-Therapy', *Lancet*, 220:5703 (17 December 1932), pp. 1322–5.

26 *'He had a powerful personality':* Ann Dally's account in this chapter is drawn from 'Biographical and Other Writings on William Sargant', part of uncatalogued material (Acc. 1521, part of PP/DAL) that was donated by Dally's family to the Wellcome Collection in 2007, after she had died. Dally's draft biography covered Sargant's early life up to and including his admission to Hanwell. Special thanks to Ann's daughter, Emma Dally, for permission to reproduce this material. And to Nicola Cook, Collections Information Librarian at the Wellcome, for helping me to locate it.

26 *Back at the Royal Society of Medicine:* The account of the meeting is taken from Proceedings of the Royal Society of Medicine ('Discussion on the Treatment of Subacute Combined Degeneration', 21 December 1933), published in *Royal Society of Medicine Journal*, 27:6 (April 1934), pp. 769–88.

27 *'He had his depression':* Ann Dally Personal Papers, Wellcome Collection, PP/DAL.

27 *no reason to doubt:* Dr Dally's daughter, Emma, confirmed to the author that her mother had told her Sargant had been a psychiatric patient.

28 *Sargant's depression:* Thanks to the anonymous author of the excellent 'ECT Statistics' blog for originally drawing attention to Michael Neve's talk at a workshop in Germany in 2004 ('The History of Illness Narratives'), which led the author to Dally's own biography ('William Sargant, Deep Sleep Treatment and ECT', 23 January 2011). Neve was senior lecturer at the Wellcome Trust Centre for the History of Medicine at UCL. At one point, he was going to take on Sargant's biography from Dally. Writing about Dally in a footnote (#22) to his talk in 2004, he said: 'Her first husband Dr Peter Dally had been Sargant's registrar and many of her sources on this episode come from such personal communications. Out of kindness and the hope that I would take the story further, she passed the MS on to me and I am indeed in the process of taking the Sargant story further.' Neve, however, later admitted to Dally that

he was never going to finish the biography and handed the manuscript back to her. He died in October 2019 (see Mike Jay's tribute to him in the *London Review of Books*, 21 November 2019).

28 *'I was very obsessed':* Hugh Freeman, 'In Conversation with William Sargant', *Bulletin of the Royal College of Psychiatrists*, 11 (September 1987), pp. 290–4.

30 *'He was able to understand':* Owen, *Time to Declare*, p. 77, and author interview.

31 *'I do not have any first-hand knowledge':* Dr Chloe Beale, 'My Illness Does Not Make Me a Better Doctor', BMJ Opinion (blogs.bmj.com/bmj/), 28 January 2021.

31 *At one party in the 1960s:* Thanks to Dr John West, Eric's son, for this recollection.

31 *R. D. Laing, 'There were rumours':* Mullan, *Mad to be Normal*, p. 256. In an appearance on BBC Radio 4's *In the Psychiatrist's Chair* (July 1985, rebroadcast in August 2015), R. D. Laing told Anthony Clare that he had suffered from clinical depression and episodic alcoholism during his life.

32 *'The full horror of Hanwell':* Sargant, *The Unquiet Mind*. p. 12.

32 *'frank and forthright': Sunday Telegraph* review quote on the cover of the Pan Books paperback edition of *The Unquiet Mind* (1971).

Chapter 4

33 *'My mother, who had eight children':* William Sargant, 'The Risks of Allowing Pornography to Grow Unchecked', *The Times*, 3 February 1976.

34 *'delusional', 'unpardonable pride':* Sargant Personal Papers, 'General Correspondence', Wellcome Collection, PP/WWS/A/4.

34 *second bishop . . . Mysore:* Sargant mistakenly referred to his brother Norman as the Bishop of Bangalore, where he was consecrated at St Mark's Cathedral on 12 April 1951. Norman was Bishop of Mysore until 1972.

34 *'thrashed time after time':* This and other details of Sargant's upbringing are from his autobiography, *The Unquiet Mind*.

35 *'For so young a boy'*: Ann Dally Personal Papers, 'Biographical and Other Writings on William Sargant', Wellcome Collection, PP/DAL.

36 *a personality type:* Vicky Long, 'Adventures in Psychiatry: Narrating and Enacting Reform in Post-War Mental Healthcare', *Studies in Literary Imagination*, 48:1 (2015), pp. 109–25.

Chapter 5

39 *'approximately 8 per cent'*: William Sargant and J. M. Blackburn, 'The Effect of Benzedrine on Intelligence Scores', *Lancet*, 228:5911 (12 December 1936), pp. 1385–7.

40 *'Imprudent people began'*: Sargant, *The Unquiet Mind*, p. 45.

40 *'remove mental fatigue'*: Erich Guttmann and William Sargant, 'Observations on Benzedrine', *BMJ*, 1:3984 (15 May 1937), pp. 1013–15.

40–1 *'By now I should have'*: 'New Superiority Drug is Tried Out', *Daily Express*, 15 May 1937.

41 *'ounce of phenobarbitone'*: Sargant, *The Unquiet Mind*, p. 32.

41 *'the greatest psychiatrist'*: Freeman, 'In Conversation with William Sargant'.

41 *disdain for the psychotherapeutic claims:* Elizabeth Roberts-Pederson, 'The Hard School: Physical Treatments for War Neurosis in Britain during the Second World War', *Social History of Medicine*, 29:3 (August 2016), pp. 611–32.

41 *Mapother was keen:* Edgar Jones, 'Aubrey Lewis, Edward Mapother and the Maudsley', *Medical History*, 47:S22 (2003), pp. 3–38.

41 *'It was not a good start'*: Sargant, *The Unquiet Mind*, p. 40.

42 *'Shamed by the advances'*: 'Brainwaves', episode 3 of *Madness: A Social History of Mental Illness*, presented by Jonathan Miller, Channel 4, broadcast 20 October 1991.

Chapter 6

43 *'heroic' therapies:* '"Heroic Therapies" in Psychiatry', Science Museum, 13 June 2019.

43 *Sakel had discovered:* Alexander Wellington, 'Dr Manfred J. Sakel: Discoverer of Insulin Shock Therapy – Psychiatry in History', *British Journal of Psychiatry*, 221:5 (November 2022), p. 682.

44 *'tempted to greet it with derision':* Sargant, *The Unquiet Mind*, p. 52.

44 *Contemporary reports of mortality rates:* Franklin G. Ebaugh, 'A Review of the Drastic Shock Therapies in the Treatment of the Psychoses', *Annals of Internal Medicine*, 18:3 (March 1943), pp. 279–96.

44 *'within about half an hour':* E. H. Larkin, 'Insulin Shock Treatment of Schizophrenia', *BMJ*, 1:3979 (10 April 1937), p. 745.

45 *'physiological lobotomy':* D. N. Parfitt, 'A Comment on Insulin Coma Therapy in Schizophrenia', *American Journal of Psychiatry*, 11:3 (1956), pp. 246–7. See also Robert Freudenthal and Joanna Moncrieff, 'A Landmark in Psychiatric Progress? The Role of Evidence in the Rise and Fall of Insulin Coma Therapy', *History of Psychiatry*, 33:1 (2022), pp. 65–78.

45 *'One unit went so far':* Sargant, *The Unquiet Mind*, p. 55.

45 *Sakel himself admitted:* 'Medicine: Insulin for Insanity', *Time*, 25 January 1937.

45 *patients probably just felt better:* Jones, *Ministering to Minds Diseased*, pp. 19–33.

46 *One conservative estimate:* Harold Bourne, 'The Insulin Myth', *Lancet*, 265:6798 (7 November 1953), pp. 964–8.

46 *'It is clear':* Sargant and Slater, *An Introduction to Physical Treatments in Psychiatry* (1st edn 1944), pp. 18 and 35.

46 *Sargant dedicated the entire opening chapter:* Although *An Introduction to Physical Treatments in Psychiatry* was co-authored by Sargant and Eliot Slater, Sargant was the driving force behind all five editions. According to Slater, in an interview in February 1981: 'Sargant said, "Come on you, you must write the introductory chapter and the section on psychotherapy in conjunction with physical treatment." He would write everything else, and I would have to take

it and see what his line of thought was and improve it in logical progression and coherence.' (Brian Barraclough, 'In Conversation with Eliot Slater', *Psychiatric Bulletin*, 5 (February 1981), pp. 158–61.)

46 *another critical article:* B. Ackner, A. Harris and A. J. Oldham, 'Insulin Treatment of Schizophrenia; A Controlled Study', *Lancet*, 272:6969 (23 March 1957), pp. 607–11.

47 *'skilful sparring with death':* Charles Burlingame, 'Insanity and Insulin Shock Treatment for Schizophrenia', *Forum* (1937), pp. 98–102.

47 *'It meant that psychiatrists':* Deborah Blythe Doroshow, 'Performing a Cure for Schizophrenia: Insulin Coma Therapy on the Wards', *Journal of the History of Medicine and Allied Sciences*, 62:2 (April 2007), pp. 213–43.

47 *'No one said anything about ethics':* Hilton and Stephenson (convenors and eds), *Psychiatric Hospitals in the UK in the 1960s*, p. 31.

48 *'it can still save years':* Sargant and Slater, *An Introduction to Physical Treatments in Psychiatry* (5th edn 1972), p. 254.

48 *'One saw people getting better':* Freeman, 'In Conversation with William Sargant'.

Chapter 7

49 *another shock treatment:* Thomas and Wilson, *Report on Cardiazol Treatment and on the Present Application of Hypoglycaemic Shock Treatment in Schizophrenia.*

49 *Today, epileptics are thought:* Antonio Metastasio and David Dodwell, 'A Translation of "L'Elettroshock" by Cerletti & Bini, with an Introduction', *European Journal of Psychiatry*, 27:4 (October–December 2013), pp. 231–9.

49 *'as if it were casting out':* Sargant, *The Unquiet Mind*, p. 53.

49 *deeply unpleasant symptoms:* Rankine Good, 'Some Observations on the Psychological Aspects of Cardiazol Therapy', *Journal of Mental Science*, 86:362 (May 1940), pp. 491–501.

50 *'roasted alive':* Ibid.

50 *the mere threat of Cardiazol:* 'Use of Metrozol [Cardiazol's

name in the US] in Sovbloc for Interrogation and Brainwashing/Negation of LSD-25 and Adrenochrome by Frenquel', Central Intelligence Agency document #0000146135, dated September 1955.

50 *gruesome physical legacy:* Phillip Polatin, Murray M. Friedman, Meyer M. Harris and William A. Horwitz, 'Vertebral Fractures Produced by Metrazol-Induced Convulsions', *Journal of the American Medical Association*, 112:17 (1939), pp. 1684–7.

50 *dislocated jaws:* William Gissane, 'Fracture Complicating Cardiazol Shock Therapy', letter, *BMJ*, 2:253 (29 July 1939), p. 253.

50 *'I have always unblushingly resorted':* Sargant, *The Unquiet Mind*, p. 54.

50 *landmark moment:* I have taken my lead here from Andrew Scull, whose fascinating book, *Desperate Remedies*, was given to me by my UK editor and has proved to be a great source of information. For the best account of the world's first ECT treatment, I agree with Scull, who recommends *Shock Therapy: A History of Electroconvulsive Treatment in Mental Illness* by Edward Shorter and David Healy, as it's based on Bini's laboratory notebooks. (See Chapter 3: Madness Cured with Electricity.) Cerletti himself later recorded what happened in several versions, which are inconsistent in minor details. I have quoted from the chapter Cerletti wrote in *The Great Physiodynamic Therapies in Psychiatry*, which, interestingly, was edited by Messrs Arthur, Mortimer and Raymond Sackler (as well as Félix Martí-Ibáñez), whose pharma empire was later rocked by the OxyContin scandal. I have also quoted from Ugo Cerletti's paper, 'Old and New Information about Electric Shock', which he wrote for the *American Journal of Psychiatry* (107:2 (1950), pp. 87–94).

51 *'In everyone's minds':* Ugo Cerletti, 'Electroshock Therapy', in Sackler, Sackler, Sackler and Martí-Ibáñez (eds), *The Great Physiodynamic Therapies in Psychiatry*, p. 92; Cerletti, 'Old and New Information about Electric Shock'.

52 *'The apnea of the spontaneous'*: Cerletti, 'Electroshock Therapy', p. 94,

53 *'Madness Cured with Electricity'*: Shorter and Healy, *Shock Therapy*, p. 43.

53 *'I think I was the second or third'*: Freeman, 'In Conversation with William Sargant'.

53 *'We generally got'*: Sargant, *The Unquiet Mind*, p. 78.

Chapter 9

66 *'utterly ridiculous'*: Sargant, *The Unquiet Mind*, p. 65.

67 *sign his dinner card:* Sargant Personal Papers, 'Personal and Biographical', Wellcome Collection, PP/WWW/A/7.

67 *'I don't think'*: Anonymous interview with Dominic Streatfeild, author of *Brainwash*, used here with kind permission of Dr Henry Rollin's widow, Dr Maria Rollin, MBE.

67 *'Passchendaele of the mind'*: 'Brainwaves', episode 3 of *Madness: A Social History of Mental Illness*, presented by Jonathan Miller.

67 *'lobotomy gets them home'*: Jack El-Hai, 'The Lobotomist', *Washington Post*, 4 February 2001.

68 *'tortured self-concern'*: William Sargant, 'Psychiatric Treatment: Here and in England', *Atlantic* (July 1964), pp. 88–95.

68 *Phineas Gage:* John M. Harlow, 'Recovery from the Passage of an Iron Bar Through the Head', *Publications of the Massachusetts Medical Society*, 2:3 (1868), pp. 329–47.

69 *The doctors had practised:* Valenstein, *Great and Desperate Cures*, p. 103.

69 *Moniz declared:* All quotations from Moniz are from Valenstein, *Great and Desperate Cures*, Chapter 6: Seven Recoveries, Seven Improvements and Six Unchanged.

70 *Moniz announced in Paris:* The findings were written up in the *Bulletin de l'Académie Nationale de Médicine* and then published as a monograph in June 1936 and in six further articles. Moniz was clearly keen to get his name and procedure out there as soon as possible, to prevent anyone else laying claim.

70 *'scarcely be overestimated':* Valenstein, *Great and Desperate Cures*, p. 101. In a letter to Fulton, Freeman also called it an 'epoch making work' (ibid., p. 112).

70 *Hammatt died five years later:* Ibid., p. 143.

70 *results were disastrous:* Scull, *Desperate Remedies*, p. 147.

71 *a pair of sharp lobotomy instruments:* The orbitoclasts are kept at the Wellcome Collection as part of Sargant's Personal Papers, including instructions on how to use them. Once the patient had been knocked out by ECT, the orbitoclast was hammered through the top of the eye socket into the brain in a swift operation that Freeman performed himself.

71 *an eccentric showman:* It's not true that the car he drove around in to perform operations was nicknamed the 'lobotomobile' – the name was given ten years after his death, according to Jack El-Hai, author of *The Lobotomist*, a biography of Freeman.

71 *troubled patients:* Irving Cooper, a student at George Washington, who went on to become a neurosurgeon, described the demonstrations as 'brilliant but . . . often chilling'. Valenstein, *Great and Desperate Cures*, p. 132.

71 *Freeman had had a nervous breakdown:* He later wrote a paper entitled 'Danger Signals: On the Advantage of a Nervous Breakdown, or a Few Neurotic Symptoms in Certain Men under Forty Years of Age'.

71 *he was on Nembutal:* Scull, *Desperate Remedies*, p. 140.

72 *'Wizardry of Surgery':* Valenstein, *Great and Desperate Cures*, p. 157.

72 *'We want a little indifference':* Waldemar Kaempffert, 'Turning the Mind Inside Out', *Saturday Evening Post*, 24 May 1941.

72 *held at the White House:* 'Mammoth White House Ball is Brilliant Backdrop for Coming Out Party of Mrs Roosevelt's Niece', *Washington Post*, 28 December 1938. 'Others at the dinner were . . . Dr William Sargant.'

72 *'seemed greatly interested':* The account of Sargant's experiences in America is drawn from *The Unquiet Mind*, Chapter 6.

Chapter 10

76 *'without telling the patient':* William Sargant and Russell Fraser, 'Inducing Light Hypnosis by Hyperventilation', *Lancet*, 232:6005 (1 October 1938), p. 778. Russell Fraser and William Sargant, 'Hyperventilation Attacks', *BMJ*, 1:4024 (19 February 1938), 378.

76 *cited in another paper:* Martin T. Orne, 'The Potential Uses of Hypnosis in Interrogation', in Albert D. Biderman and Herbert Zimmer (eds), *The Manipulation of Human Behaviour* (New York: Wiley, 1961), pp. 169–215. Orne wrote: 'This paper is based in part upon work under a grant from the Society for the Investigation of Human Ecology, Inc.' Also known as the Human Ecology Fund, the society was a front organisation for the CIA, which used it to channel funds into relevant research – see Chapter 33.

76 *'I made a most valuable':* Sargant, *The Unquiet Mind*, p. 72.

76 *'the Versailles of the New York rich':* Conant, *Tuxedo Park*, p. 5.

76 *'a secret discussion':* Sargant, *The Unquiet Mind*, p. 72.

77 *published various papers:* Papers included 'Potential Rhythms of the Cerebral Cortex During Sleep' (*Science*, 1935) and 'Search for Changes in Direct-Current Potentials of the Head During Sleep' (*Journal of Neurophysiology*, 1939).

77 *'sleeping room':* Conant, *Tuxedo Park*, p. 109.

77 *Loomis' array of distinguished guests:* Ibid., p. 108.

78 *'mark certain confidential documents':* Ibid., pp. 173–5.

78 *'the most valuable cargo':* Baxter, *Scientists Against Time*, p. 142.

78 *continued to seek his advice:* Conant, *Tuxedo Park*, p. 288.

79 *'thorough knowledge of the Soviet Union':* CIA memorandum, 10 May 1951 (approved for release, 30 August 2000): https://www.cia.gov/readingroom/docs/CIA-RDP80-01446R000100140048-0.pdf

79 *his son Henry:* Henry Loomis' report for the PSB in 1951 is entitled 'Social Science Research in Cold War Operations'. He worked for the CIA between 1949 and 1951: Navy.togetherweserved.com.

79 *'Loomis moved in intelligence circles':* Author interview.

Chapter 11

81 *'I remain remarkably free'*: Letter to Dr Alexander Walk, 3 March 1976, Sargant Personal Papers, 'Personal and Biographical', Wellcome Collection, PP/WWS/A13.

81 *Dr Eric Strauss:* It's not clear whether Sargant ever met Dr Strauss, but he would go on to play an interesting role in the Kim Philby affair, at one point trying to help Philby's second wife, Aileen, who had severe mental health issues. Strauss abandoned patient confidentiality to pass on to the intelligence services Aileen's growing suspicions about her husband's treachery. According to David Cornwell, aka John le Carré, Philby's friend and MI6 colleague Nicholas Elliott used to refer to Strauss as the 'office shrink'. See John le Carré's Afterword in Ben Macintyre's book on Philby, *A Spy Among Friends*, for more.

81 *'medical bureaucratic obstructionism'*: Sargant, *The Unquiet Mind*, p. 81.

82 *'of relative unimportance'*: Ibid.

82 *seemed remarkably ambivalent:* Covering letter from Sargant to Leslie Hohman, and a letter from Sargant to Hohman's colleague, 7 May 1963, Leslie Benjamin Hohman Papers, Duke Medical Center Archives.

82 *St Ebba's:* Sargant, *The Unquiet Mind*, pp. 81–2.

83 *instructions in 1944:* Sargant and Slater, *An Introduction to Physical Treatments in Psychiatry* (1st edn 1944), pp. 64–9.

Chapter 13

96 *Belmont:* For more about Sargant and his wartime work at Belmont, see *Battle for the Mind: Dr William Sargant in Conversation with Dr Ernesto Spinelli*, Channel 4, 1987, Sargant Personal Papers, Wellcome Collection, closed stores: 1492V.

96 *'intelligent Boston ex debutantes', 'intelligent Sutton girls':* Sargant, *The Unquiet Mind*, p. 99.

97 *'After some difficulty'*: Sargant, *The Mind Possessed*, p. 118.

98 *'The sound of falling bombs'*: Sargant, *The Unquiet Mind*, p. 100.

98 *Dunkirk changed everything:* William Sargant, 'Some Physical

Treatments of War Neuroses', *Medical Press and Circular* (February 1941), pp. 145–8. Sargant Personal Papers, 'War', Wellcome Collection, PP/WWS/E/2/5.

99 *'Opportunities of treatment':* William Sargant, 'Aims and Methods of Treatment (From 'Addresses Given in the USA in 1947 and 1948'), p. 198, Sargant Personal Papers, 'General Psychiatry', Wellcome Collection, PP/WWS/C1/7.

99 *'War time was a tremendous experience':* 'Profile: Dr William Sargant', *St Thomas' Hospital Gazette*, 65:1 (spring 1967), pp. 18–21, Sargant Personal Papers, 'Personal and Biographical', Wellcome Collection, PP/WWS/A/9.

99 *One of the earliest Dunkirk casualties:* Sargant, *The Unquiet Mind*, p. 87.

100 *'acute shell shock':* William Sargant and Eliot Slater, 'Acute War Neuroses', *Lancet*, 236:6097 (6 July 1940), pp. 1–2.

101 *'It was like the surgical rule':* Sargant, *The Unquiet Mind*, p. 90.

101 *'No psychiatrist can yet':* Ibid., p. 183.

Chapter 14

103 *letter from Colonel John Rawlings Rees:* 12 July 1940, Sargant Personal Papers, 'War', Wellcome Collection, WWS/PP/E/1/1.

103 *Rees had been appointed:* Nafsika Thalassis, 'Treating and Preventing Trauma: British Military Psychiatry during the Second World War', PhD thesis, University of Salford, 2004, p. 83.

103 *various government agencies:* Streatfeild, *Brainwash*, p. 35.

104 *'In an hour':* J. Stephen Horsley, 'Narco-analysis', *Lancet*, 227:5862 (4 January 1936), p. 55.

104 *on the needle:* Streatfeild, *Brainwash*, p. 33.

105 *'deeper into obscure episodes':* Gilbert Debenham, Denis Hill, William Sargant and Eliot Slater, 'Treatment of War Neurosis', *Lancet*, 237:6126 (25 January 1941), pp. 107–9.

105 *A few months later:* Proceedings of the Royal Society of Medicine, Section of Psychiatry ('Amnesic Syndromes in War', 24 June 1941, with Eliot Slater), published in *Royal Society of Medicine Journal*, 34:12 (October 1941) pp. 757–64.

105 *On 1 February 1942:* The letter only includes the day and

month, but the year is most likely to have been 1942. Clayton-Jones was an assistant editor on the *Lancet* at the time and Sargant refers in his letter to his work of 'the past three years', presumably a reference to his work at Belmont since war broke out in 1939. Sargant Personal Papers, 'War', Wellcome Collection, PP/WWS/E/1/2.

105 *potential of barbiturates:* Alfred W. McCoy, 'Science in Dachau's Shadow: Herb, Beecher, and the Development of CIA Psychological Torture and Modern Medical Ethics', *Journal of the History of the Behavioural Sciences*, 43:4 (Fall 2007), pp. 401–17.

105 *Rees oversaw:* See John Rawlings Ress and Henry Victor Dicks, *The Case of Rudolf Hess: A Problem in Diagnosis and Forensic Psychiatry* (London: William Heinemann, 1947).

106 *According to Ann Dally:* Holden, *Shell Shock*, p. 81.

106 *'He'd bring him back':* Quote taken from an interview with Ann Dally by Dominic Streatfield for *Brainwash*, kindly shared with the author and published here with permission of Ann's daughter, Emma.

106 *'The treatment must be stopped':* W. S. Dawson and M. Barkas, 'Somnifen Treatment in the Psychoses', *Lancet*, 208:5388 (4 December 1926), pp. 1155–6.

106 *'considerable risk':* Ibid.

106 *In February 1936:* D. N. Parfitt, 'Treatment of Psychoses by Prolonged Narcosis', *Lancet*, 227:5869 (22 February 1936), pp. 424–6.

107 *'acutely ill anxiety neurotic':* Sargant and Slater, *An Introduction to Physical Methods of Treatment in Psychiatry* (1st edn 1944), Chapter VI: Continuous Sleep Treatment.

108 *'not very exciting ritual':* Sargant and Slater, *An Introduction to Physical Methods of Treatment in Psychiatry* (3rd edn 1954), p. 176.

108 *'agitated indecisive patient':* Ibid.

Chapter 15

109 *'artificially fattening them up':* Sargant, *The Unquiet Mind*, p. 91.

109 *Mitchell . . . curing patients:* Mitchell, *Fat and Blood*, pp. 107–74.

110 *'There is no need for flurry':* Sargant and Slater, *An Introduction to Physical Methods of Treatment in Psychiatry* (1st edn 1944), p. 48.

110–11 *'The aim is to stabilise':* Ibid., pp. 48–51.

113 *writing an article:* Slater's contribution to the Festschrift, published in *Allgemeine Zeitschrift für Psychiatrie und ihre Grenzgebiete* (vol. 112, April 1939, pp. 148–52), was called 'On the Concept and Applicability of the Probability of Manifestation' ('Über *Begriff und Anwendbarkeit der Manifestationswahrscheinlichkeit*'). For a more detailed analysis of Slater's relationship with Nazi Germany, see Volker Roelcke, 'Eugenic Concerns, Scientific Practices: International Relations in the Establishment of Psychiatric Genetics in Germany, Britain, the USA and Scandinavia, c. 1910–60', *History of Psychiatry*, 30:1 (2019), pp. 19–37.

113 *'pathfinder in the field of hereditary hygiene':* Jay Joseph and Norbert A. Wetzel, 'Ernst Rüdin: Hitler's Racial Hygiene Mastermind', *Journal of the History of Biology*, 46:1 (2013), pp. 1–30. According to Joseph and Wetzel, Rüdin received numerous awards for his work for Nazi Germany, including a Goethe Medal of Arts and Sciences in 1939. The medal that Hitler gave him in 1944 ('*Adlerschild des Deutschen Reiches*') bore the Nazi eagle.

113 *'We all arrived':* 'Autobiographical Sketch' in Shields and Gottesman (eds), *Man, Mind, and Heredity*, pp. 1–23.

114 *Britain's first lobotomy:* There were conflicting claims between the Burden Neurological Institute and Warlingham Park Hospital about who performed the first leucotomy in the UK. In a letter to the *BMJ* (7 July 1951), Golla confirmed that it was at the Burden, citing the original *Lancet* article from 1941.

114 *'close upon':* Professor Geoffrey Jefferson in 'Obituary', *BMJ*, 1:4334 (29 January 1944), p. 165.

114 *using a paper knife:* F. Wilfred Willway, 'The Technique of Prefrontal Leucotomy', *Journal of Mental Science*, 89:375 (April 1943), pp. 192–3.

114 *'My feeling at the moment':* Ibid.

114 *'brutal and bloody operation':* F. L. Golla, 'The Range and Technique of Prefrontal Leucotomy', *Journal of Mental Science*, 89:375 (April 1943), pp. 189–91.

114 *written up in the* Lancet*:* E. Lilian Hutton, G. W. T. H. Fleming and F. E. Fox, 'Early Results of Prefrontal Leucotomy', *Lancet*, 238:6149 (5 July 1941), pp. 3–7.

115 *'The was what the New Testament':* Sargant, *The Unquiet Mind*, p. 85.

115 *'Our earliest experiments':* William Sargant, 'Ten Years' Clinical Experience of Modified Leucotomy Operations', *BMJ*, 2:4840 (10 October 1953), pp. 800–3.

115 *Terry Gould . . . estimated: The Lobotomists*, presented by Hugh Levinson, BBC Radio 4, first broadcast 7 November 2011.

116 *'amnesia, confusion, somnolence':* Wylie McKissock, 'The Technique of Pre-Frontal Leucotomy', *Journal of Mental Science*, 89:375 (April 1943), pp. 194–201.

116 *twelve thousand lobotomies:* Tooth and Newton, *Leucotomy in England and Wales*, pp. 2–4.

117 *'There is a tract':* Peter Evans, 'Sargant at Arms', *General Practitioner*, 7 October 1977.

117 *quest to discover biomarkers:* Leonardo Tozzi, Xue Zhang, Adam Pines et al., 'Personalized Brain Circuit Scores Identify Clinically Distinct Biotypes in Depression and Anxiety', *Nature Medicine*, 30 (2024), pp. 2076–87.

117 *no physical test for depression: Breaking Depression: The SANE Guide to Major Depressive Disorder* (November 2022), co-created with Janssen Neuroscience.

117 *the brain of someone with schizophrenia:* The most consistent and reproduced finding in schizophrenia is that sufferers have slightly smaller brains and larger brain cavities, but such differences have now been shown to be caused, in large part, by drug treatment. (J. Moncrieff, 'A Systematic Review of the Effects of Antipsychotic Drugs on Brain Volume', *Psychological Medicine*, 40:9 (September 2010), pp. 1409–22.)

117 *limitations in diagnosis:* Some symptoms associated with schizophrenia can be caused by general medical conditions such as brain tumours, malaria, syphilis, high fever or

lead or mercury poisoning. Alzheimer's, Parkinson's and brain arteriovenous malformations (AVMs) can also trigger psychosis. The author Susannah Calahan suffered terrifying psychotic episodes and catatonia before she was diagnosed with anti-NMDA receptor autoimmune encephalitis. She was eventually cured by a neurologist, an experience she described in her bestselling memoir, *Brain on Fire*.

117 *'We've been telling patients':* Statement by David Kupfer, MD, American Psychiatric Association press release, 3 May 2013. Dr Lucy Johnstone, a clinical psychologist, quoted Kupfer in her talk, 'Against Psychiatric Diagnoses', at the Institute of Art and Ideas in March 2019.

Chapter 16

Sargant wrote about Pavlov in three of his books and all are quoted in this chapter: *Battle for the Mind* (principally from the Introduction, Chapter 1: Experiments in Animals and Chapter 2: Animal and Human Behaviour Compared; *The Unquiet Mind* (Chapter 12: Pavlov's Impact on Modern Psychiatry); and *The Mind Possessed* (Chapter 1: The Mind under Stress).

118 *'I remember about the third':* 'Profile: Dr William Sargant'.

121 *'worse than an atomic explosion':* Joost A. M. Merloo, 'Pavlovian Strategy as a Weapon of Menticide', *American Journal of Psychiatry*, 110:11 (May 1954), pp. 809–13.

122 *more sinister intent:* Professor William Douglas Woody of the University of Northern Colorado has written extensively about the links between Sargant's take on Pavlov and its use in interrogation. See 'William Sargant: Pavlov, Interrogation and Narcosis Therapy', paper presented by Woody at the American Psychological Association convention 'What We Can Learn from the Histories of Trauma and Interrogation', Denver, August 2016.

122 *Aldous Huxley:* Later, in *Brave New World Revisited* (1958), Huxley wrote of other drugs in the 'pharmacopoeia'. Pentothal, for example, was popular with the police for extracting confessions. 'Stresses amply sufficient to cause a

complete cerebral breakdown can be induced by methods which, though hatefully inhuman, fall short of physical torture ... For the dictator and his policemen, Pavlov's findings have important practical implications.' And in the appendix to his 1952 novel, *Devils of Loudun*, Huxley wrote about a 'mysterious poison' that induced a heightened state of suggestibility 'resembling that which follows an injection of sodium amytal ... While in this state they will believe any nonsense bawled at them, will act upon any command or exhortation, however senseless, mad or criminal.' See Jay, 'Over the Edge' (via mikejay.net) and Streatfeild, *Brainwash* for more about Huxley's endorsement of Sargant's theories. Some scholars, including Professor William Douglas Woody, also wonder if it is possible to recognise an early variation of Sargant's and Cameron's sleep labs in Huxley's orgy-porgy scene in *Brave New World*.

Chapter 17

124 *'soullessly one-sided':* Sargant, *The Unquiet Mind*, p. 120.

124 *'cruel and irresponsible':* Ibid., p. 121.

125 *'suddenly famous':* Ibid., p. 123.

125 *'I morbidly imagined myself':* Ibid., p. 129.

126 *'The upper eyelid':* Walter Freeman, 'Transorbital Leucotomy', *Lancet*, 252:6523 (4 September 1948), pp. 371–3.

126 *the action of a windscreen wiper:* Dr Adam Rutherford used this vivid description in 'The Boy with an Ice Pick in his Brain', an episode of *The Human Subject* on BBC Radio 4, first broadcast 25 August 2024.

127 *'Over my dead body':* Michael M. Phillips, 'An Operation's Champion and the Vets Left Behind', part 2 of 'The Lobotomy Files: One Doctor's Legacy' special report, *Wall Street Journal*, 13 December 2013.

127 *'The whole Negro-rescue plan':* Sargant, *The Unquiet Mind*, p. 130.

127 *another notorious experiment:* The study involved 399 people who had syphilis and 201 who did not have the disease. In 1997, President Clinton gave a formal apology and $10 million was paid out in compensation.

127 *lobotomised 228 patients:* de Young, *Encyclopedia of Asylum Therapeutics*, p. 291.

128 *'wiping the slate clean for God':* Sargant, *The Unquiet Mind*, p. 135.

Chapter 18

131 *'We are having a good ending':* Letter to Leslie Hohman, Professor of Psychiatry at Duke University School of Medicine, 9 August 1948, Leslie Benjamin Hohman Papers, Duke Medical Center Archives.

132 *'Two tigers cannot live':* Letter from Edward Hare, editor of the *British Journal of Psychiatry*, 21 January 1976, Sargant Personal Papers, 'Geneal Correspondence', Wellcome Collection, PP/WWS/A/13.

132 *'at the Lord's end':* Letter to Robert Graves, 18 August 1955, Sargant Personal Papers, 'General Correspondence/Robert Graves', Wellcome Collection PP/WWS/A/21/1.

133 *Nightingale nurses:* To become a state registered nurse (SRN) typically required three years of training. Nurses at St Thomas' did a fourth year, after which they became a Nightingale nurse, complete with distinctive blue badge and lace hat. The title was phased out in the mid 1990s, but since 2017, Guy's and St Thomas' NHS Foundation Trust has awarded annual 'Nightingale Nurse' and 'Nightingale Midwife' awards.

134 *Attendances shot up:* 'Report on the Department of Psychological Medicine, St Thomas's Hospital, 1948–1965', Wellcome Collection, PP/WWS/B/2/5.

134 *'It was a completely isolated unit':* Hilton and Stephenson (convenors and eds), *Psychiatric Hospitals in the UK in the 1960s*, p. 31.

134 *manage their own endowment funds:* The details of St Thomas' endowment funds, bank accounts and donations come from the following records, kept at the London Metropolitan Archives: Board of Governors minutes and papers, 1948–1974 (H01/ST/A/128/001-019); General Purposes and Finance Committee minutes and papers, 1948–1974

(H01/ST/A/129/001-035); Local Hospitals Committee minutes and papers, 1948–1969 (H01/ST/A/133/001-003); Endowment Fund Sub-Committee minutes, 1949–1969 (H01/ST/A/149/001-003).

134 *duly set up in 1948:* Another account, the St Thomas' Hospital Royal Waterloo Account, was set up in 1948, at the National Provincial Bank. It was for day-to-day maintenance but was closed on 17 July 1949 and all funds were transferred to St Thomas' main account.

135 *Between 1950 and 1953:* Twenty-two weekly sessions were allocated to senior registrars, five to registrars and eleven to house physicians.

135 *A consulting room:* According to Nita Mitchell-Heggs, Sargant's colleague Dr Desmond Kelly used this room in the early 1970s for plethysmographic tests. One of them involved measuring blood flow while sodium lactate infusions were used to induce panic attacks. The control group, with no psychiatric history, was drawn from friends and family of the staff.

136 *'not being treated as lunatics':* 'Report on the Department of Psychological Medicine, St Thomas's Hospital, 1948–1965', Wellcome Collection, PP/WWS/B/2/5.

137 *psychopharmacological revolution:* Thomas A. Ban, 'Fifty Years Chlorpromazine: A Historical Perspective', *Neuropsychiatric Disease and Treatment*, 3:4 (August 2007), pp. 495–500.

137 *'We must provisionally accept':* Sargant and Slater, *An Introduction to Physical Methods of Treatment in Psychiatry* (5th edn 1972), p. 22.

137 *'in massive doses':* Sargant, *The Unquiet Mind*, p. 150.

138 *'psychic indifference':* Anton Stephens carried out a trial at Warley Hospital, Essex, cited in Fennell, *Treatment Without Consent*, p. 155.

138 *'nearly all psychiatric patients':* Sargant, *The Unquiet Mind*, p. 161.

138 *'most problematic':* Sargant and Slater, *An Introduction to Physical Methods of Treatment in Psychiatry* (1st edn 1944), p. 100.

138 *Sargant later revealed:* C. J. S. Walter, Nita Mitchell-Heggs and William Sargant, 'Treatment with Modified Narcosis: A Retrospective Controlled Study of 106 Patients', draft paper, *c.* 1973, Sargant Personal Papers, 'Post War Work', Wellcome Collection, PP/WWS/F/8/3.

139 *Between 1948 and 1955:* Tooth and Newton, *Leucotomy in England and Wales*, pp. 2–4.

139 *'She worshipped him':* Hilton and Stephenson (convenors and eds), *Psychiatric Hospitals in the UK in the 1960s*, p. 31.

Chapter 19

140 *a controversial paper:* William Sargant, 'The Mechanism of "Conversion"', *BMJ*, 2:4727 (11 August 1951), pp. 311–16.

141 *'mental enema':* R. C. Lewontin, letter to the editor, *New York Review of Books*, 30 June 1983.

142 *'abnormal emotion':* Sargant, 'The Mechanism of "Conversion"'.

142 *letters pages of the* BMJ: 'Correspondence', *BMJ*, 2:4731 (8 September 1951), pp. 606–7.

143 *Directed by Ken Loach:* Tim Snelson, 'From *In Two Minds* to MIND: The Circulation of "Anti-Psychiatry" in British Film and Television during the Long 1960s', *History of the Human Sciences*, 34:5 (2001), pp. 53–81.

143 *'severe and on the defensive':* Author email exchange with Joan Bakewell.

143 *'the way a General addresses a Major':* Mullan, *Mad to be Normal*, p. 256.

144 *Western observers:* Streatfeild, *Brainwash*, pp. 3–5.

144 *'some unknown force':* Marks, *The Search for the 'Manchurian Candidate'*, p. 21.

144 *'Somehow they took his soul apart':* Streatfeild, *Brainwash*, p. 6.

144 *According to a declassified CIA document:* CIA memorandum, 3 October 1952, ref. 0000144746, theblackvault.com

145 *apparent confessions of American pilots:* Albarelli, *A Terrible Mistake*, p. 197.

145 *'The words were mine':* Streatfeild, *Brainwash*, p. 17.

146 *'I began to wonder':* Sargant, *The Unquiet Mind*, p. 118.

146 *'Wesley, Pavlov':* Ibid., p. 119.
146 *very nearly got cancelled:* Khaleelah Jones, 'Making the Political Popular: The Early Days of the BBC's *Panorama*', *Historical Journal of Film, Radio and Television*, 38:3 (2018), pp. 622–41.
147 *play the recording backwards:* Lindley, *Panorama*, p. 10.
147 *'Here is a physician':* Sargant Personal Papers, 'BBC', Wellcome Collection (PP/WWS/J/1/6).
148–9 *'to consult us':* The National Archives of the UK (TNA): FO 371/106283; NH 1052/215.
149 *'murkier side of the Foreign Office':* Lindley, *Panorama*, p. 10.
149 *confession that he was a spy:* TNA: FO 371/106283; NH 1052/215.
149 *While in Budapest:* Dorril, *MI6*, p. 176. See also TNA: FO 371/106283.
149 *ideal intelligence asset:* Gábor Bátonyi, 'Diplomacy by Show Trial: The Espionage Case of Edgar Sanders and British-Hungarian Relations, 1949–53', *Slavonic and East European Review*, 93:4 (2015), pp. 692–731.

Chapter 20

151 *three antibiotics:* Harman put Sargant on streptomycin, para-aminosalicylic acid and isonicotinic acid.
151 *'What a difference it makes':* Sargant, *The Unquiet Mind*, p. 170.
151 *'incapable of work':* Harman signed him off sick at 7 p.m. on 8 July 1954. Sargant Personal Papers, 'General Correspondence', Wellcome Collection, PP/WWS/A/4.
151–2 *Friends corresponded:* Ibid.
152 *'William couldn't put two words':* Hilton and Stephenson (convenors and eds), *Psychiatric Hospitals in the UK in the 1960s*, p. 30.
152 *'godlike':* Sargant, *The Unquiet Mind*, p. 176.
153 *'if activities slightly off the normal path':* Sargant, 'The Risks of Allowing Pornography to Grow Unchecked'.
153 *'an outstanding exception':* Sargant, *The Unquiet Mind*, p. 177.
154 *'a charming man':* Jay, 'Over the Edge'.
154 *'for all your kindness':* Letter to Robert Graves, 8 June 1955,

Sargant Private Papers, 'General Correspondence/Robert Graves', Wellcome Collection, PP/WWS/A/21/1.

154 *'Dear Will'*: Letter to William Sargant, 10 June 1955, ibid.

154 *'re-English'*: Letters from Robert Graves to Spike Milligan, 10 April and 3 July 1966, Robertgravesletters.org. Graves also told Sargant that he did 'a lot of re-Englishing' but he didn't actually write *Battle for the Mind*, as Sargant liked to tell people. See letter from Graves to Sargant, 18 April 1959, Sargant Private Papers, 'General Correspondence/Robert Graves', Wellcome Collection, PP/WWS/A/21/1.

154 *'which should butter a few carrots'*: Letter from Robert Graves to Ricardo Sicre Cedrá, aka Richard Stickler, a former counter intelligence officer with the Office of Strategic Services, forerunner of the CIA. 10 October 1955, Robertgravesletters.org.

155 *'I am Public Enemy No. 1'*: Letter from Robert Graves to Sargant, 18 November 1955, Sargant Private Papers, 'General Correspondence/Robert Graves', Wellcome Collection, PP/WWS/A/21/1.

155 *'This had the immediate result'*: Letter from Sargant to Graves, 9 December 1957, ibid.

155 *Sargant's glowing review:* 'Chemical Mysticism', *BMJ*, 1:4869 (1 May 1954), p. 1024.

155 *'absorbingly interesting'*: Quoted in Jay, 'Over the Edge'.

155 *'We shall find out'*: Ibid.

156 *'how beliefs, whether good or bad'*: Sargant, *Battle for the Mind*, p. xxiv.

156 *'When I hear any talk'*: Ibid., p. 108 fn. The Wesley quote comes from Tyerman's *Life of Wesley*.

156 *'high emotional tension'*: Sargant, *Battle for the Mind*, p. 78.

156–7 *'It seems very difficult'*: Ibid, p. 165.

157 *'potential harm of the subject'*: Otterman, *American Torture*, p. 24.

157 *published in a declassified version:* Lawrence E. Hinkle, Jr and Harold G. Wolff, 'Communist Interrogation and Indoctrination of "Enemies of the States": Analysis of Methods Used by the Communist State Police (A Special

Report)', *Archives of Neurology and Psychiatry*, 76:2 (1956), pp. 115–74.

157 *an earlier, classified version:* According to John Marks, Hinkle and Wolff's study on brainwashing appeared in classified form on 2 April 1956 as a CIA Technical Services Division publication co-authored by Hinkle and entitled *Communist Control Techniques*. See *The Search for the 'Manchurian Candidate'*, notes to Chapter 8, p. 223.

158 *Maresfield Camp:* Thomas, *Secrets & Lies*, p. 68.

158 *new Psychological Warfare Centre:* Lee Richards, 'The Rainbow in the Dark: Assessing a Century of British Military Information Operations', *Defence Strategic Communications*, 1:1 (winter 2015), p. 61; Streatfeild, *Brainwash*, pp. 380–1; 'Brainwashing Shocks: War Office Admits Grilling Tests on Elite Troops', *Daily Mail*, 9 March 1960; James Meek, 'Nobody is Talking', *Guardian*, 18 February 2005.

159 *KUBARK's central approach:* McCoy, *A Question of Torture*, p. 51.

159 *'a sort of policeman's guide':* Evans, 'Sargant at Arms'.

159 *'Recent Ulster revelations':* Letter to *The Times*, 3 May 1974.

Chapter 21

167 *'When you change':* Lyrics to 'Ruby Tuesday' by Keith Richards and Mick Jagger. Copyright © Abkco Music Inc., BMG Rights Management.

Chapter 22

176 *in* Lobster *magazine:* Anthony Frewin, 'The Dr Strangeloves of the Mind', *Lobster*, 59 (summer 2010), pp. 4–29.

176 *'Britain's leading medical expert':* Thomas, *Journey into Madness*, p. 122.

176 *'strip patients of their selfhood', 'Whatever you manage':* Ibid., p. 189.

176 *editorial in the* Lancet*:* Notes and News, *Lancet*, 332:8616 (15 October 1988), pp. 917–20.

177 *less scrupulously researched:* Sargant's death, for example, is

given as 27 August 1986, two years before he died. And he was visiting Langley long before the CIA was headquartered there in late 1961.

177 *'To discover all this':* Thomas, Secrets & Lies, p. 386.

178 *cocktail party in Washington:* Gordon Thomas' dates are inconsistent. *Battle for the Mind* was published in America in 1957, making it unlikely that Sargant had a proof copy in 1954, the year he began working on the book. In *Journey into Madness*, the date of the Dulles cocktail party is given as early March 1953. The discrepancies, however, don't undermine the basic essence of the anecdote, that Sargant, a supreme self-publicist and networker, gave the wife of the Director of the CIA a signed proof copy of his book. He was a frequent visitor to Washington and might have attended more than one cocktail party. Thomas also later said that he had continued to meet with Sargant after *Journey into Madness* had first been published in October 1988, even though Sargant had died two months earlier.

178 *'Clover Dulles, a gracious lady':* Thomas, *Secrets & Lies*, p. 178.

178 *'swinger parties':* Ibid., p. 69.

179 *'this was not to be':* Gordon Thomas, memorandum sent to Eric Olson, 30 November 1998.

179 *'potty':* Interview with Peggy Sargant by Dominic Streatfeild, 2 April 2004, which he kindly shared. Peggy's work in prisons was with Nacro, a social justice charity.

179 *'We didn't in those days':* Interview with Peter Dally by Dominic Streatfield, 3 September 2004, which he kindly shared. Reproduced here with permission of Peter Dally's daughter.

179 *'Regardless of whether':* Author interview.

179 *'hitherto unsuspected insights':* Thomas, *Journey into Madness*, p. 364.

Chapter 23

181 *upholding medical ethics:* At some point in the early sixties, Beecher clearly had a change of heart, prompted by guilt or expedience (or both). Either way, he set a new high bar for

ethical testing, establishing standards for informed consent that are still adhered to today. The Beecher Prize continues to be awarded annually at Harvard Medical School to students working in medical ethics.

182 *engaged in clandestine work:* We only know of the dark chapter in Beecher's life thanks to the forensic work by the American historian Alfred W. McCoy, J. R. W. Smail Professor of History at the University of Wisconsin, and the German documentary maker Egmont Koch, who made a programme for ARD-TV in which Beecher's role came to light. For the account of Beecher and his journeys to Europe, I have drawn on Beecher's own account: a covering letter to Colonel John R. Wood, Surgeon General, Department of the Army, dated 21 October 1951, and his accompanying report. Koch kindly sent me a copy of the 'Beecher Report'; he has also made it available on Wikimedia Commons (https://commons.wikimedia.org/wiki/Category:Beecher_Report) Other valuable sources include McCoy's book *Torture and Impunity* as well as Ulf Schimdt's *Secret Scien*ce and John Lancaster and James P. Rathwell's article about Beecher, 'The Moralist', *Delacorte Review*, 14 July 2016.

182 *summarised a trip he made to Europe:* According to Professor Ulf Schmidt, Beecher represented 'the US Army's Assistant Chief of Staff Intelligence Branch, G-2, and the Medical Research and Development Board at the Office of the Surgeon General': *Secret Science*, p. 326.

182 *'a Manhattan Project of the mind':* McCoy, *A Question of Torture*, p. 7.

183 *Between 1953 and 1973:* 'Project MKULTRA, the CIA's Program of Research in Behavioral Modification: Joint Hearing before the Select Committee on Intelligence and the Subcommittee on Health and Scientific Research of the Committee on Human Resources, United States Senate, Ninety-fifth Congress, First Session, August 3, 1977'.

183 *the Josiah Macy Jr. Foundation:* Interestingly, the Josiah Macy Jr. Foundation had distributed copies of a paper by Sargant at a US National Research Council conference in 1940. Cited

in Dimsdale, *Dark Persuasion*, p. 88, referencing Christopher Tudico, *The History of the Josiah Macy Jr Foundation*. At the meeting, according to Tudico, organisers of the conference circulated Sargant and Slater's *Lancet* paper on acute war neuroses at Dunkirk to the Committee on Neuropsychiatry and to the liaison officers from the armed services and Selective Service.

183 *Some of the questions:* Albarelli, *A Terrible Mistake*, p. 29.

184 *1959 novel:* In a weird twist worthy of *The X-Files*, in 1998 Condon was accused by a software engineer of plagiarising sections of *I, Claudius* by none other than Robert Graves. Condon: 'Johnny knew in his superstitious heart of hearts that his marriage to Raymond's mother was an impious thing and this knowledge, it seems, affected him nervously, putting an inner restraint upon his flesh.' Graves: 'He knew that the marriage was impious: this knowledge, it seems, affected him nervously, putting an inner restraint on his flesh.' See Adair Lara, 'Has a Local Software Engineer Unmasked "The Manchurian Candidate"? Menlo Park Woman Says Author Richard Condon Plagiarized', SFGate, 4 October 2003.

184 *Another document stated:* Streatfeild, *Brainwash*, p. 26.

184 *'"black psychiatry"':* Hank Albarelli and Jeffrey Kaye, in a 2010 article for Truthout, quoted a CIA official who defined black psychiatry as referring to 'psychiatric methods used by trained and licensed physicians on subjects. These methods may not be in the best interest of the subject's wellbeing and health.' H. p. Albarelli Jr and Jeffrey Kaye, 'Cries from the Past: Torture's Ugly Echoes', Truthout, 23 May 2010.

184 *'of considerable note':* ARTICHOKE document dated 3 December 1951, cited in Ross, *The CIA Doctors*, p. 52.

185 *'excruciating pain':* Ibid.

185 *'electric shock', 'neurosurgical techniques':* Marks, *The Search for the 'Manchurian Candidate'*, p. 26.

185n *'And then he asked':* Author interview.

186 *pillar of Boston society:* Lancaster and Rathwell, 'The Moralist'.

186 *'an acquaintance of longstanding':* Beecher Report, p. 4.

186 *a special symposium:* Section of Psychiatry, Royal Society of Medicine Archives. 'Two Days Symposium by United States Speakers', 1 Wimpole Street, London W1, 12 and 13 September 1949, followed by dinner 'in honour of American guests' at the Hyde Park Hotel. Toasts were made to the King and the President of the United States of America.

187 *erstwhile Nazi scientists:* Schreiber was given a visa to America as part of Operation Paperclip, a controversial US intelligence progamme to recruit former Nazis for their scientific knowledge. He had to be hastily relocated from Texas to Argentina when the press got wind of his appointment in America. 'Escape from Justice: Nazi War Criminals in America', *ABC News Close-Up*, 13 January 1980.

187 *'intelligent and helpful':* Beecher Report, p. 8.

Chapter 24

189 *wide range of LSD experiments:* 'MKULTRA 101: The Basics', *Stuff They Don't Want You to Know* podcast.

189 *overseen by Sidney Gottlieb:* Kinzer, *Poisoner in Chief*, p. 51. According to Kinzer, 'The TSS was responsible for developing, testing, and building the tools of espionage. Its Chemical Division was Gottlieb's to shape as he wished.'

190 *'Where else could a red-blooded':* Marks, *The Search for the 'Manchurian Candidate'*, p. 101.

190 *both took LSD:* Kinzer, *Poisoner in Chief*, p. 188.

190 *desire to weaponise LSD:* Marks, *The Search for the 'Manchurian Candidate'*, p. 121.

190 *'We must always remember to thank':* Interview by David Sheff with John Lennon and Yoko Ono, *Playboy* (January 1981).

190 *A rumour:* Streatfeild, *Brainwash*, p. 77; Marks, *The Search for the 'Manchurian Candidate'*, p. 66.

191 *video footage:* Edited highlights of the video have been watched on YouTube more than five million times. The area on the 15,000-acre Porton estate in Wiltshire where the exercise took place is known among staff to this day as Happy Valley.

191 *'The stakes are simply too high':* Schmidt, *Secret Science*, p. 332.

191 *'sound, progressive'*: Beecher Report, p. 4.
191 *Schmidt believes:* Schmidt, *Secret Science*, p. 332.
191 *rare admission of guilt:* Ibid., p. 335.
191 *'extensive trials'*: Wright, *Spycatcher*, p. 160 (first noted by Rob Evans in 'Drugged and Duped', *Guardian*, 14 March 2002).
192 *'all the same family'*: Saul Hormats, interview with Observer Films (1994), cited by Rob Evans in *Gassed: British Chemical Warfare Experiments on Humans at Porton Down* (London: House of Stratus, 2000). Evans has donated his research for the book to King's College London. See https://archives.kingscollections.org/index.php/gassed for a full description of all thirty-nine boxes. The Hormats interview is in a box called 'Observer 1': Transcripts of interviews conducted by Observer Films for ITV programme 'Secrets of Porton Down', broadcast on October 11 1994.
193 *'truth drug' interrogation:* Dr Harry Cullumbine, unpublished autobiography, reproduced with kind permission from his family.
193 *'Quite a lot of interesting work'*: Letter to Gordon Wasson, 8 November 1955, Sargant Personal Papers, 'General Correspondence', Wellcome Collection, PP/WWS/A/21/1.
193 *'We were experimenting'*: Interview with Peter Dally by Dominic Streatfeild.
193 *'psychosis in miniature'*: McCoy, 'Science in Dachau's Shadow'.
194 *'humdrum' work:* Streatfeild, *Brainwash*, p. 70.

Chapter 25

195 *'Ten shillings'*: Eric Gow's recollections in this chapter are from author interviews, with some quotes from Rob Evans' articles in the *Guardian* and the Imperial War Museum's 'oral history' interviews with Gow (iwm.org.uk/collections/item/object/80029992).
198 *'inadequately controlled'*: Evans, 'Drugged and Duped'.
198 *'They told us'*: Dominic Webb's quotes are from an interview with Dominic Streatfield and *Revealing the Mind Bender General*, presented by James Maw, BBC Radio 4, first broadcast 1 April 2009.

199 *'walls melting':* Rob Evans, 'MI6 Pays Out Over Secret LSD Mind Control Tests', *Guardian*, 24 February 2006.

200 *Porton resented MI6:* Rob Evans, 'MI6 Ordered LSD Tests on Servicemen', *Guardian*, 22 January 2005.

200 *'People from MI6':* Cullumbine, unpublished autobiography.

201 *publishing a joint paper:* 'Leukaemia and Neoplastic Processes Treated with Langat and Kyasanur Forest Disease Viruses: A Clinical and Laboratory Study of 28 Patients', *BMJ*, 1:5482 (29 January 1966), pp. 258–66. The authors were H. E. Webb (consultant neurologist and senior lecturer, St Thomas' Hospital and Medical School, London), G. Wetherley-Mein (Professor of Haematology, St Thomas' Hospital and Medical School, London), C. E. Smith (director, Microbiological Research Establishment, Porton Down) and Dolores McMahon (senior scientific officer, Microbiological Research Establishment, Porton Down). See also Robert Harris and Jeremy Paxman, *A Higher Form of Killing*, p. 102.

201 *migrating birds:* Lewis, *Inventing Global Ecology*, Chapter 4: Scientists or Spies. At one point, the Indian ornithologist Salim Dhar was accused (and later cleared) of being funded by the CIA.

202 *'old coaching inn':* Thomas, *Secrets & Lies*, p. 123. Thomas alleged that 'the patients had no idea they were being used as medical guinea pigs'. In the 1966 *BMJ* article, the authors stated: 'The nature of the treatment was carefully explained to each of them and to their relatives by one of us and their full consent was obtained.' Thomas also suggested that the visit happened in 1957; the trials ran from 1960 to 1966. Once again, however, he got a lot right too.

202 *'I wouldn't be a bit surprised': Revealing the Mind Bender General.*

202 *'I'm sure he was linked':* Author interview.

Chapter 26

203 *'He's a very significant person':* Eric Olson's quotes in this chapter are from his interview for *The CIA Murdered my Dad*,

a Financial Eyes/London Conversation podcast, 23 October 2018.

204 *'quite agitated'*: Kinzer, *Poisoner in Chief*, p. 115, quoting Olson's boss, Vincent Ruwet.

204 *'was uncharacteristically moody'*: Sworn affidavit by Alice Olson, submitted to the courts in Canada to help former patients of Ewen Cameron successfully win $750,000 compensation from the CIA in October 1988. Alice's evidence was used by lawyers for the eight plaintiffs to portray the 'negligence' and 'incompetence' of Sidney Gottlieb and Robert Lashbrook. See turnerhome.org/jct/anat-2.html.

204 *'messed up'*: Kinzer, *Poisoner in Chief*, p. 115.

205 *Gadgets included:* Thomas, *Journey into Madness*, p. 174.

205 *'He'd come to work'*: Kinzer, *Poisoner in Chief*, p. 112.

205 *'new path'*: Jeffrey Steinberg, 'It Didn't Start with Abu Ghraib: Dick Cheney – Vice President for Torture and War', *Executive Intelligence Review*, 11 November 2005.

205 *According to his diplomatic passport:* A copy of Olson's passport was kindly supplied to the author by Egmont Koch.

206 *'He came back'*: *Das Gehirnwäsche-Programm der CIA Deckname Artischocke*, a TV documentary first broadcast in Germany and America in 2002, now available on YouTube. Directed by Egmont R. Koch and Michael Weck.

206 *CIA documents reveal:* Ibid.

206 *A CIA memorandum:* Egmont R. Koch and Michael Weck, *Deckname Artischocke: Die Geheimen Menschenversuche der CIA* (Munich: C. Bertelsmann, 2002), p. 113 (the book based on their TV documentary – see above.) The memorandum was addressed to Director Central Intelligence and headed 'Artichoke cases, June 1952'.

206 *'Disposal of the body'*: Marks, *The Search for the 'Manchurian Candidate'*, p. 38.

207 *'in consultation with SOD researchers'*: Albarelli, *A Terrible Mistake*, p. 247.

207 *until spring 1953:* Koch and Weck, *Deckname Artischocke*, p. 203. Olson stepped down as head of SOD after complaining of ulcers and the stress of work.

207 *'quintessential' American abroad:* Thomas, *Secrets & Lies*, p. 153.
207 *'come face to face':* Thomas, memorandum, 30 November 1998.
208 *'He sounded different': Das Gehirnwäsche-Programm der CIA Deckname Artischocke.*
208 *'soul-searching':* Thomas, memorandum, 30 November 1998.
208 *'someone who could go':* Ibid.
208 *'He came so close':* Ronson, *The Men Who Stare at Goats*, p. 254.
208 *'I don't know what he said exactly':* In December 2022, Eric emailed the author to say: 'He knew Sargent [*sic*] personally, so there's no doubt that this report was correct, even though there is no further verification.'
208 *'joined at the hip':* Thomas, *Secrets & Lies*, p. 156.
208 *'could only have been murdered':* Thomas, memorandum, 30 November 1998.
208 *'bad business':* Thomas, *Secrets & Lies*, p. 225.
209 *'been rendered unable': A Study of Assassination* (1953), released by the CIA after a Freedom of Information request in 1997. The file was related to the Guatemalan Destabilisation Programme.
209 *'locked up in his lab mentality':* Thomas, memorandum, 30 November 1998.

Chapter 27

211 *'A survey of the existing literature':* D. Ewen Cameron, J. G. Lohrenz and K. A. Hancock, 'The Depatterning Treatment of Schizophrenia', *Comprehensive Psychiatry* (Official Journal of the Psychopathological Society), 3:2 (April 1962), pp. 66–7.
212 *'We had already found':* Ibid.
212 *'Many patients':* Sargant and Slater, *An Introduction to Physical Methods of Treatment in Psychiatry* (5th edn 1972), p. 89.
212 *the sound of screams:* Marks, *The Search for the 'Manchurian Candidate'*, p. 135.
212 *'There are marked memory deficits':* Cameron, Lohrenz and Hancock, 'The Depatterning Treatment of Schizophrenia'.
213 *his own Maudsley Bequest paper:* William Sargant, 'The Present Treatment of Schizophrenia', Maudsley Bequest

Lecture (draft), February 1963, Sargant Personal Papers, 'Post War Work', Wellcome Collection, PP/WWS/F/10/5.

213 *keener than Cameron:* Cameron had dismissed insulin coma treatment in his opening comments, acknowledging a 'demonstrable measure of success' but its 'degree of effectiveness' had left 'much to be desired'.

Chapter 28

215 *'authoritarian':* 'MK Ultra: CIA Mind Control Program in Canada', *The Fifth Estate*, CBC TV documentary, 1980.

216 *'Girlie, we're going to cure':* Collins, *In the Sleep Room*, p. 165.

216 *the effect of dehydration:* D. Ewen Cameron, 'The Dehydration Method in Epilepsy', *American Journal of Psychiatry*, 88:1 (July 1931), pp. 123–30.

216 *patients became increasingly desperate:* Jordan Torbay, 'The Work of Donald Ewen Cameron: From Psychic Driving to MK Ultra', *History of Psychiatry*, 34:3 (March 2023), pp. 320–30.

216 *'not insane at the present time':* Donald Ewen Cameron Collection, 'Papers Concerning Rudolf Hess', McGill University Archives, file 15.

216 *'bastion':* D. Ewen Cameron, 'The Process of Remembering', *British Journal of Psychiatry*, 109:460 (May 1963), pp. 325–40. The Thirty-Seventh Maudsley Lecture, delivered before the Royal Medico-Psychological Association, 14 November 1962.

216 *'Nuremberg was that moment':* David Pratt, '"Scotland's Mengele": The Truth about Dr Ewen Cameron', *The National*, 17 February 2019.

217 *pushing things:* Naomi Klein, *The Shock Doctrine*, p. 35.

217 *'Psychic Driving':* D. Ewen Cameron, 'Psychic Driving', *American Journal of Psychiatry*, 112:7 (January 1956), pp. 502–9.

217 *John Gittinger:* McCoy, *A Question of Torture*, p. 42; Kinzer, *Poisoner in Chief*, p. 127.

217 *'If you don't keep quiet':* Cameron, 'Psychic Driving'.

218 *'ten to thirty minutes' driving':* D. Ewen Cameron, 'Psychic Driving: Dynamic Implant', *Psychiatric Quarterly*, 31:1 (January 1957), pp. 703–12.

218 *they were played through headphones:* It was a particularly

invasive form of therapy, literally creating voices in someone's head, as Jacob Kingsbury Downs highlighted in his doctoral thesis, 'Headphone Listening Space, Embodiment, Materiality', Department of Music, Faculty of Arts and Humanities, University of Sheffield, 2021.

218 *'You are a tease':* Collins, *In the Sleep Room*, p. 173.

218 *'move out of the area of exposure':* D. Ewen Cameron, Leonard Levy and Leonard Rubenstein, 'Effects of Repetition of Verbal Signals upon the Behaviour of Chronic Psychoneurotic Patients'. Read by D. Ewen Cameron at the Annual Meeting of the Royal Medico-Psychological Association, Glasgow, July 1959.

219 *Cerebrophone:* Streatfeild, *Brainwash*, p. 216.

219 *cure people of bad habits:* Collins, *In the Sleep Room*, p. 122.

219 *'A special mechanism':* Cameron, Levy and Rubenstein, 'Effects of Repetition of Verbal Signals upon the Behaviour of Chronic Psychoneurotic Patients'.

219 *'If this thing worked':* Collins, *In the Sleep Room*, p. 130.

219 *Previous sleep treatments:* H. Azima, 'Prolonged Sleep Treatment in Mental Disorders (Some New Psychopharmacological Considerations)', *Journal of Mental Science*, 101:424 (July 1955), pp. 593–603.

220 *In Cameron's Sleep Room:* Collins, *In the Sleep Room*, p. 160.

220 *'heightened awareness':* Ibid., p. 126.

220 *'You let your mother':* The negative and positive messages are taken from Marks, *The Search for the 'Manchurian Candidate'*, pp. 136–7.

220 *James Monroe:* Jack Anderson and Dale Van Atta, 'Subproject 68: The Case Continues', *Washington Post*, 27 October 1985.

220 *Peter Roper:* 'Stunning Tale of Brainwashing, the CIA and an Unsuspecting Scots Researcher', *Scotsman*, 2 August 2006.

221 *According to Gordon Thomas:* Thomas, *Journey into Madness*, pp. 152–3. Thomas also claimed that Allen Dulles believed the Rudolf Hess awaiting trial was an impostor – the real Hess had been executed on the orders of Churchill. Dulles could prove this because Hess had a scar on the left side of

his torso. Later, when Cameron went to assess Hess' mental state, he asked for his shirt to be removed, but the prison guard refused.

221 *'In 1957 a close inspection'*: Collins, *Inside the Sleep Room*, p. 137

221 *'study the effects'*: Class Action in Superior Court, Quebec, Montreal, Canada, 2019 (#500-06-000972-196): J. Tanny vs Royal Victoria Hospital and McGill University, and Attorney General of Canada and United States Attorney General, p. 34.

221 *MKULTRA Subproject 68:* See CIA document #0000017468 for full details of payments.

222 *'invaluable' help:* Letter from Dr Ewen Cameron, dated 12 April 1960, ibid.

222 *'good cover'*: Anderson and Van Atta, 'Subproject 68'.

222 *probably have continued:* Rebecca Lemov, 'Brainwashing's Avatar: The Curious Career of Dr Ewen Cameron', *Grey Room*, 45 (2011), pp. 61–87.

222 *written up in 1956:* Cameron, 'Psychic Driving'.

222 *'applying galvanic stimulation'*: D. Ewen Cameron, Leonard Levy and Leonard Rubenstein, 'Effects of Repetition of Verbal Signals Upon the Behaviour of Chronic Psychoneurotic Patients', *Journal of Mental Science*, 106: 443 (1960), pp. 742–54.

222 *'repeated depatterning'*: Marks, *The Search for the 'Manchurian Candidate'*, p. 138.

223 *'personality pattern'*: D. Ewen Cameron, Leonard Levy and Leonard Rubenstein, 'A Further Report on the Effects of Repetition of Verbal Signals upon Human Behaviour', *Canadian Journal of Psychiatry*, 6:4 (August 1961), pp. 210–21.

Chapter 29

224 *weren't 'tortured enough'*: Harvey Cashore, Lisa Ellenwood and Bob McKeown, 'Trudeau Government Gag Order in CIA Brainwashing Case Silences Victims, Lawyer Says', CBC News, 15 December 2017.

225 *'Sargant told me'*: Kevin Dowling and Phillip Knightley, 'The Olson File: A Secret That Could Destroy the CIA', *Night & Day: Mail on Sunday Review*, 23 August 1998.

225 *'What was being done':* Thomas, *Secrets & Lies*, p. 227.
225 *'long-lost friends':* Streatfeild, *Brainwash*, p. 242.
226 *'to attend and read a paper':* Endowment Fund Sub-Committee minutes, 1959, London Metropolitan Archives, H01/ST/A/149/002.
226 *the conference's opening paper:* H. E. Lehmann, 'Psychiatric Concepts of Depression: Nomenclature and Classification', *Canadian Psychiatric Association Journal*, 4:Special Supplement (1959), pp. S1–12.
226 *'The work on this project':* Cameron, Levy and Rubenstein, 'Effects of Repetition of Verbal Signals upon the Behaviour of Chronic Psychoneurotic Patients' was subsequently published in the *Journal of Mental Science*, 106 (April 1960), pp. 742–54.
227 *'blacker than black':* Dowling and Knightley, 'The Olson File'.
227 *'We have shown':* 'AGM: 1959; programme, copies of summaries of papers, correspondence with speakers', Noel Gordon Harris Personal Papers, Wellcome Collection, PP/NGH/27.
227 *In June 1961:* Minutes of the Annual General Meeting, Canadian Psychiatric Association, 4 June 1961. 'The Organizing Committee for the World Congress of Psychiatry had asked if CPA would consider bestowing Honorary Membership on several distinguished psychiatrists during the Congress.' Thanks to Ben Spears for alerting the author to this appointment.
227 *'My last patient was a deviant':* Álvaro Corazón Rural, 'Gais, lesbianas y transg*énero* durante el franquismo', Jot Down, 1 September 2015.
227 *'a great personal friend':* Letter to Gregson Ellis at AP Watt literary agency, 21 June 1961, suggesting López-Ibor could help with a Spanish translation of *Battle for The Mind*. Sargant Personal Papers, 'Conversion, Religion and Brainwashing', Wellcome Collection G/2/9.
227 *'The atomic stalemate':* 'Brainwashing Technique Described', *The Gazette* (Montreal), 20 May 1964.

228 *'It was terrifying'*: Marks, *The Search for the 'Manchurian Candidate'*, pp. 139–40.

229 *'about 20 per cent of her capacity'*: David Remnick, '25 Years of Nightmares', *Washington Post*, 28 July 1985.

229 *'It was noted'*: St Thomas' Local Hospitals Committee minutes and papers, 1948–1969, July 1960, London Metropolitan Archives, H01/ST/A/133/001-003.

229 *'for the purpose'*: Endowment Fund Sub-Committee minutes, 1949–1969, May 1952, London Metropolitan Archives, H01/ST/A/149/001-003.

230 *'We have explored'*: Ewen Cameron, 'The Transition Neurosis', delivered at the Fifth Annual Neuropsychiatric Meeting in North Little Rock, Arkansas, February 1953. Cited by Harvey M. Weinstein in *Father, Son, CIA* and kept in the American Psychiatric Association Archives. Discovering the paper was a breakthrough for Weinstein, who was on his last day of a forensic search through Cameron's papers at the APA when he came across it. It was the evidence he needed that Cameron had been brainwashing his patients, including Harvey's father, at the Allan Memorial.

231 *converted into a pub:* Author interview. John Pollitt also alludes to a bar on Ward Five. 'If his favourite setting is the public house bar, this can be crudely reproduced,' he wrote in *Psychological Medicine for Students*, p. 98.

Chapter 31

243 *front-page story:* 'Private Institutions Used in Cal Effort to Control Behavior', *New York Times*, 2 August 1977. The article named two other front organisations, the Geschickter Fund for Medical Research in Washington DC and the Josiah Macy, Jr. Foundation.

243 *ten from 'Ewen' to 'Will':* The majority of the letters between Sargant and Cameron are in Folder 71 of Ewen Cameron's personal papers at the American Psychiatric Association; there are a couple in Folder 68 too. Other correspondence relating to the World Psychiatric Association can be found in Folders 65 and 67.

243 *They settled on:* Circular WPA letter, signed by Sargant, to foreign psychiatric journals, undated, Ewen Cameron Personal Papers, APA Archives, folder 71.

243 *'turning up trumps':* Letter from Sargant to Cameron, 10 August 1965, ibid.

243 *Sargant was delighted:* Letter from Sargant to Cameron, 21 September 1965, ibid.

243 *Cameron was also keen:* Letter from Cameron to Sargant, 8 October 1965, ibid.

244 *According to Peggy:* Interview with Peggy Sargant by Dominic Streatfeild.

244 *'The thing to do':* If Sargant's explanatory tone suggests that Cameron might not be aware of narcosis treatment (which he clearly was, having run a CIA-funded sleep room in Montreal), it's because Sargant had attached a copy of part of the letter for Cameron to pass on to the patient's parents. In other words, he was outlining the basics of narcosis treatment combined with ECT not for Cameron's benefit, but for theirs.

245 *'It is difficult to think':* 'Obituary Notices', *BMJ*, 3:5568 (23 September 1967), pp. 803–4.

Chapter 32

MKULTRA documents can be accessed via a variety of online sites, including the Internet Archive (archive.org), The Black Vault (blackvault.com) and the CIA Reading Room (cia.gov/readingroom/home). Their availability today is a legacy of John Marks' extraordinary investigative work in the 1970s. The easiest way to find documents is by searching for 'MKULTRA' and the relevant file numbers, given below.

248 *He even convinced:* St Thomas' Endowment Fund Sub-Committee minutes, February 1961, London Metropolitan Archives, H01/ST/A/149/002.

248 *'the grant of £1,200':* St Thomas' General Purposes and Finance Committee minutes and papers, 1948–1974, London Metropolitan Archives, H01/ST/A/129/010.

248 *a long letter:* St Thomas' Research Advisory Committee minutes, 16 June 1959; letter dated 27 February 1959, ibid.

249 *'Experimentation took place':* Streatfeild, *Brainwash*, p. 40.

249 *not before attending:* Dally's travel and subsistence was paid for out of endowment funds. Initially, the Royal Medico-Psychological Association was going to charter a plane, but the plans fell through. Minutes of the Endowment Fund Subcommittee, 28 February 1962, London Metropolitan Archives, H01/ST/A/149/002.

249 *'[Peter] saw an awful lot of spies':* Interview with Dominic Streatfeild, shared with the author.

249 *'A candidate would be invited':* Thomas, *Inside British Intelligence*, p. 75.

250 *'It was only occasional':* Interview with Ann Dally in 2005 by Dominic Streatfeild, shared with the author.

250 *'Many senior officers':* Wright, *Spycatcher*, pp. 275–6.

251 *'I never knew the name':* Author interview.

251 *'I do, however, remember':* Author interview.

252 *'Every patient needs psychotherapy':* Ann Dally, 'Obituaries: Peter Dally', *BMJ*, 10:1136 (2 February 2006), p. 332.

252 *'under heavy sedation':* 'Greville Wynne in Hospital', *Guardian*, 28 April 1964; 'Greville Wynne in Hospital "2 or 3 Weeks"', *Guardian*, 28 April 1964.

252 *'Sargant was undoubtedly on the X list':* Author interview.

252 *one of three:* On the advice of the medical committee, a grant for a research registrar was extended for eight months from 1 August 1960; Rohde's appointment as a locum research registrar was extended by a month to September 1960; and Pollitt, who had returned from a one-year Rockefeller fellowship in the US, was appointed research registrar, on a personal grading of senior registrar, from September 1960 to the end of March 1961.

252 *'working on a grant':* Peter Rohde and William Sargant, 'Treatment of Schizophrenia in General Hospitals', *BMJ*, 2:5244 (8 July 1961), pp. 67–70. 86 per cent of the original ninety-five patients were out of hospital, and 75 per cent appeared to be 'free from evidence of active schizophrenia';

results were better in the group treated with chlorpromazine, modified insulin treatment and ECT, compared to the group treated with insulin coma and ECT.

252 *based in Hong Kong:* Peter Rohde Personal Papers, uncatalogued archive (108 boxes), Wellcome Collection, PP/ROH.

253 *The donor had also indicated:* St Thomas' Research Advisory Committee minutes, September 1963, London Metropolitan Archives, H01/ST/A/129/015.

253 *'As soon as the research registrar':* Ibid.

253 *'full time research psychiatrist':* MKULTRA document #0000017468. Marks, *The Search for the 'Manchurian Candidate'*, p. 136.

253 *'A number of the grants':* David H. Price, 'Buying a Piece of Anthropology, Part One: Human Ecology and Unwitting Anthropological Research for the CIA', *Anthropology Today*, 23:3 (June 2007), pp. 8–13.

254 *'would continue to act as liaison':* Thomas, *Secrets & Lies*, p. 72.

254 *'indebted':* H. J. Eysenck and R. A. Willett, 'The Measurement of Motivation through the Use of Objective Indices', *Journal of Mental Science*, 107:450 (September 1961), pp. 961–8.

254 *'As long as somebody pays':* Peter Pringle, 'Eysenck Took £800,000 Tobacco Funds', *Independent*, 31 October 1996.

254 *Monroe had heard:* Significantly, Abrams had initially contacted the Behavioural Science Division of the US Air Force Office of Scientific Research, who passed on his details to Monroe.

254 *'support the research in Oxford':* MKULTRA document #0000017395.

255 *who his real paymasters were:* David Luke, 'Steve Abrams: Psychedelic Trickster', *Paranthropology*, 4:1 (2013), pp. 36–40.

255 *His personal papers:* Steve Abrams' personal papers can be found at the Wellcome Collection, ref. PP/SAB. For more on his meeting with Robert Lashbrook, see PP/SAB/B/1/5/14.

255 *opened in 1964:* For more on the possible significance of 1964, see Robert Miller's blog, *The Eye Wink at the Hand.* robertmiller-octspan.co.nz/moderntragedy.

256 *'We are very sorry':* Statement from a spokesperson for Guy's and St Thomas' NHS Foundation Trust, sent to the author on 15 August 2024.

256 *Writing in 1965:* 'Report on the Department of Psychological Medicine, St Thomas's Hospital, 1948–1965', Wellcome Collection, PP/WWS/B/2/5.

256 *'generous donation':* D. H. W. Kelly, C. J. S. Walter and William Sargant, 'Modified Leucotomy Assessed by Forearm Blood Flow and Other Measurements', *British Journal of Psychiatry*, 112:490 (1966), pp. 871–81.

256 *'no official outside research support':* Sargant, *The Unquiet Mind*, p. 226.

257 *'Sargant may well have':* Author interview.

257n *Patrick Pakenham:* Peter Stanford, 'Obituary: Patrick Pakenham', *Guardian*, 24 June 2005.

Chapter 33

258 *'studies of the mechanics of indoctrination':* 'Award for Londoner', *Sunday Times*, 18 October 1959.

260 *'splendid relationship':* Letter from Stewart Kipling to Cameron, 8 November 1965, Ewen Cameron Personal Papers, APA Archives, folder 71.

260 *'Geigy have really gone to town':* Letter from Sargant to Cameron, 14 March 1966, ibid.

260 *'We do hope':* Letter from Stewart Kipling to Sargant, 14 January 1966, ibid.

261 *undertook a one-year study:* 'Native Doctors Lauded', *The Gazette* (Montreal), 16 March 1965.

262 *'I couldn't imagine why the CIA':* 'MK Ultra: CIA Mind Control Program in Canada'.

262 *the CIA had funded:* David H. Price, 'Buying a Piece of Anthropology, Part Two: The CIA and Our Tortured Past', *Anthropology Today*, 23:5 (October 2007), pp. 17–22.

262 *'run amok in Indonesia':* 'MK Ultra: CIA Mind Control Program in Canada'.

262 *a number of papers:* 'Witch Doctoring, Zar and Voodoo: Their Relation to Modern Psychiatric Treatments', *Journal of the*

Royal Society of Medicine, 60:10 (1 October 1967), given at the Section of Psychiatry Meeting, 11 April 1967.

262 *'complete control':* Letter to Cameron, 1 October 1965, Ewen Cameron Personal Papers, APA Archives, Folder 71.

Chapter 34

265 *'This was dangerous':* St Thomas' General Purposes and Finance Committee minutes and papers, 'Ward V – additional lavatory', 1966, London Metropolitan Archives, H01/ST/A/129/018.

266 *'a tremendous psychotherapeutic boost':* 'Report on the Department of Psychological Medicine, St Thomas's Hospital, 1948–1965', Wellcome Collection, PP/WWS/B/2/5.

267 *'Doses of up to 3,000mg':* Sargant and Slater, *An Introduction to Physical Methods of Treatment in Psychiatry* (5th edn 1972), pp. 21–2. The passage on chlorpromazine remained largely unchanged from the 1964 edition.

267 *Cameron had administered:* Collins, *In the Sleep Room*, p. 160. Cameron suggested that if the patient was restless during the night, a further 50mg of chlorpromazine could be given; milk of magnesia (30cc) was also given with the night sedation. He also sometimes added Phenergan, a sedative, to the chlorpromazine.

267 *later he dropped the tricyclics:* Sargant and Slater, *An Introduction to Physical Methods of Treatment in Psychiatry* (5th edn 1972), p. 94.

267–8 *'Although anxiety was greatly reduced':* Ibid.

268 *on a par with heroin:* p. R. Smith, 'Prescribing Mandrax', letter, *BMJ*, 2:5865 (2 June 1973), p. 552.

269 *'good previous personality':* Sargant and Slater, *An Introduction to Physical Methods of Treatment in Psychiatry* (5th edn 1972), p. 61.

269 *'lead the world':* Sargant, *The Unquiet Mind*, p. 49. See also Fennell, *Treatment Without Consent*, p. 169.

269 *'one of the central paradoxes':* Fennell, *Treatment Without Consent*, pp. 161–2; Claire Hilton, 'Changes Between the 1959 and 1983 Mental Health Acts (England & Wales),

with Particular Reference to Consent to Treatment for Electroconvulsive Therapy', *History of Psychiatry*, 18:2 (June 2007), pp. 217–29.

270 *'intensively used':* 'Report on the Department of Psychological Medicine, St Thomas's Hospital, 1948–1965', Wellcome Collection, PP/WWS/B/2/5.

270 *'for some resistant patients':* Sargant and Slater, *An Introduction to Physical Methods of Treatment in Psychiatry* (5th edn 1972) p. 90.

270 *'well cleaned head':* Ibid., p. 81.

270 *'inhalation of the vomitus':* Ibid., p. 84.

271 *'Normally, however':* Ibid., p. 85.

271 *'for some special reason':* Ibid., pp. 79–82.

271 *'open to abuse':* Fennell, *Treatment Without Consent*, p. 179.

271 *'special canvas restraining sheet':* Ibid., p. 80.

Chapter 35

274 *Nurses assigned to the Sleep Room:* Most of the interviews in this chapter (Christine, Shelley, Catherine Mountain, Julia Ross, Ann Rowland, Tish) were with the author. Two interviews, one with Jane, a Nightingale nurse, and another with an anonymous senior ward sister, were conducted in 2005 by Dominic Streatfeild, who kindly shared them.

274 *'horrendous':* Streatfeild, *Brainwash*, p. 249.

275 *'She was the nurse in charge':* Mullan, *Mad to be Normal*, p. 176.

276 *'like a spoilt child':* Author interview. See also Owen, *Time to Declare*, pp. 75–81.

276 *His 1972 legacy paper:* Walter, Mitchell-Heggs and Sargant, 'Modified Narcosis, ECT and Antidepressant Drugs'.

277 *'There has been one further death':* Sargant and Slater, *An Introduction to Physical Methods of Treatment in Psychiatry* (5th edn 1972), p. 96.

277 *Anticipating such criticism:* Thanks to Robert Miller, author of *The Eye Wink at the Hand*, for drawing my attention to Sargant's promise of a second paper. See robertmiller-octspan.co.nz for a detailed study of deep sleep therapy in New Zealand and elsewhere.

280 *'It was a series of one-off': Revealing the Mind Bender General.*
281n *'To be quite frank':* Ibid.

Chapter 36

284 *under Sargant's supervision:* Walter, Mitchell-Heggs and Sargant, 'Treatment with Modified Narcosis'.
288 *'William . . . would not have survived':* Hilton and Stephenson (convenors and eds), *Psychiatric Hospitals in the UK in the 1960s*, p. 34.
290 *'Dr Sargant initiated':* GMC response to the author's two Freedom of Information requests.

Chapter 38

305 *'He would sit down':* Streatfeild, *Brainwash*, pp. 253–4 and from his interview with Mo Harvey, kindly shared with the author.
306n *'a strange high-pitched voice':* Peter Gladstone Smith, 'MI5 Indignant Over Tkachenko Affair Haste', *Sunday Telegraph*, 24 September 1967.
307 *'semi-conscious':* John Miller, 'Moscow Conference Called', *Daily Telegraph*, 18 September 1967.
307 *'secret nursing home':* Adam Raphael, 'Russians Say Scientist is Held Forcibly', *Guardian*, 18 September 1967.
307 *subsequent Royal Society report:* 'Correspondence and Papers Regarding Russian Exchange Scientist V. I. Tkachenko and Diplomatic Incident between Russia and Britain', September 1967, Professional Papers of Harold Warris Thompson, The Royal Society Archives, HWT/24/6/11.
307 *'beetle-browed 59-year-old physician':* John Stevenson, 'Kachenko: And the Man Who Closed the Dossier', *Daily Sketch*, 21 September 1967.
308 *arranged for the prime minister:* Letter from Harold Wilson to Mrs Tkachenko, 22 September 1967, Prime Minister's Office: Correspondence and Papers, 1967–1970, TNA: PREM 13/1844.
307 *'MI5 indignant':* Gladstone Smith, 'MI5 Indignant Over Tkachenko Affair Haste'. The article also made pointed

reference to a talk given by Sargant three years earlier to the British Academy of Forensic Sciences, at which he had upset Special Branch by suggesting that police interrogation methods could lead to false confessions. See 'The Mechanism of Police Confessions', June 1964, Sargant Personal Papers, 'Conversion, Religion and Brainwashing', Wellcome Collection, PP/WWS/G/7/3: 'There are, unfortunately, quite a number of instances of provenly false confessions being obtained by current police methods in this country in recent years,' Sargant said. He had given a similar talk to the British Society of Criminology in May 1963 (PP/WWS/G/7/1).

Chapter 39

309 Your Life in Their Hands*:* The episode, on depression, also featured Sargant's colleagues Peter Dally and John Pollitt.

310 *'From the Stone Age to Hitler':* Sargant, *The Mind Possessed*, p. 244. He would go on to compare Beatles fans to the trancelike state of the Samburu dancers in Kenya: 'Many of the other dancers approached very near trance, and showed states of increased suggestibility at the end of a long and intensive period of repetitive and monotonous dancing. They looked very much like fans of the Beatles or other "pop groups" after a long session of dancing.'

311 *Neighbours remember:* Quotes from the current owner of Sargant's former home in East Woodyates and neighbours who knew Sargant at the time are from interviews with the author.

Chapter 40

314 *'Perhaps he was too individualistic':* 'William Sargant', *Psychiatric Bulletin*, 12:12 (December 1988), p. 556.

315 *'In medicine':* William Sargant, 'Eat All the Humble Pie You Can', *World Medicine* (18 June 1975), pp. 22–3.

315 *Foundation Fellow:* 'William Sargant', *Psychiatric Bulletin*. The obituary, which described him as 'Emeritus Consultant, St

Thomas' Hospital, London' was signed 'PD', most probably Peter Dally.

315 *'He wanted to be'*: Author interview.

315 *distanced himself from the college:* Joanne Li Shen Ooi, 'How Loud is the Unquiet Mind? William Sargant (1907–88) and British Psychiatry in the Mid-20th Century', *Journal of Medical Biography*, 20:2 (May 2012), pp. 71–8.

315 *publicly accusing the 'talkers'*: Letter to *The Times*, 25 August 1976.

315 *'one of the most extraordinary'*: Bixley, *Inside the Priory*, p. 117.

315 *'the Narcosis room'*: Lady Seebohm visited the Royal Waterloo Hospital on 14 September 1971. St Thomas' General Purposes and Finance Committee minutes and papers, 1948–1974, London Metropolitan Archives, H01/ST/A/129/031.

315 *'his Ward V fund'*: Ibid.

316 *'like a living mortuary'*: 'V Argent, Friston, United Kingdom' posted his comment more than a decade ago on an online version of an article published in the *Daily Mail* (Barbara Davies, 'The Zombie Ward', 7 August 2013).

317 *his 1973 book:* Pollitt, *Psychological Medicine for Students*, pp. 241–66.

317 *'Pollitt was not a natural ally'*: Author interview.

Chapter 41

321 *'The minute I left'*: Freeman, 'In Conversation with William Sargant'.

321 *'The trouble is'*: Letter to Kurt Fleischmann, 19 September 1975, Sargant Personal Papers, 'General Correspondence', Wellcome Collection, PP/WWS/A13.

321 *'narcosis ward'*: William Sargant, 'Looking After Schizophrenics', letter, *BMJ*, 2:5918 (8 June 1974), p. 557.

322 *'several thousands of patients'*: William Sargant, 'Prescribing Mandrax', letter, *BMJ*, 2:5868 (23 June 1973), p. 716.

322 *'Modified narcosis as a term'*: Author interview.

325 *'plenty of beds'*: Letter to Eric Cunningham Dax, 20 June 1975, Sargant Personal Papers, 'General Correspondence', Wellcome Collection, PP/WWS/A/13.

325 *'drug traffickers in central London':* Quoted in Jay, 'Over the Edge'.

325 *'Jesus Christ might simply':* William Sargant, 'The Movement in Psychiatry Away from the Philosophical', *The Times*, 22 August 1974.

325–6 *'we are never going to learn':* William Sargant, 'Antidepressant Drugs', letter, *BMJ*, 1:5448 (5 June 1965), p. 1495.

326 *'"statistical" experiment':* William Sargant, 'Should Patients be Tortured in the Name of Progress?', *The Times*, 29 August 1975.

326 *'Should patients be tortured':* Ibid.

326 *'Whenever [Sargant] met me':* Li Shen Ooi, 'How Loud is the Unquiet Mind?'

326 *'I wouldn't let myself':* 'People Like US', an episode of the BBC documentary strand *Towards Tomorrow*, 1968.

326 *a stinging article:* Anthony Clare, 'Will Sargant and the Double Blind', *World Medicine* (3 December 1975).

327 *Franz Mesmer:* Thanks to Professor Roger Luckhurst of Birkbeck, University of London, who gave a fascinating talk about the puzzling history of states of unnatural sleep, including Franz Mesmer's claims to put patients into a state of suspended animation. (London Fortean Society, February 2024.)

327 *white middle-class Americans:* Burrough, *Days of Rage*, p. 277.

327 *'Death to the fascist insect':* Dimsdale, *Dark Persuasion*, p. 137.

327 *'You're kinda like the pet chicken':* Hearst, *Every Secret Thing*, p. 86.

328 *'suddenly and dramatically':* William Sargant, 'When the Mind is Pushed to Breaking Point', *The Times*, 3 May 1974.

328 *'Jolly' West:* Marks, *The Search for the 'Manchurian Candidate'*, p. 59. West's tragic experiment with Tusko was partly funded by the Foundations Fund for Research in Psychiatry, which the *New York Times* revealed was a CIA conduit.

328 *Martin Orne:* Ibid., p. 177. According to Marks, Orne was a 'longtime MKULTRA consultant'.

328 *Robert Jay Lifton:* Albarelli, *A Terrible Mistake*, p. 195.

328 *another article for* The Times*:* William Sargant, 'The Gentle Art of Brainwashing', *The Times*, 12 November 1975.

328 *'As you know'*: 'Stress Expert Examines Patty', *Press-Courier*, 16 November 1975.

328 *'She's pathetic now'*: Dimsdale, *Dark Persuasion*, p. 147.

329 *'tall, craggy faced physician'*: *Independent* (San Francisco), 17 November 1975.

329 *'She is not being difficult'*: 'Brainwash Expert Sees Miss Hearst', *Daily Telegraph*, 17 November 1975.

329 *'I found her'*: 'Patty is Not Fit', *Guardian*, 22 November 1975.

329 *'There will never be any doubt'*: William Sargant, 'How 60 Days in the Dark Broke Patty', *The Times*, 29 January 1976.

329 *'moral outrage'*: William Sargant, 'Should Patty Hearst be Set Free?', *The Times*, 20 July 1976.

Chapter 42

331 *'atrocities', 'brutality'*: 'The Citizens' Commission on Human Rights', *Freedom*, UK no. 69 (1981), p. 2. The full mission statement reads: 'CCHR is a social reform group set up in 1969 and sponsored by the Church of Scientology. Its purpose is the exposure of atrocities and the eradication of brutality in the field of mental health.'

332 *a series of articles:* Ibid., pp. 1–2. The GMC could only confirm one complaint, made in 1987.

333 *According to the* News of the World: *Freedom*, UK no. 70, 1981, citing the *News of the World*, 20 April 1975.

333 *'All true'*: Author interview.

333 *'took a very serious view'*: Letter from the Medical Defence Union to Sargant, 17 December 1981, Wellcome Collection PP/WWS/A16.

334 *'The scientologists are torturing me'*: David Rose, 'Doctor in Distress', *Time Out*, 6 November 1981.

334 *Brian Bromberger:* See Bromberger and Fife-Yeomans, *Deep Sleep*.

335 *'supporting the prosecution'*: *Revealing the Mind Bender General.*

335 *'I've had enough'*: 'Deep Sleep Therapy', broadcast in the UK as part of Channel 4's *Secret History* series, 1992, and drawing on material from two earlier ABC documentaries in Australia.

335 *a series of lectures:* The lectures were introduced by Professor David Goldberg, University of Manchester. Topics included: 'The Anatomy of Healing' (Dr Desmond Kelly, medical director, Priory Hospital); 'Physical Treatment as an Indication of Concern for the Patient' (Dr Jim Birley, dean, Royal College of Psychiatrists); 'Therapeutic Effects of the Medical Encounter' (Professor David Goldberg); 'The Classification and Treatment of Anxiety' (Dr Peter Tyrer, consultant psychiatrist, Mapperley Hospital); 'Sexual Dysfunction – Organic or Psychiatric?' (Dr Peter Gautier-Smith, consultant physician, The National Hospital, Queen Square).

336 *'We had a turnout':* Bixley, *Inside the Priory*, p. 117.

336 *'the most important figure':* Ibid.

336 *'All of us':* Ibid.

336 *'dominating personality':* Streatfeild, *Brainwash*, pp. 233 and 245.

336 *'not an apologist':* Author interview.

336 *'embarrassed being seen':* Interview with Dominic Streatfeild, kindly shared with the author.

337 *annual William Sargant Lecture:* Sargant left money in his will to the RCP, on condition that they held an annual lecture. 'The College acknowledges with much gratitude the bequest from the late William Sargant on the condition that there should be an annual lecture named as the "William Sargant Lecture" which will be attached to a particular Quarterly Meeting' ('The College: The Eighteenth Annual Meeting, 1989', *Psychiatric Bulletin*, 13 (1989), pp. 709–16).

337 *re-released by an Indian publisher:* William Sargant, *Battle for the Mind: Overcoming Limiting Beliefs and Embracing Personal Empowerment* (New Delhi: Prabhat Prakashan, 2019).

337 *'He had a very lucky streak':* Streatfeild, *Brainwash*, p. 235.

337 *end the era:* John Beard, 'Dr William Sargant (1907–88) and the Emergence of Physical Treatments in British Psychiatry', *Journal of Medical Biography*, 17:1 (2009), pp. 23–9.

337 *to almost two thousand people:* According to the Royal College of Psychiatrists, '1,835 adults received acute ECT

from eighty-five mental health clinics across England, Wales and Ireland between January and December 2021', under general anaesthetic and with a muscle relaxant. Two out of three patients were women. ('New Data Shows More Than a Thousand People Benefit from Life-Saving Electroconvulsive Therapy, Majority of Which are Women', Royal College of Psychiatrists press release, 19 December 2023.)

337 *wasn't the only doctor:* Deep sleep therapy with ECT was also given elsewhere in the UK in the 1960s and 1970s, including at Park Prewett, a psychiatric hospital in Hampshire; St Augustine's Hospital, formerly the East Kent County Asylum; Hill End Hospital, a mental health facility in Hertfordshire; Farnborough Hospital in Kent; St John's Hospital, a mental health facility in Stone, Buckinghamshire; and Stone House Hospital, formerly the City of London Mental Hospital, in Dartford, Kent. It was also thought to have been given at St John of God Hospital in Dublin, Ireland in the 1970s.

338 *died on 27 August 1988:* Dally, 'William Walters Sargant'. Wealth at death: £753,558 (probate 30 January 1989).

Index